Acute Trauma and Trauma Care in Orthopedics

Acute Trauma and Trauma Care in Orthopedics

Guest Editors

Pietro Maniscalco
Gianfilippo Caggiari

MDPI

Basel • Beijing • Wuhan • Barcelona • Belgrade • Novi Sad • Cluj • Manchester

Guest Editors
Pietro Maniscalco
Orthopedics and
Traumatology Department
Guglielmo da Saliceto
Hospital
Piacenza
Italy

Gianfilippo Caggiari
Orthopaedic and
Traumatology Department
Università degli Studi di
Sassari
Sassari
Italy

Editorial Office
MDPI AG
Grosspeteranlage 5
4052 Basel, Switzerland

This is a reprint of the Special Issue, published open access by the journal *Journal of Clinical Medicine* (ISSN 2077-0383), freely accessible at: https://www.mdpi.com/journal/jcm/special_issues/470IL9R42Q.

For citation purposes, cite each article independently as indicated on the article page online and as indicated below:

Lastname, A.A.; Lastname, B.B. Article Title. *Journal Name* **Year**, *Volume Number*, Page Range.

ISBN 978-3-7258-4617-7 (Hbk)
ISBN 978-3-7258-4618-4 (PDF)
https://doi.org/10.3390/books978-3-7258-4618-4

Contents

Journal of
Clinical Medicine

MDPI

Article

Functional Postoperative Outcome for 92 Cases of Radial Head Fractures: A PROM-Based Retrospective Study

Michael Müller *, Verena Mann, Julian Zapf, Konstantin Kirchhoff, Michael Zyskowski, Peter Biberthaler, Chlodwig Kirchhoff and Markus Wurm

Department of Trauma Surgery, Hospital Rechts der Isar, Technical University of Munich, 81675 Munich, Germany; julian.zapf@mri.tum.de (J.Z.); michael.zyskowski@mri.tum.de (M.Z.); markus.wurm@mri.tum.de (M.W.)
* Correspondence: michael.mueller@mri.tum.de

Abstract: Background: Fractures of the radial head are common injuries, whereas, in the case of displaced fractures, surgical treatment using screw or plate osteosynthesis, excision, or replacement of the radial head is required. However, data about patient-related outcomes (PROM) for different types of radial head fractures is limited in the current literature. Therefore, this study was conducted to evaluate the functional outcome after operatively treated radial head fractures and to further correlate these results with the initial modified Mason classification. **Methods**: In this retrospective study, all suitable patients with surgical treatment of a radial head fracture were identified. Only patients with Mason II-IV fractures were included. All patients completed the Elbow Self-Assessment Score (ESAS) questionnaire. Data on fracture classification, type of surgery, and revision operations (if needed) were assessed. **Results**: A total of 92 patients suffering from fractures of the radial head (57 Mason II, 35 Mason III-fractures) who were operatively treated at our institution were enrolled. There were 42 (47.7%) female and 50 (54.3%) male patients with an average age of 47.5 ± 14.1 years. Screw osteosynthesis was performed in 67 patients, plate osteosynthesis in 20 patients, and five patients received radial head arthroplasty. The average ESAS score accounted for 89.7 ± 16.7. Mason II fractures showed significantly better functional results with higher ESAS scores (92.3 ± 13.9 vs. 85.4 ± 20.1) as well as significantly lower rates of necessary implant removal (0 vs. 5 (14.3%) than Mason III fractures. Screw osteosynthesis showed significantly better functional ESAS scores, 91.0 ± 16.5, than plate osteosynthesis, with 85.3 ± 17.6 (p = 0.041), but was predominantly used in Mason II fractures. **Conclusions**: Surgical treatment using screw- and plate osteosynthesis of radial head fractures provides a good overall outcome. The postoperative function is associated with the initial Mason classification as the patients' reported outcome was worse in Mason III fractures compared to Mason type II fractures. In this context, the ESAS score can be considered a useful tool for the assessment of the patient-based functional outcome.

Keywords: proximal radius; patient-reported outcome; ESAS

1. Introduction

Fractures of the radial head are common injuries with an incidence of 12.4/100,000 people [1], typically occurring at an average age of 48 years. Female patients are, on average, 10 years younger than the male cohort [2]. A fall on the outstretched hand with the elbow in a slightly flexed and pronated position presents the typical trauma mechanism. However, radial head fractures also appear as part of complex dislocation injuries of the elbow [3].

The most established classification system was originally published by Mason in 1954 [4]. Today's most commonly used classification is the modified Mason classification described by Hotchkiss [5]. In addition, a treatment algorithm is derived from this modified classification. Mason type I fractures show minimal displacement (<2 mm) and mostly present with an undiminished range of motion. In these cases, conservative treatment is broadly accepted. Conservatively treated fractures of the radial head with a short immobilization of only 48 h provide good clinical results [6]. Fractures with a displacement of 2 mm or more without signs of comminution are classified as type II fractures. In these cases, motion may be mechanically blocked. The best treatment regime for Mason type II fractures is still controversially discussed. If surgery is decided upon, a screw osteosynthesis is usually performed. However, conservative therapy for Mason II fractures also provides comparable results, although the rate of postoperative radiological signs of osteoarthritis is higher [7]. Multiple fragments, along with severe comminution is considered as a type III fracture, which can only be treated by excision according to Hotchkiss' publication in 1997 [5].

Over the years, surgical treatment options have improved, and not every comminuted radial head needs to undergo excision. Nonetheless, it is still common sense that Mason type III and IV fractures should be treated with open reduction and internal fixation (ORIF) using screw or plate osteosynthesis. Irreparable fractures can be treated by radial head prosthesis or resection of the radial head, depending on the extent of concomitant ligamentous injuries [8].

The overall outcome after radial head fractures shows good results not only for conservatively treated Mason I fractures [9] but also for complex Mason III types treated with radial head resection, prosthesis, or reconstruction [10,11]. However, the number of studies evaluating the functional outcome following radial head fractures is limited. In particular, not enough attention has been paid to patient-reported outcomes, which are nowadays considered an increasingly important benchmark [9,12]. Most studies compare the results between different treatment options for one fracture type (Mason classification), but different fracture types, according to Mason, were not compared.

For this reason, the aim of this study was to evaluate and compare the patient-reported functional outcome of surgically treated Mason type II and type III radial head fractures. As a hypothesis, it can be assumed that the surgical treatment of radius head fractures provides good results overall.

Mason type II fractures are probably associated with better functional outcomes than Mason III fractures. In addition, a correlation between the necessary treatment method (plate or screws) and the outcome is to be expected.

2. Materials and Methods

2.1. Study Population and Data Collection

In this single-center cohort study, the in-house fracture register was investigated for patients suffering from radial head fractures treated surgically between the years 2003 and 2016. Only isolated radial head fractures were included in the study. Patients suffering from complex injuries, including concomitant ligamentous injuries such as monteggia-like lesions or elbow dislocations, were excluded. Ligament stability is tested intraoperatively after the completion of the osteosynthesis. The width of the joint space under varus and valgus stress is assessed under fluoroscopic control. In the event of instability, this was addressed using reconstruction with suture anchors. Furthermore, multiple trauma was also considered an exclusion criterion.

2.2. Data Collection (Parameters)

Epidemiologic baseline information (age, gender) of enrolled patients was obtained from the hospital's data management program (SAP SE, Walldorf, Germany). Based on the preoperative X-rays and CT scans, all fractures were classified according to the Hotchkiss modification of the Mason classification system. Whenever the Mason classification is mentioned in this paper, it refers to the modification by Hotchkiss [5]. Further information on follow-up operations, such as surgery for revision or elective implant removal, was assessed. In case the patient gave his informed consent, they were asked to complete the Elbow self-assessment score (ESAS) questionnaire.

The ESAS is a patient-reported outcome measure (PROM) that allows patients to rate their subjective elbow function [13]. The questionnaire was developed and validated by Beirer et al. in 2016. It includes illustrative photos, useful for the patient to determine the objective range of motion. Questions on pain level and functionality are also part of the ESAS. In addition to the subjective function, the questionnaire can also be used to objectively assess the range of motion in order to be able to determine a persisting postoperative flexion contracture of the elbow.

2.3. Surgical Technique

All patients underwent surgery via a lateral approach modified according to Kaplan [14]. The type of treatment was based on the instability and complexity of the fractures according to the Hotchkiss modification of the Mason classification. Simple 2-part fractures were stabilized using 2 mm lag screws (Medartis AG, Basel, Switzerland), whereas multi-fragmentary fractures were treated with 2.4 mm LCP radial head plates (DePuy Synthes GmbH, Oberdorf, Switzerland) as well as with 2.0 mm TriLock Radial Head Plates (Medartis AG, Basel, Switzerland). In case of irreparable fractures, radial head arthroplasty (RHA) was performed (MoPyC, Tornier SAS, Montbonnot Saint Martin, France). Figure 1 shows typical cases with pre- and postoperative x-rays of a mason type II fracture treated with screw osteosynthesis and a mason type III fracture treated with plate osteosynthesis

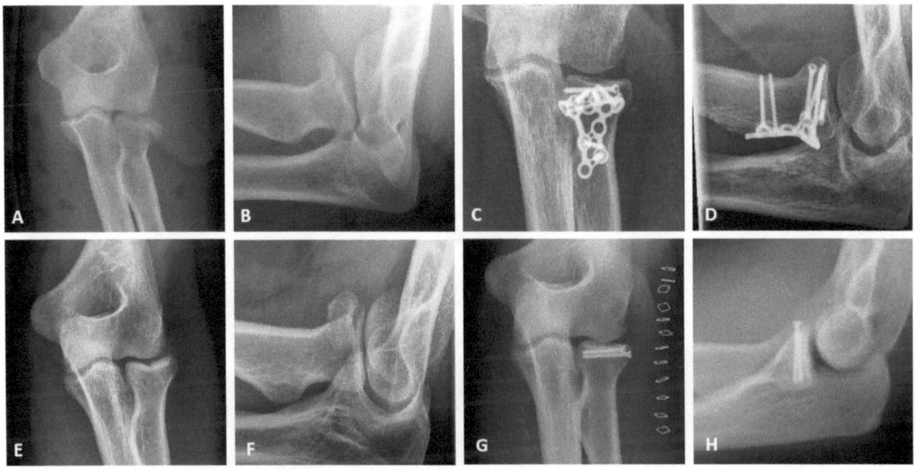

Figure 1. X-ray diagnostics; (**A**,**B**) Mason type II fracture in AP and lateral oblique view; (**C**,**D**) Mason type III fracture postoperatively after plate osteosynthesis in AP and lateral oblique view; (**E**,**F**) Mason type II fracture in AP and lateral oblique view; (**G**,**H**) Mason type II fracture postoperatively after screw osteosynthesis in AP and lateral view.

2.4. Postoperative Treatment

The initial cast immobilization was terminated on day two after the surgery. Early functional exercising under physiotherapeutic assistance with a free range of motion was subsequently started. The prevention of postoperative stiffness of the elbow is essential in the aftercare of any type of radius head fracture. This applies to conservative therapy as well as to all surgical procedures such as screw osteosynthesis, plate osteosynthesis, and radial head prostheses. Therefore, all patients are instructed to start physiotherapeutic exercise at an early stage. Lifting weights was not allowed for six weeks until clinical and radiological control in our outpatient clinic took place.

2.5. Statistics

Frequencies of variables were specified with the number and the percentage share. For bivariate analyses, continuous variables were described using mean ± standard deviation. Binary variables were compared with percentages in cross-tables. Pearson's-Chi-Square test was used to validate significance. Continuous variables were compared using the Student's *t*-tests. Differences of not normally distributed variables were assessed using the Mann–Whitney-U Test. The level of significance was defined as $p < 0.05$. Statistics were calculated using SPSS (IBM SPSS Statistics for Windows, Version 22; Armonk, NY, USA).

3. Results

3.1. Baseline Epidemiological Data

A total of 92 patients met the inclusion criteria and returned the ESAS questionnaire: 42 (45.7%) of those patients were female and 50 (54.3%) were male. The average age was 47.5 ± 14.1 years, with a minimum of 17 years and a maximum of 77 years. The average time to follow up was 49.9 ± 37.1 months. Classification of the fracture morphology revealed 57 (62%) Mason type II fractures and 35 (38%) Mason type III fractures. The left elbow was affected more often (n= 49, 53.3%)) compared to the right side (n= 42, 45.7%). Analysis of the distribution of accidents over one calendar year showed a seasonal concentration in the summer months along with a peak in August (n = 16) (see Figure 2).

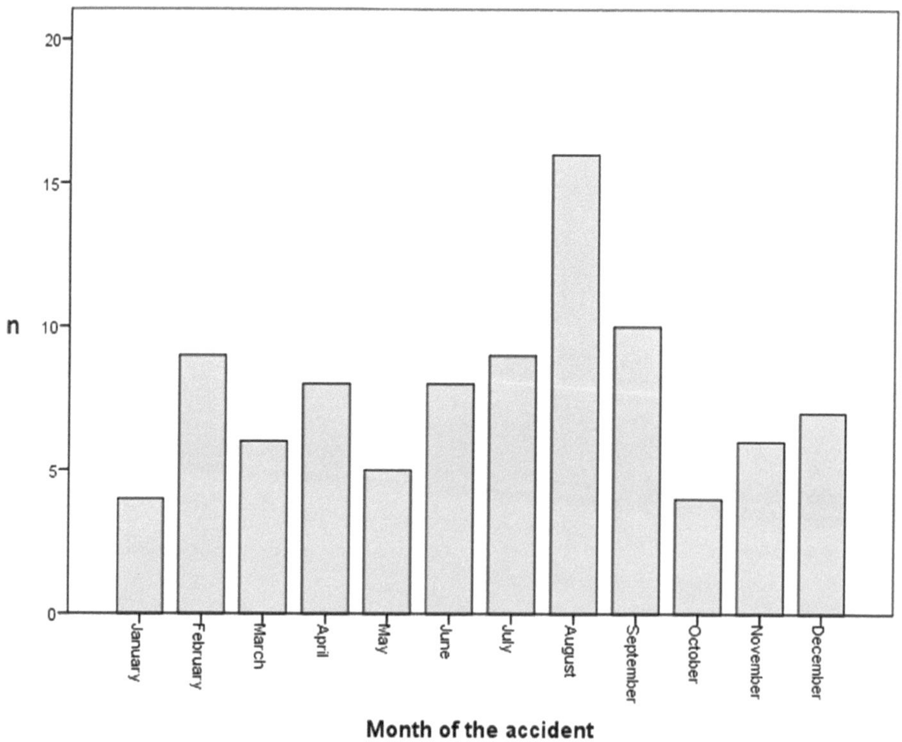

Figure 2. Monthly incidence of operatively treated radial head fractures.

3.2. Treatment and Revisions

The majority of 67 (72.8%) fractures were treated using screw osteosynthesis, 20 (21.7%) patients underwent plate osteosynthesis, and for 5 (5.4%) patients the fracture was found to be irreparable, resulting in the implantation of a radial head prosthesis.

In three cases (3.3%), revisional surgery was indicated. Two patients suffered from secondary dislocation of the fragments after screw osteosynthesis. One patient suffered from persistent postoperative elbow instability, so a ligament reconstruction in terms of a revision was indicated as well. Elective implant removal was performed in 5 (5.4%) patients due to subjective irritation from the implant. Four (4.3%) of those implant removals were performed after plate osteosynthesis.

3.3. Outcome

Functional outcome was obtained using the ESAS PROM. The average functional outcome score reached 89.7 ± 16.7 points. There was no gender difference regarding the functional outcome. Female patients had an average ESAS Score of 89.7 ± 17.2 points, male patients of 89.7 ± 16.5 points. The patients' age had no statistically relevant influence on the ESAS value (Pearson correlation coefficient −0.013 ($p = 0.900$).

Restriction of full extension of the elbow could be observed in 20 (20.7%) patients. Flexion was limited in 19 (20.7%) patients. Two (2.2%) patients reported a maximum flexion of 90° or less. Another 17 patients (18.5%) were able to bend to a maximum of 120°. All other 73 (79.3%) patients reported full ability of flexion, as shown in the elbow self-assessment questionnaire. Complications leading to revision surgery occurred in only 3 (3.3%) patients. Two patients who had been treated with screw osteosynthesis showed secondary dislocation of the fracture in the postoperative X-ray control. Therefore, revision with conversion to plate osteosynthesis was necessary in one of these patients and conversion to radial head prosthesis in the other. The third patient showed persistent ligamentous instability during the postoperative follow-up, so stabilization was carried out after 4 weeks using suture anchors.

3.4. Comparison of Mason Type II and III Fractures

Table 1 presents the differences between the Mason classification types. Looking at the epidemiological baseline data, no significant differences in age and gender were found. Since Mason III fractures are defined as unstable and presented with multiple fragments, these fractures were more likely to be treated using plate osteosynthesis. In this context, it should be mentioned that revision surgery and implant removal were only performed in cases of type III fractures. The difference in implant removal between Mason classification types reached significance ($p = 0.007$) but missed it regarding revision surgery ($p = 0.052$). The Elbow Self-Assessment Score was significantly lower for Mason type III fractures, indicating a poorer postoperative function (see Figure 3). This is also reflected in the range of motion, especially for the full extension of the elbow. Restricted range of motion could be observed in 9 (15.8%) cases of Mason type II fractures and 11 (34%) cases among type III fractures.

Table 1. Baseline characteristics and outcome for Mason type II and type III fractures.

	Mason II	Mason III	*p*-Value
n (%)	57 (62%)	35 (38%)	
Age [years]	46.6 ± 11.9	49.1 ± 17.1	0.243
Gender female	27 (47.4%)	15 (42.9%)	0.419
Surgery type			**<0.01** *
Screw osteosynthesis	56 (98.2%)	11 (31.4%)	
Plate osteosynthesis	1 (1.8%)	19 (54.3%)	
arthroplasty	0 (0%)	5 (14.3%)	
Flexion contracture	9 (15.8%)	11 (31.4%)	0.067
ESAS Score	92.3 ± 13.9	85.4 ± 20.1	**0.022** *
Revision surgery	0 (0%)	3 (8.6%)	0.052
Implant removal	0 (0%)	5 (14.3%)	**0.007** *

Data presented as mean ± SD or *n* (%); * = statistically significant.

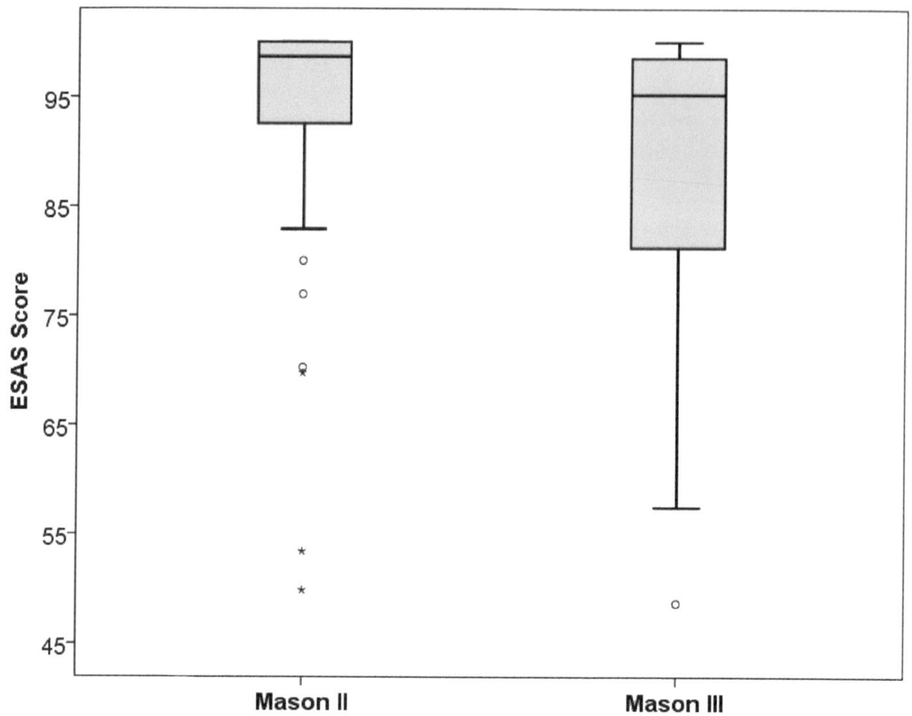

Figure 3. Boxplot diagram of ESAS scores in Mason type II and Mason type III fractures. (circles and stars mark outliers and extreme outliers).

3.5. Screw vs. Plate Osteosynthesis

Besides the modified Mason classification, the type of ORIF was investigated in relation to the postoperative functional outcome. In total, 67 patients were treated with screw osteosynthesis, and 20 patients received plate osteosynthesis. Patients who received screw osteosynthesis showed significantly better functional outcome scores in the ESAS (91.0 ± 16.5) compared to patients treated with plate osteosynthesis (85.3 ± 17.6; $p = 0.041$). Furthermore, the rate of postoperative restricted ROM was significantly higher in the screw ORIF group ($n = 10$; 14.9%) compared to the plate ORIF group ($n = 9$; 45.0%) ($p = 0.007$). Implant removal was performed in 1.5% ($n = 1$) of patients treated with screws and in 20% ($n = 4$) of patients treated with plate osteosynthesis ($p = 0.009$).

Table 2 presents the analysis of functional outcomes in the group of Mason type III fractures. There was no difference between screw osteosynthesis and plate osteosynthesis in terms of functional outcome as measured using the ESAS score and the prevalence of restricted ROM. RHA, however, showed better functional ESAS scores without reaching the level of significance due to the small number of cases in the sample.

Table 2. Functional outcome in Mason III fractures treated with different types of surgery.

	Surgery Type			
	Screw ORIF $n = 11$	**Plate ORIF** $n = 19$	**RHA** $n = 5$	***p*-Value**
ESAS	84.6 ± 25.6	84.9 ± 17.9	89.1 ± 17.3 (18.2%)	0.887
Restricted ROM	2 (18.2%)	8 (42.1%)	1 (20%)	0.332

Data presented as mean ± SD or *n* (%); RHA = radial head arthroplasty; ORIF open reduction internal fixation.

A multivariant linear regression analysis was performed using age, gender, fracture type according to the modified Mason classification, and type of surgery as variables, whereas the ESAS score was considered as the dependent outcome variable. This analysis did not reveal any of the mentioned variables as independent predictors, showing the following p-values: age $p = 0.952$; gender $p = 0.898$; Mason fracture type $p = 0.071$ and type of surgery $p = 0.607$.

4. Discussion

The presented study demonstrates a good overall postoperative functional outcome after operative treatment of Mason type II and III radial head fractures. Regardless of the type of operation, surgical therapy provides good results in the ESAS score with a low complication rate of only 3.3 percent.

There are several studies investigating the outcome after radial head fractures. Nevertheless, most studies only compare different treatment options for the same fracture type according to the Mason classification [7,11,15–17]. Sufficient data about the functional outcome comparing different Mason fracture types are still lacking in the current literature. The importance of patient-reported outcomes is constantly increasing in the evaluation process of postoperative outcomes. For this reason, this study was conducted to evaluate the overall postoperative outcome based on the patient-reported ESAS questionnaire in cases of displaced fractures of the radial head, including different types of fractures and treatment.

In his original publication describing the modification of the Mason classification, Hotchkiss also provided management guidelines, including a recommendation for treating Mason III fractures with excision or arthroplasty [5]. These recommendations can be repeatedly found in current literature [16,18–20]. In the presented sample of patients, only five cases were considered irreparable radial head fractures and, therefore, treated using RHA. All other enrolled fractures underwent surgical reconstruction using either screw or plate osteosynthesis showing good clinical results with an average ESAS score of 85.4 points in the Mason type III group. The continuous development in the field of implants with a special focus on anatomically preformed plates and interlocking screws for angular stability has led to a distinct improvement in the quality of radial head reconstructions so that arthroplasty or radial head resections are performed less frequently.

Despite the improvement in surgical methods and implants, Mason type III fractures remain challenging for upper extremity surgeons, usually resulting in poorer postoperative function. This is underlined by the results of this study, showing a lower average ESAS score of 85.4 ± 20.1 in the Mason III fracture group compared to an ESAS score of 92.3 ± 13.9 in the Mason II fracture group.

Although these facts may be self-evident to the experienced surgeon, there is no publication in the current literature that scientifically demonstrates this based on patient-reported outcome measures.

To the best of our knowledge, the presented study used the Elbow Self-Assessment score for the investigation of function after radial head fractures for the first time since its publication and validation in 2017 [13]. As of today, only a few studies have used the ESAS, which is why only a little evidence regarding the practical feasibility of this score exists [21,22]. The results of this study demonstrate that the ESAS can detect clinical differences in elbow functionality with high sensitivity. Furthermore, the quality of the clinical use of this PROM is confirmed using the presented results.

Lee et al. conducted a similar study on radial head fractures in 2018 [23]. Functional outcome and range of motion were investigated in a clinical examination by two Board-certified orthopedic surgeons using the QuickDASH score [24]. The authors found comparable results to this study with worse overall functional scores for Mason type III (QuickDASH 18 Range 0–68.2) compared to Mason type II fractures (QuickDASH 26.2 Range 0–86.4). This coherence with the QuickDASH score further demonstrates that the ESAS PROM is a useful tool for examiner-independent follow-up investigations of patients with elbow pathologies and is particularly suitable for use in register studies with high case numbers. The detection of the range of motion, which is not possible using other established scores like the DASH [24] or MEPS (Mayo Elbow Performance Score) [25], is an advantage of the ESAS.

Plate osteosynthesis provided worse functional results compared to screw osteosynthesis with regard to the ESAS score when the two procedures were compared independently of the fracture severity. Since plate osteosynthesis is used almost exclusively for Mason III fractures, it is only reasonable to look at this subgroup separately. Within the Mason III fracture group, no functional differences were found between plate and screw osteosynthesis. This suggests that the outcome is rather defined by the severity of the injury than by the type of surgery chosen. Nevertheless, the modified Mason classification could not be identified as an independent predictor of the functional outcome. Hereby, further investigations, including higher patient numbers, would be required.

Wu et al. also compared the outcome of screw-osteosynthesis with those of plate osteosynthesis, as well as with those of arthroplasty in 3-part radial head fractures and found functional outcomes comparable to our results but with a higher complication rate for plate osteosynthesis [15]. However, in their trial, no prospective, randomized study design was presented, so no reliable statements about the best treatment method can be derived.

In this study, Mason II fractures were very often treated surgically, which corresponds to the individual therapeutic algorithm of the authors. In general, however, there are still controversial opinions on the optimal treatment of isolated Mason type II radial head fractures. Guzzini et al. examined 50 patients with conservative treatment after mason type II fractures and described excellent functional outcome scores (DASH) and only marginal persistent limitations in range of motion [7].

In a systematic review of the literature, Lazerath et al. found that there were no differences in functional outcomes at mid-term follow-up when comparing Mason type II fractures treated surgically or conservatively. Nevertheless, the rate of osteoarthritis was higher in conservatively treated patients even though the mean follow-up period was shorter for the nonoperative cohort [26]. In our approach, we, therefore, favor surgical therapy for young patients to reconstruct the radiocapitellar joint surface as anatomically as possible, as the late effects of osteoarthritis are more evident in these patients.

The choice of the best possible osteosynthesis method always requires a precise preoperative analysis of the fracture. The final decision, however, depends on the intraoperative fracture assessment of the surgeon. A general statement regarding a superior osteosynthesis technique cannot be derived from the data.

Limitations

This study is potentially subject to several biases. First, there is a possible selection bias between the patients who participated in the survey and those who declined to participate. Since the presented study is not a randomized trial, the choice of treatment was made by the surgeon. Therefore, no independent conclusion about the best surgical procedure can be derived from the present study results. Another limitation is the relatively low international application of the ESAS score. Even if the score is sufficiently validated, there are only limited studies that allow comparability.

5. Conclusions

This study demonstrates positive postoperative clinical outcomes of surgically treated radial head fractures with low rates of revision surgery. The higher complexity of Mason III fractures is reflected in slightly worse functional outcomes compared to Mason II fractures. Furthermore, this study shows good clinical applicability of the ESAS PROM whereby subjective function and gross range of motion can be measured in a valid way and independent of the examiner.

Author Contributions: M.M., P.B. and M.W. were responsible for the conception and design of the study. J.Z. and V.M. conducted the data collection. M.M. and M.W. performed data analysis and interpretation. M.M. wrote the main manuscript text. M.Z., K.K. and C.K. assisted with literature research and performed proofreading. All authors read, revised, and approved the final manuscript. All authors have read and agreed to the published version of the manuscript.

Funding: This research received no external funding.

Institutional Review Board Statement: The study protocol was approved by the Ethics Committee of the Medical Faculty, Technical University of Munich (study number 71/15 S).

Informed Consent Statement: Informed consent was obtained from all participating individuals. This study was performed in accordance with the established ethical guidelines, including the Helsinki Declaration.

Data Availability Statement: The data set can be made available on individual request to the corresponding author.

Conflicts of Interest: The authors declare no conflict of interest.

Abbreviations

AP	anteroposterior
DASH	disabilities of the arm, shoulder and hand
ESAS	elbow self-assessment score
MEPS	mayo elbow performance score
ORIF	open reduction internal fixation
PROM	patient reported outcome measure
RHA	radial head arthroplasty
ROM	range of motion

References

1. Rupp, M.; Walter, N.; Pfeifer, C.; Lang, S.; Kerschbaum, M.; Krutsch, W.; Baumann, F.; Alt, V. The incidence of fractures among the adult population of germany—An analysis from 2009 through 2019. *Dtsch. Arztebl. Int.* **2021**, *118*, 665–669.
2. Kaas, L.; van Riet, R.P.; Vroemen, J.P.; Eygendaal, D. The epidemiology of radial head fractures. *J. Shoulder Elb. Surg.* **2010**, *19*, 520–523. [CrossRef] [PubMed]
3. Jackson, J.D.; Steinmann, S.P. Radial head fractures. *Hand Clin.* **2007**, *23*, 185–193, vi. [CrossRef] [PubMed]
4. Mason, M.L. Some observations on fractures of the head of the radius with a review of one hundred cases. *Br. J. Surg.* **1954**, *42*, 123–132. [CrossRef] [PubMed]
5. Hotchkiss, R.N. Displaced fractures of the radial head: Internal fixation or excision? *J. Am. Acad. Orthop. Surg.* **1997**, *5*, 1–10. [CrossRef] [PubMed]
6. de Muinck Keizer, R.J.; Walenkamp, M.M.; Goslings, J.C.; Schep, N.W. Mason type i fractures of the radial head. *Orthopedics* **2015**, *38*, e1147–e1154. [CrossRef]
7. Guzzini, M.; Vadalà, A.; Agrò, A.; Di Sanzo, V.; Pironi, D.; Redler, A.; Serlorenzi, P.; Proietti, L.; Civitenga, C.; Mazza, D.; et al. Nonsurgical treatment of mason type ii radial head fractures in athletes. A retrospective study. *G. Chir.* **2017**, *37*, 200–205.
8. van Riet, R.P.; van den Bekerom, M.; Van Tongel, A.; Spross, C.; Barco, R.; Watts, A.C. Radial head fractures. *Shoulder Elb.* **2020**, *12*, 212–223. [CrossRef]
9. Herbertsson, P.; Josefsson, P.O.; Hasserius, R.; Karlsson, C.; Besjakov, J.; Karlsson, M.K. Displaced mason type i fractures of the radial head and neck in adults: A fifteen- to thirty-three-year follow-up study. *J. Shoulder Elb. Surg.* **2005**, *14*, 73–77. [CrossRef] [PubMed]
10. Avisar, E.; Persitz, J.; Shohat, N.; Tamir, E.; Assaraf, E.; Keren, T. Does radial head resection impair hand and wrist function? A long-term follow-up. *J. Orthop. Trauma* **2021**, *35*, e486–e490. [CrossRef]
11. Scoscina, D.; Facco, G.; Luciani, P.; Setaro, N.; Senesi, L.; Martiniani, M.; Gigante, A.P. Mason type iii fractures of the radial head: Orif, resection or prosthetic replacement? *Musculoskelet. Surg.* **2022**, *107*, 223–230. [CrossRef]
12. Herbertsson, P.; Josefsson, P.O.; Hasserius, R.; Karlsson, C.; Besjakov, J.; Karlsson, M. Uncomplicated mason type-ii and iii fractures of the radial head and neck in adults. A long-term follow-up study. *J. Bone Jt. Surg. Am.* **2004**, *86*, 569–574. [CrossRef]
13. Beirer, M.; Friese, H.; Lenich, A.; Cronlein, M.; Sandmann, G.H.; Biberthaler, P.; Kirchhoff, C.; Siebenlist, S. The elbow self-assessment score (esas): Development and validation of a new patient-reported outcome measurement tool for elbow disorders. *Knee Surg. Sports Traumatol. Arthrosc.* **2017**, *25*, 2230–2236. [CrossRef]
14. Kaplan, E.B. Surgical approaches to the proximal end of the radius and its use in fractures of the head and neck of the radius. *JBJS* **1941**, *23*, 86–92.

15. Wu, P.H.; Shen, L.; Chee, Y.H. Screw fixation versus arthroplasty versus plate fixation for 3-part radial head fractures. *J. Orthop. Surg.* **2016**, *24*, 57–61. [CrossRef] [PubMed]
16. Dou, Q.; Yin, Z.; Sun, L.; Feng, X. Prosthesis replacement in mason iii radial head fractures: A meta-analysis. *Orthop. Traumato Surg. Res.* **2015**, *101*, 729–734. [CrossRef]
17. Mulders, M.A.M.; Schep, N.W.L.; de Muinck Keizer, R.O.; Kodde, I.F.; Hoogendoorn, J.M.; Goslings, J.C.; Eygendaal, D. Operative vs. Nonoperative treatment for mason type 2 radial head fractures: A randomized controlled trial. *J. Shoulder Elb. Surg.* **2021**, *30*, 1670–1678. [CrossRef]
18. Eyberg, B.A.; McKee, M.D. Indications and clinical results of radial head replacement: Has anything changed? *J. Orthop. Trauma* **2019**, *33* (Suppl. 8), S1–S6. [CrossRef]
19. Ring, D.; Quintero, J.; Jupiter, J.B. Open reduction and internal fixation of fractures of the radial head. *J. Bone Jt. Surg. Am.* **2002**, *84*, 1811–1815. [CrossRef] [PubMed]
20. Rosenblatt, Y.; Athwal, G.S.; Faber, K.J. Current recommendations for the treatment of radial head fractures. *Orthop. Clin. N. Am.* **2008**, *39*, 173–185. [CrossRef] [PubMed]
21. Willinger, L.; Siebenlist, S.; Lenich, A.; Liska, F.; Imhoff, A.B.; Achtnich, A. Arthroscopic arthrolysis provides good clinical outcome in post-traumatic and degenerative elbow stiffness. *Knee Surg. Sports Traumatol. Arthrosc.* **2018**, *26*, 312–317. [CrossRef] [PubMed]
22. Geyer, S.; Lacheta, L.; Seilern Und Aspang, J.; Willinger, L.; Lutz, P.M.; Lappen, S.; Imhoff, A.B.; Siebenlist, S. Patient satisfaction, joint stability and return to sports following simple elbow dislocations: Surgical versus non-surgical treatment. *Arch. Orthop. Trauma. Surg.* **2022**, *143*, 1481–1489. [CrossRef] [PubMed]
23. Lee, Y.S.; Kang, Y.H.; Chung, Y.G.; Shin, S.H. Open reduction and internal fixation for mason type iii radial head fractures: Is it different from that for mason type ii fractures? *J. Orthop. Surg.* **2018**, *26*, 1560–1568. [CrossRef]
24. Hudak, P.L.; Amadio, P.C.; Bombardier, C. Development of an upper extremity outcome measure: The dash (disabilities of the arm, shoulder and hand) [corrected]. The upper extremity collaborative group (uecg). *Am. J. Ind. Med.* **1996**, *29*, 602–608. [CrossRef]
25. Morrey, B.; An, K.-N.; Chao, E.Y.S. Functional evaluation of the elbow. In *The Elbow and Its Disorders*; Elsevier Health Sciences: Amsterdam, The Netherlands, 2009; pp. 80–91.
26. Lanzerath, F.; Hackl, M.; Wegmann, K.; Müller, L.P.; Leschinger, T. The treatment of isolated mason type ii radial head fractures: A systematic review. *J. Shoulder Elb. Surg.* **2021**, *30*, 487–494. [CrossRef]

Journal of
Clinical Medicine

MDPI

Article

Vertebral Fractures in Pediatric Suicidal Jumpers: A Retrospective Study with Epidemiological and Clinical Analysis before and after the COVID-19 Pandemic

Marco Crostelli [1], Osvaldo Mazza [1,*], Francesca Manfroni [1], Federico Tundo [1], Valeria Calogero [1], Marianna Mazza [2], Roberto Averna [3] and Stefano Vicari [2,3]

1 Spine Surgery Department, Bambino Gesù Children's Hospital IRCCS, 00168 Rome, Italy; marco.crostelli@opbg.net (M.C.); francesca.manfroni@opbg.net (F.M.); federico.tundo@opbg.net (F.T.); valeria.calogero@opbg.net (V.C.)

2 Institute of Psychiatry and Psychology, Fondazione Policlinico Universitario A. Gemelli IRCCS, Università Cattolica del Sacro Cuore, 00168 Rome, Italy; marianna.mazza@policlinicogemelli.it (M.M.); stefano.vicari@opbg.net (S.V.)

3 Childhood and Adolescent Neuropsychiatric Unit, Neuroscience Department, Bambino Gesù Children's Hospital IRCCS, 00168 Rome, Italy; roberto.averna@opbg.net

* Correspondence: osvaldo.mazza@opbg.net

Abstract: Background: From the beginning of the COVID-19 pandemic, reports in the literature confirm a significant increase in suicide attempts in children and adolescents. At the Bambino Gesù Pediatric Hospital Emergency Department (Rome, Italy), there was a dramatic increase in suicidal jumpers. Many of these presented vertebral fractures. Methods: This retrospective study includes all suicidal jumpers with vertebral fractures treated from April 2017 to March 2023. We collected and compared data from three years before to three years after the pandemic, analyzing vertebral fractures. Results: From April 2019 to March 2020, 141 cases of suicide attempt arrived at the emergency department. Five of these were suicidal jumpers without vertebral fractures. From April 2020 to March 2023, 362 cases of suicide were hospitalized and 19 were suicidal jumpers; 12 reported vertebral fractures (mean age 14 years). Seven patients were treated by percutaneous pedicle fixation. Three patients needed an open spinal surgery by posterior approach. One case with cervical fractures was treated by Halo-Vest. Conclusions: This is the first report that shows a sharp increase in vertebral body fractures due to suicide jumping attempts in children and adolescents. This could be a new epidemiological phenomenon persisting or even increasing over time in the pediatric population as a consequence of the COVID-19 pandemic.

Keywords: pediatric spine fractures; suicidal jumpers; spine fracture surgery; COVID-19; suicidal attempts

1. Introduction

Suicide is a relatively rare event in pediatric population, but its prevalence increases during adolescence and it is highly lethal [1]. The World Health Organization states that suicide is a social problem, and prevention is particularly important for managing suicide attempts in the youngest population, which has longest life expectancy [2]. According to the World Health Organization, suicide is the fourth leading cause of death among 15- to 29-year-olds [2] and the United Nations International Children's Emergency Fund in "The State of the World's Children 2021" highlights that suicide is the second leading cause of death among 15- to 19-year-olds in Europe [3]. Almost 1200 youth between the ages of 10 and 19 years die by suicide every year in Europe [3]. According to the Centers for Disease Control and Prevention (CDC), 2018 suicide is the second most common cause of death among 10- to 14-year-olds and 20- to 34-year-olds in USA [4]. Suicide in youths is globally recognized as an important public health problem [2].

Poisoning by pesticides represents the 20% of suicides in low- and middle-income countries [2], but there are large differences between countries and genders in suicide attempt methods [5,6]. In an analysis of 15 European countries, Värnik et al. [6] claimed that hanging and jumping from height were, respectively, the first and the second suicide method for both genders in people between 15 and 24 years of age, followed by using a moving vehicle for males and poisoning for females. According to Kolves et al., the most frequent suicide method in children and adolescent aged 10–19 years in different countries worldwide is hanging. Jumping from height is also an important alternative method [5].

Many recent studies reported in the literature confirm a significant increase in mental health disease in children and adolescents from the beginning of the COVID-19 pandemic, with a rise in suicidal ideation and suicide attempts [7–17].

From the beginning of the COVID-19 pandemic, admission of patients with mood disorders, self-injurious behaviors, and suicidal ideation significantly increased in our hospital [16]. We noted a significant increase in suicidal attempts by jumping from height in adolescent patients, compared with pre-COVID data. Many of these suicidal jumper attempts resulted in vertebral fractures.

There are few studies on the type of injuries associated with falls from heights in pediatric patients. In general, traumatic spinal injuries in the pediatric population are uncommon and are frequently related to motor vehicle crashes [18,19]. In patients younger than 4 years in age, most vertebral fractures involve the upper cervical spine (C0–C4) [20], and this is due to anatomical age-related conditions. Thoracic spine is the most common localization of spine fractures in the general pediatric population, followed by lumbar spine [21,22]. Conservative treatment, for 6 to 8 weeks with a thoraco-lumbo-sacral orthosis, is the gold standard for stable fractures [21,23]. Neurological impairment is reported in about 5% of cases [21] and is considered a risk factor for progressive spinal deformity [23].

The care of vertebral fractures in suicidal jumpers is peculiar and must consider the issue of patients' mental health.

This work highlights the new and widespread epidemiological phenomenon of a high frequency of suicidal attempts with an uncommon modality in adolescents following the COVID-19 pandemic. It is particularly important to analyze the treatment of numerous complex vertebral fractures in polytrauma pediatric patients who committed suicide attempts by jumping from heights.

2. Material and Methods

In this retrospective study, we reviewed all patients treated at Bambino Gesù Children's Hospital Emergency Department in Rome from 1 April 2017 to 31 March 2023 for suicidal attempt.

We compared the three-year post-COVID 19 pandemic beginning with the three-year period before pandemic. Italian government imposed a national lockdown on 9 March 2020, but in this study we decided to start the pandemic period from 1 April, about 1 month after, to better highlights the effects.

In our hypothesis, the dramatic increase in suicidal attempts by jumping from height within the pediatric and adolescent population in Italy, and consequent increase in incidence of vertebral fractures, is the direct consequence of pandemic restrictions and limitations of everyday life and normal social interaction on the mental health of the youngest part of the Italian population.

To our knowledge, this is the first work specifically focusing on the increase in the occurrence of suicidal jumpers' vertebral fractures within the pediatric population during the COVID-19 pandemic.

Only patients with vertebral fractures for a suicidal attempt were included. Fracture classification, treatment, and midterm follow-up were analyzed.

Thoracolumbar, subaxial cervical, and sacropelvic fractures were classified according to AO spine [24–26] and cervical fractures were classified using the Anderson–D'Alonso classification [27].

The fracture pattern in these jumpers is not different from other nonsuicidal high-energy spine fractures treated in patients of similar age, but particular consideration has been given to the choice of treatment, which to some extent is different from the treatment for patients without suicidal attempt issues. We decided treatment according to the grade of fracture instability, neurological impairment, and psychiatric treatment needed. Usually, patients who attempted suicide require immediate and prolonged psychiatric treatment with a long hospitalization period in dedicated wards. Since the possibility of early mobilization of the patient without orthosis is paramount to begin successful psychiatric rehabilitation treatment, in many "borderline" spine fractures (vertebral fractures without neurological impairment that in a patient without psychiatric issues could be treated with a prolonged orthosis or cast immobilization), we opted for percutaneous surgical treatment to avoid long bracing treatment.

The study received approval from the local ethical committee (Ethics Committee of the Bambino Gesù Pediatric Hospital, Rome, Italy, ID 2426-OPBG-2021). Written informed consent was obtained from all participants and/or their parents for minors.

3. Results

At Bambino Gesù Children Hospital, there were 141 cases of suicidal attempts from 1 April 2017 to 31 March 2020 and 5 (2.8%) of these were suicidal jumpers; none of them reported vertebral fractures.

From 1 April 2020 to 31 March 2023, there were 362 suicidal attempts with 19 (5.2%) suicidal jumpers. Twelve (63.2%) of the suicidal jumpers had a vertebral fracture (M:F = 4:8) (Table 1).

Table 1. Patients involved in the study.

	Patient	Age	Sex	Vertebral Fracture—AO Classification	Other Fractures	Other Injuries	Spine Treatment	Hospitalization Days	Follow-Up
1	V.C.G.C.	15 y 9 m	F	L1 (A4), L4 (A1), Coccyx (A0)	right distal tibia, right fibula, left proximal humerus, left ulnar styloid process	pneumothorax, splenic injury, subdural hematoma, diffuse axonal injury	T12 to L2 Percutaneous pedicle fixation	118	22 months No deficit Implant removal
2	**A.M.**	14 y 1 m	M	L1 (A3)	right ankle		T12 to L2 Percutaneous pedicle fixation	20	21 months No deficit Implant removal
3	Z.P.E.	14 y 11 m	M	L3 (A1), L4(A4)	right acetabulum, right ischiopubic branch, right tibia, bilateral wrist, bilateral heels	pneumothorax, aortic isthmus lesion, right peroneal nerve injury	L3 to L5 Percutaneous pedicle fixation	37	17 months No deficit Implant removal
4	B.T.M.A	12 y 7 m	F	D11 (A1)	multiple ribs		Conservative	15	17 months No deficit
5	R.S.M.	16 y 1 m	F	D8 (A0), D11 (A1), L1 (A1), L4 (A1)	right ankle, left distal radius		Conservative	12	11 months No deficit

Table 1. *Cont.*

	Patient	Age	Sex	Vertebral Fracture—AO Classification	Other Fractures	Other Injuries	Spine Treatment	Hospitalization Days	Follow-Up
6	L.G.G.	10 y 5 m	F	C2 (AD 2), C5 (A4), C6 (A1), L1 (A1), L2 (A3), L3 (A0), L4 (A0), Right sacroiliac joint	multiple ribs, right acetabulum, ilio-ischiopubic bilateral branch, left heel	liver injury, splenic injury, pleural effusion	Halo-Vest and L1 to L3 Percutaneous pedicle fixation	64	10 months No deficit
7	H.B.	15 y 5 m	F	L5 (A0), Sacral U-Shaped Fracture (C3)	right acetabulum, bilateral olecranos, right femural shaft	paraplegia, complete neurogenic bowel and bladder dysfunction	L4 to Pelvis posterior open fusion, left sacral plate and L4 to S1 decompression	30	8 months complete neurogenic bowel and bladder dysfunction; motor deficit of the right limb partial recovered
8	**D.G.**	12 y 10 m	F	D6 (A1), D7 (A1)	multiple right ribs	pneumothorax	D5 to D8 Percutaneous pedicle fixation	210	9 months No deficit Implant removal
9	M.D.	16 y 5 m	M	D12 (A1), L1 (A3)		anal injury	T10 to L2 Percutaneous pedicle fixation	56	6 months No deficit
10	G.A.	16 y 6 m	M	L2 (A4), L5 (A4)	right orbital maxilla surface, right open tibia and fibula		L1 to S1 Percutaneous pedicle fixation	40	6 months No deficit
11	B.V.	15 y 3 m	F	L1 (A4)		pulmonary contusion, complete neurogenic bowel and bladder dysfunction	T11 to L3 open pedicle screw fixation and posterior L1 decompression	14	1 month Urinary retension
12	P.E.	12 y	F	L5 (A0), Sacral fracture (B3)	orbital floor, bilateral nose bones, ilio-ischiopubic left branch, pubic symphysis diastasis		L4 to ilium left open fixation and iliosacral screw	33	1 month No deficit

Legend: Bold text for patients with previous neuropsychiatric diagnosis. Underlined text is for lesions surgically treated. A, B, and C (AO classification), AD (Anderson–d'Alonso classification).

The mean age was 14 years (range 10 to 16). Only two patients had a neuropsychiatric diagnosis before the suicide attempt (16.6%). The most common level of fracture was L1 (six cases). Thoracic spine was involved in four cases and lumbar spine in ten. Hospitalization period ranged from 12 to 210 days, with high variability mostly due to neuropsychiatric care.

Vertebral fractures are a direct consequence of the impact of jumpers' bodies with soil. Owing to the pandemic lockdown restrictions in Italy, data for suicidal attempt circumstances from first emergency teams that rescued patients are not available; thus, it is not possible to determine a relationship between the height of the jump or nature of the impact surface and severity or pattern of fractures.

According to AO spine thoracolumbar classification [24], there were five A0, ten A1, three A3, and five A4 vertebral fractures, alone or in association (Table 1). Moreover, there was an "U shaped sacral fracture" (C3 AO spine) [26], a transforaminal sacral fracture (B3 AO spine) [26], a coccyx fracture (A1 AO spine) [26] and an Anderson–D'Alonso C2 type II fracture [27].

In the latter case, a burst C5 fracture (A4 AO spine) and a compression C6 fracture (A1 AO spine) [25] were associated with the C2 fracture and she was conservatively treated with a Halo-Vest for 3 months.

Only two patients with thoracolumbar A0 and A1 types of fractures (cases 4 and 5, Table 1) were conservatively treated with a rigid thoracolumbar orthosis for 3 months with good compliance and results. Percutaneous pedicle fixation was applied in seven patients with an indirect decompression and to restore and improve sagittal balance (Figures 1 and 2; Table 1, case 6 and 10). Only in two cases we observed neurological impairment. In both cases, an open spinal decompression and posterior spinal fusion was performed. All surgically treated patients used a soft spine orthosis for 1 month to facilitate early mobilization and to reduce muscular pain.

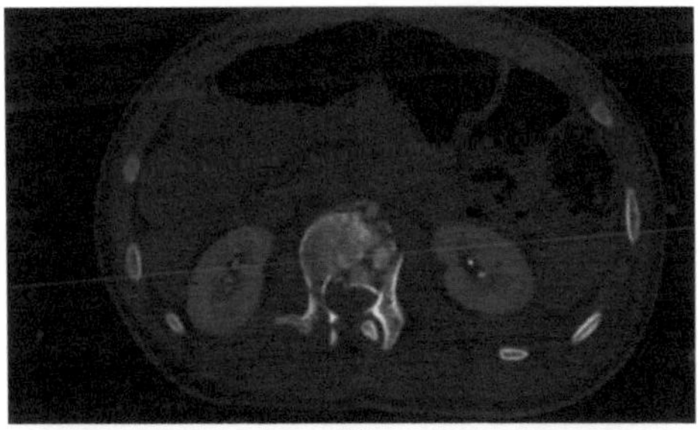

(A)

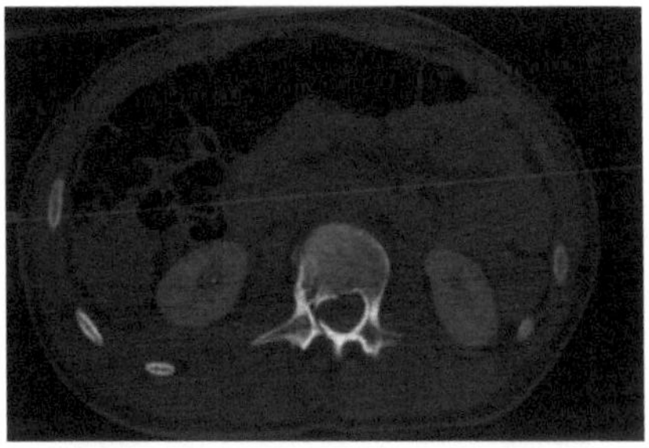

(B)

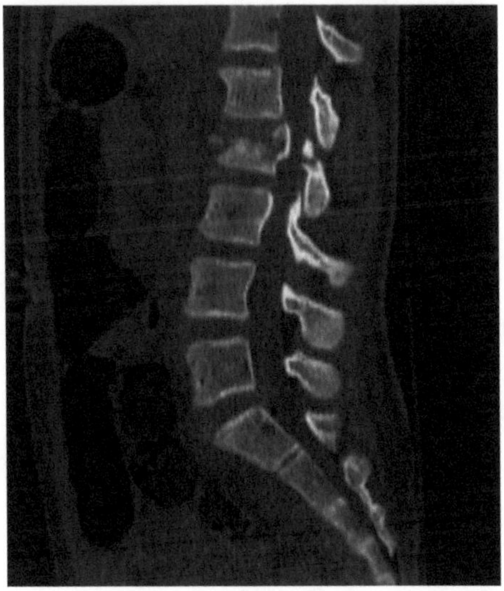

(C)

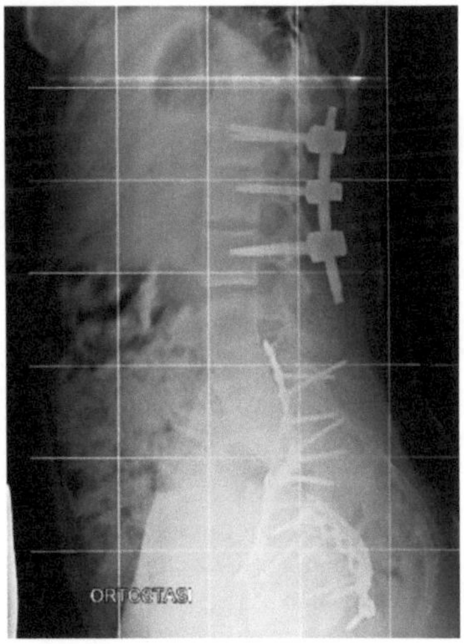

(D)

Figure 1. *Cont.*

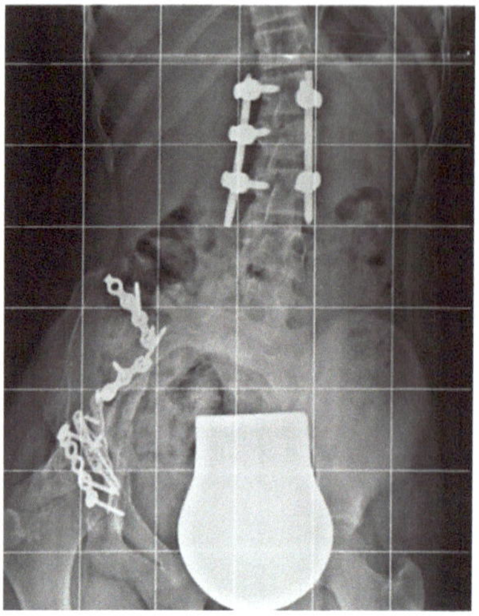

(**E**)

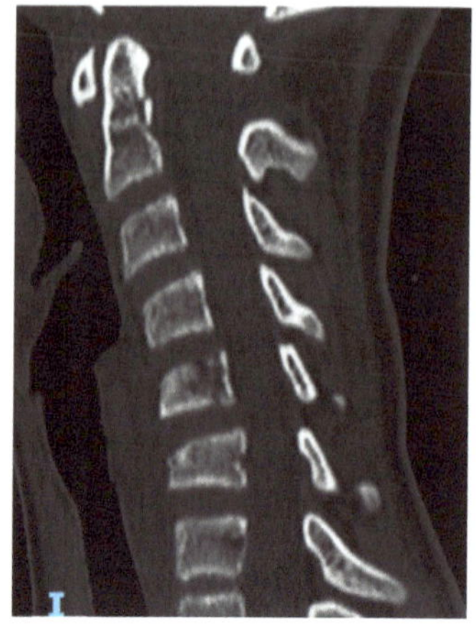

(**F**)

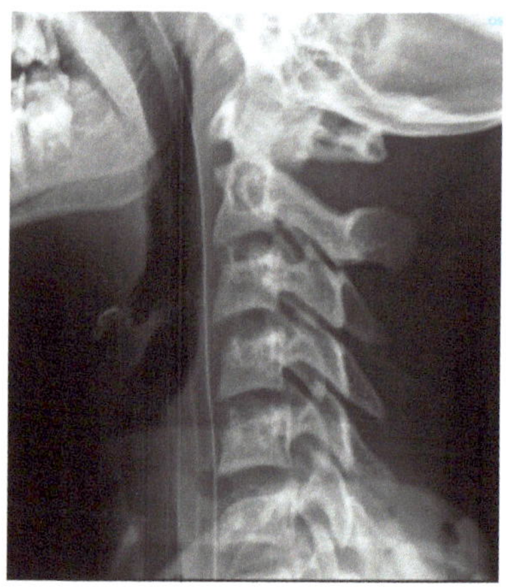

(**G**)

Figure 1. Case 6 (Table 1): (**A**,**B**) preoperative axial CT scan of L1 and L2; (**C**) preoperative sagittal CT scan of lumbar spine; (**D**,**E**) anteroposterior and lateral X-ray of lumbar spine after surgery; (**F**) sagittal CT scan of post-traumatic cervical spine; (**G**) X-ray lateral view in Halo-Vest.

All patients had other appendicular fractures or other injuries that in some cases needed surgical treatment. Eight patients underwent other procedures: seven orthopedic surgeries for appendicular fractures, one maxillofacial surgery for an orbital floor fracture, and one vascular and one proctological surgery. Many different medical specialties were involved in these patients' care.

Four patients had preoperative neurologic deficits. The first patient (case 1, Table 1) presented with a diffuse axonal injury and a left hemiparesis that completely recovered in 4 months. The second (case 3, Table 1) had a transitory right peroneal nerve palsy. The third (case 6, Table 1) had a paraplegia and complete neurogenic bowel and bladder dysfunction; the latter had a complete neurogenic bowel and bladder dysfunction which improved during the last month (case 12, Table 1).

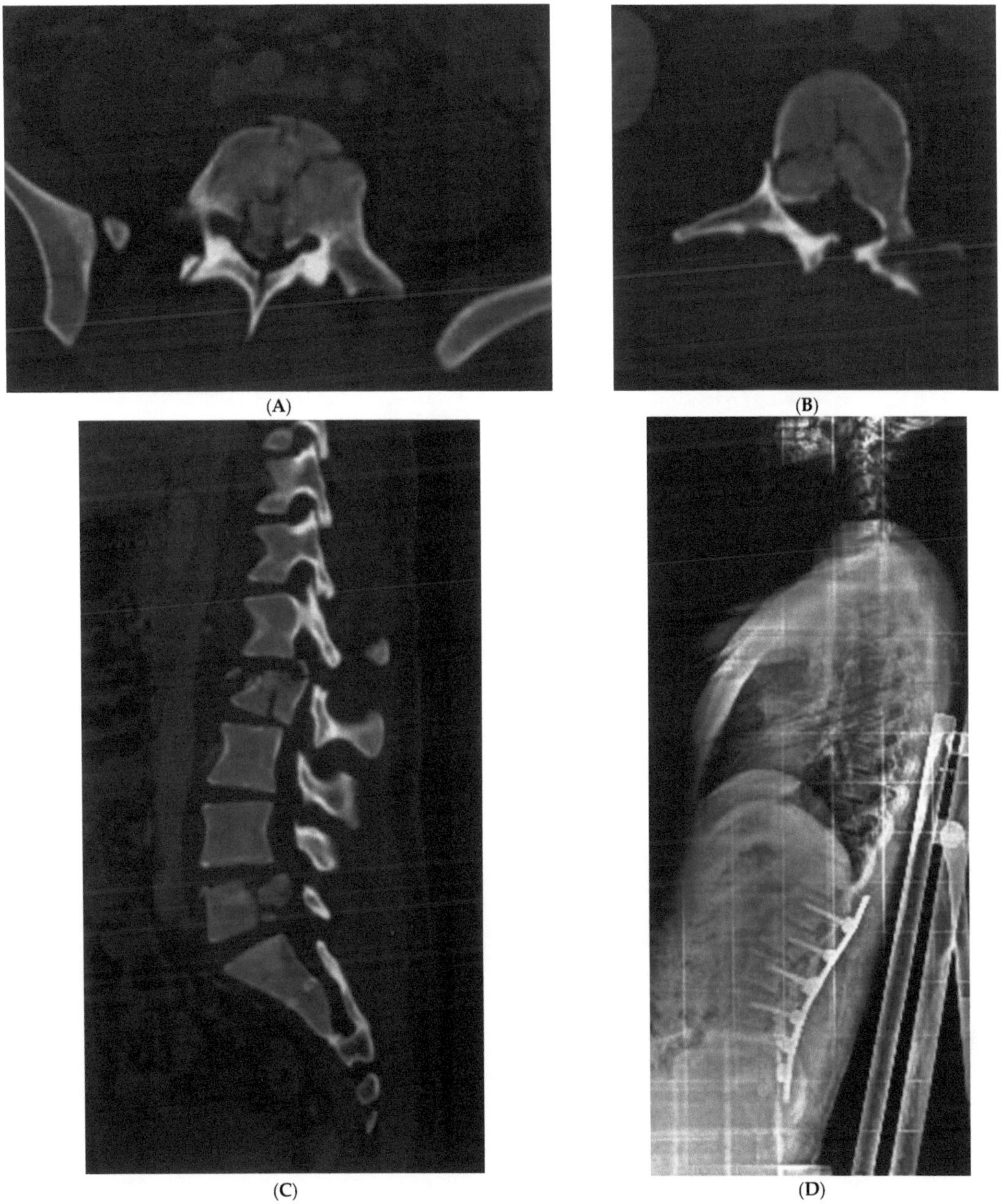

Figure 2. Case 10 (Table 1): (A) preoperative axial CT scan of L5; (B) preoperative axial CT scan of L2; (C) preoperative sagittal CT scan of lumbar spine; (D) postoperative X-ray lateral view in sitting position.

At last follow-up, the third patient showed a persistent complete sphincter deficiency and a partial recovery of paraplegia. Nowadays, she can walk with crutches for short distances. Otherwise, the latter patient only has a urinary retention.

One year after trauma, four patients underwent implant removal surgery (cases 1, 2, 3, and 8, Table 1) with excellent clinical and radiological results. All these patients resumed their daily activities, including sports.

4. Discussion

Recent literature highlights concern about the consequences of the COVID-19 pandemic on pediatric population mental health [7–16]. In this study, the comparison between 3 years before and 3 years after pandemic demonstrates an increase in suicidal attempts. Comparing the two periods, suicidal attempts after the pandemic increased by 61.1% and suicidal jumpers increased by 73.7%. In the 3 years before the pandemic, no vertebral fractures in suicidal jumpers were noted. Otherwise, in the other 3 years analyzed, during the pandemic, 63.2% of suicidal jumpers reported vertebral fractures.

The purpose of our study was to analyze this new and dramatic phenomenon and, in particular, to report the peculiarity of vertebral fracture treatment in young suicidal jumpers during the pandemic.

To our knowledge, this is the first study that shows a significant increase in suicide jumping attempts and a related increase in vertebral fractures in pediatric patients after the pandemic.

Regarding the twelve patients included in the study and according to concerns reported in the literature on the increase in neuropsychiatric diseases, only 16.6% had a previous neuropsychiatric diagnosis. Even if it is not statistically significant, considering the limited timeframe and low number of patients involved, in our opinion, these raw data show the devastating effect of the COVID-19 crisis on the social environment and behavioral habits of youngest Italian population.

Before the COVID-19 pandemic, jumping from heights was an unusual suicide attempt behavior in our country's adolescent population, and experience with surgical treatment of spine fractures in adolescent patients involved in these suicidal attempts was almost inexistent.

In this study, different types of vertebral fractures were found and most were surgically treated (83.3%). The pattern of fractures presented in this study are similar to high-energy spine fractures due to other kinds of injuries (e.g., motor vehicle crash), but their frequent recurrence in a relatively short period of time is a new finding. Some of the fractures treated are rare in the pediatric population (i.e., spinopelvic dissociation) and are more frequent in adults who jumpèd from heights. Sacral fractures are about 0.16% of all pediatric trauma [28] and cervical fractures are also rare and different according to age [29]. Only 1.5% of pediatric trauma cause cervical spine injury, but 60 to 80% of vertebral pediatric injuries involve the cervical spine [29].

In the literature, conservative treatment with orthosis for 6 to 8 weeks is suggested for stable vertebral fractures without neurologic impairment [21,23]. Nonsurgical treatment is also indicated in the case of burst fractures without neurologic impairment, since no significant differences have been demonstrated in functional outcomes compared to operative treatment [30,31].

In this study, surgery was performed not only to decompress or to restore a better sagittal balance but also to achieve a faster recovery. Conservative spine treatment with rigid orthosis or casts for a long period following a suicide attempt could be an additional burden for these patients. Surgical percutaneous treatment for thoracolumbar fractures allows early mobilization, and this can ensure to the patient a quick resumption of daily activities. Suicidal jumper patients are usually adolescents, with multiple injuries and severe mental health diseases, who face long periods of psychiatric and multidisciplinary treatments. Surgery can be considered a temporary internal fixation as an alternative to conservative treatment with a rigid orthosis, which could be a hitch to the patient's therapeutic path.

However, cervical spine surgery is much more invasive and the only case with multiple cervical fractures and good results was conservatively treated with a Halo-Vest. In this patient, neurological impairment was not observed, and a surgical treatment had no real advantage over conservative treatment to obtain better fracture reduction and stabilization. In this case, surgery could have a potential higher risk of complications (i.e., surgical site infection, vascular and nervous iatrogenic damage, blood loss) and instrumentation spread on more levels. Patients and relatives occasionally experience difficulty in complying with Halo-Vest treatment, even if Halo is somehow preferable to collar bracing or casting; during long treatment, patient discomfort is less when using Halo-Vest, particularly regarding alimentation and hygiene. In our case, patient and parents showed good compliance with Halo-Vest, and the orthopedic treatment did not impair her psychiatric therapy.

In this study, four patients had neurologic lesions and two with severe outcomes. Treatment of these patients was challenging, especially when they were isolated from relatives and friends. Moreover, spinal treatments had to be coordinated with the need for treatment of other associated injuries. A multidisciplinary team has been essential to optimize the management of these patients and avoid major complications.

The main limitation of this study is the low number of involved patients; a multicenter study at European level, where there were similar pandemic conditions and restrictions, could certainly widen the cohort of patients with the aim to define the best treatment guidelines.

In future research, we could expand these preliminary results in order to clarify if this dramatic phenomenon and related injuries will remain as a grim result of postpandemic changes in social behavior or if suicidal jumper attempts in adolescents will return to prepandemic incidence.

5. Conclusions

This study shows an exponential increase in pediatric vertebral fractures due to suicide jumping attempts after the COVID-19 pandemic. These are high-energy fractures that are rather unusual in adolescents, and rarely observed in specific cases (such as spinopelvic dissociation). The unusual high frequency of suicidal attempts with an uncommon modality in adolescents is a new epidemiological phenomenon after the COVID-19 pandemic. The high number of complex vertebral fractures, in polytrauma pediatric patients who committed a self-harm act, could be a big issue for a spine surgeon. The choice of treatment must be guided by biological and biomechanical knowledge, but also by the mental health condition of young patients and by other necessary treatments. In our experience, percutaneous surgery was the treatment strategy used most and allowed for fast recovery. Suicidal jumper patients must be handled by a multidisciplinary team to optimize and personalize therapeutic management. In future studies, we could clarify if suicidal jumper attempts in adolescents will return to prepandemic incidence or, conversely, if this dramatic phenomenon will remain as a long-term consequence of COVID-19 pandemic.

Author Contributions: Conceptualization: M.C., O.M. and M.M.; methodology: M.C.; software: M.C. and F.T.; validation: M.C.; formal analysis: M.C. and M.M.; investigation: M.C. and F.T.; data curation, M.C., V.C. and R.A.; writing—original draft: F.M. and O.M.; writing—review and editing: O.M. and M.M.; visualization: M.C. and S.V.; supervision: M.C. All authors have read and agreed to the published version of the manuscript.

Funding: This research received no external funding.

Institutional Review Board Statement: The study received approval from the local ethical committee (Ethics Committee of the Bambino Gesù Pediatric Hospital, Rome, Italy, ID 2426-OPBG-2021).

Informed Consent Statement: Informed consent was obtained from all subjects involved in the study.

Data Availability Statement: Data are unavailable due to privacy restrictions.

Conflicts of Interest: The authors declare no conflict of interest.

References

1. Theodorou, C.M.; Yamashiro, K.J.; Stokes, S.C.; Salcedo, E.S.; Hirose, S.; Beres, A.L. Pediatric suicide by violent means: A cry fo help and a call for action. *Inj. Epidemiol.* **2022**, *9*, 13. [CrossRef]
2. WHO. *Preventing Suicide: A Global Imperative*; WHO: Geneva, Switzerland, 2014; p. 92. Available online: https://www.who.int publications/i/item/9789241564779 (accessed on 8 April 2022).
3. UNICEF. *The State of the World's Children 2021*; On my Mind: Promoting, Protecting and Caring for Children's Mental Health UNICEF: New York, NY, USA, 2021; Available online: https://www.unicef.org/reports/state-worlds-children-2021 (accessed or 8 April 2022).
4. CDC. C for DC and PNC for HS. National Vital Statistics System, Mortality 2018–2021 on CDC WONDER Online Database Released in 2023. 2023. Available online: http://wonder.cdc.gov/mcd-icd10-expanded.html (accessed on 8 April 2022).
5. Kõlves, K.; de Leo, D. Suicide methods in children and adolescents. *Eur. Child Adolesc. Psychiatry* **2017**, *26*, 155–164. [CrossRef]
6. Värnik, A.; Kõlves, K.; Allik, J.; Arensman, E.; Aromaa, E.; van Audenhove, C.; Bouleau, J.-H.; van der Feltz-Cornelis, C.M. Giupponi, G.; Gusmão, R.; et al. Gender issues in suicide rates, trends and methods among youths aged 15–24 in 15 European countries. *J. Affect. Disord.* **2009**, *113*, 216–226. [CrossRef]
7. Bera, L.; Souchon, M.; Ladsous, A.; Colin, V.; Lopez-Castroman, J. Emotional and Behavioral Impact of the COVID-19 Epidemic in Adolescents. *Curr. Psychiatry Rep.* **2022**, *24*, 37–46. [CrossRef] [PubMed]
8. Gracia, R.; Pamias, M.; Mortier, P.; Alonso, J.; Pérez, V.; Palao, D. Is the COVID-19 pandemic a risk factor for suicide attempts in adolescent girls? *J. Affect. Disord.* **2021**, *292*, 139–141. [CrossRef]
9. Yard, E.; Radhakrishnan, L.; Ballesteros, M.F.; Sheppard, M.; Gates, A.; Stein, Z.; Hartnett, K.; Kite-Powell, A.; Rodgers, L. Adjemian, J.; et al. Emergency Department Visits for Suspected Suicide Attempts Among Persons Aged 12–25 Years Before and During the COVID-19 Pandemic—United States, January 2019–May 2021. *MMWR Morb. Mortal. Wkly. Rep.* **2021**, *70*, 888–894 [CrossRef] [PubMed]
10. COVID-19 Mental Disorders Collaborators. Global prevalence and burden of depressive and anxiety disorders in 204 countries and territories in 2020 due to the COVID-19 pandemic. *Lancet* **2021**, *398*, 1700–1712. [CrossRef] [PubMed]
11. Sivertsen, B.; Knapstad, M.; Petrie, K.; O'Connor, R.; Lønning, K.J.; Hysing, M. Changes in mental health problems and suicidal behaviour in students and their associations with COVID-19-related restrictions in Norway: A national repeated cross-sectional analysis. *BMJ Open* **2022**, *12*, e057492. [CrossRef] [PubMed]
12. Gilsbach, S.; Herpertz-Dahlmann, B.; Konrad, K. Psychological Impact of the COVID-19 Pandemic on Children and Adolescents with and Without Mental Disorders. *Front. Public Health* **2021**, *9*, 679041. [CrossRef] [PubMed]
13. Carison, A.; Babl, F.E.; O'Donnell, S.M. Increased paediatric emergency mental health and suicidality presentations during COVID-19 stay at home restrictions. *Emerg. Med. Australas.* **2022**, *34*, 85–91. [CrossRef] [PubMed]
14. Mayne, S.L.; Hannan, C.; Davis, M.; Young, J.F.; Kelly, M.K.; Powell, M.; Dalembert, G.; McPeak, K.E.; Jenssen, B.P.; Fiks, A.G. COVID-19 and Adolescent Depression and Suicide Risk Screening Outcomes. *Pediatrics* **2021**, *148*, e2021051507. [CrossRef] [PubMed]
15. Hill, R.M.; Rufino, K.; Kurian, S.; Saxena, J.; Saxena, K.; Williams, L. Suicide Ideation and Attempts in a Pediatric Emergency Department Before and During COVID-19. *Pediatrics* **2021**, *147*, e2020029280. [CrossRef] [PubMed]
16. Vicari, S.; Pontillo, M. Developmental Psychopathology in the COVID-19 period. COVID-19 Pandemic Impact on Children and Adolescents' Mental Health. *Psychiatr. Danub.* **2021**, *33*, 33–35.
17. Maina, C.; Cioffi, S.P.B.; Altomare, M.; Spota, A.; Virdis, F.; Bini, R.; Ragozzino, R.; Renzi, F.; Reitano, E.; Corasaniti, L.; et al. Increasing Trend in Violence-Related Trauma and Suicide Attempts among Pediatric Trauma Patients: A 6-Year Analysis of Trauma Mechanisms and the Effects of the COVID-19 Pandemic. *J. Pers. Med.* **2023**, *13*, 128. [CrossRef] [PubMed]
18. Cirak, B.; Ziegfeld, S.; Knight, V.M.; Chang, D.; Avellino, A.M.; Paidas, C.N. Spinal injuries in children. *J. Pediatr. Surg.* **2004**, *39*, 607–612. [CrossRef] [PubMed]
19. Crostelli, M.; Mazza, O.; Mariani, M.; Persiani, P.; Ranaldi, F.M.; Mascello, D.; Iorio, C. T7 vertebral burst fracture with left pedicle separated from vertebral body and displaced in vertebral canal without neurologic deficits in a 12 years old motorbike competition rider. *Glob. Surg.* **2018**, *5*, 2–5. [CrossRef]
20. Knox, J.B.; Schneider, J.E.; Cage, J.M.; Wimberly, R.L.; Riccio, A.I. Spine trauma in very young children: A retrospective study of 206 patients presenting to a level 1 pediatric trauma center. *J. Pediatr. Orthop.* **2014**, *34*, 698–702. [CrossRef] [PubMed]
21. Payr, S.; Schuller, A.; Dangl, T.; Chocholka, B.; Binder, H.; Tiefenboeck, T.M. Spine Fractures in Children and Adolescents-Frequency, Causes, Diagnostics, Therapy and Outcome-A STROBE-Compliant Retrospective Study at a Level 1 Trauma Centre in Central Europe. *Child* **2021**, *8*, 1127. [CrossRef]
22. Reddy, S.P.; Junewick, J.J.; Backstrom, J.W. Distribution of spinal fractures in children: Does age, mechanism of injury, or gender play a significant role? *Pediatr. Radiol.* **2003**, *33*, 776–781. [CrossRef]
23. Parisini, P.; Di Silvestre, M.; Greggi, T. Treatment of spinal fractures in children and adolescents: Long-term results in 44 patients. *Spine* **2002**, *27*, 1989–1994. [CrossRef]
24. Vu, C.; Gendelberg, D. Classifications in Brief: AO Thoracolumbar Classification System. *Clin. Orthop. Relat. Res.* **2020**, *478*, 434–440. [CrossRef] [PubMed]
25. Canseco, J.A.; Schroeder, G.D.; Paziuk, T.M.; Karamian, B.A.; Kandziora, F.; Vialle, E.N.; Oner, F.C.; Schnake, K.J.; Dvorak, M.F.; Chapman, J.R.; et al. The Subaxial Cervical AO Spine Injury Score. *Glob. Spine J.* **2022**, *12*, 1066–1073. [CrossRef] [PubMed]

26. Kweh, B.T.S.; Tee, J.W.; Oner, F.C.; Schnake, K.J.; Vialle, E.N.; Kanziora, F.; Rajasekaran, S.; Dvorak, M.; Chapman, J.R.; Benneker, L.M.; et al. Evolution of the AO Spine Sacral and Pelvic Classification System: A systematic review. *J. Neurosurg. Spine* **2022**, *37*, 914–926. [CrossRef]
27. Anderson, L.D.; D'Alonzo, R.T. Fractures of the odontoid process of the axis. *J. Bone Jt. Surg. Am.* **1974**, *56*, 1663–1674. [CrossRef]
28. Hart, D.J.; Wang, M.Y.; Griffith, P.; McComb, J.G. Pediatric sacral fractures. *Spine* **2004**, *29*, 667–670. [CrossRef] [PubMed]
29. Montalbano, M.; Fisahn, C.; Loukas, M.; Oskouian, R.J.; Chapman, J.R.; Tubbs, R.S. Pediatric Hangman's Fracture: A Comprehensive Review. *Pediatr. Neurosurg.* **2017**, *52*, 145–150. [CrossRef] [PubMed]
30. Vander Have, K.L.; Caird, M.S.; Gross, S.; Farley, F.A.; Graziano, G.A.; Stauff, M.; Segal, L.S. Burst fractures of the thoracic and lumbar spine in children and adolescents. *J. Pediatr. Orthop.* **2009**, *29*, 713–719. [CrossRef]
31. Siebenga, J.; Leferink, V.J.M.; Segers, M.J.M.; Elzinga, M.J.; Bakker, F.C.; Haarman, H.J.T.M.; Rommens, P.M.; ten Duis, H.-J.; Patka, P. Treatment of traumatic thoracolumbar spine fractures: A multicenter prospective randomized study of operative versus nonsurgical treatment. *Spine* **2006**, *31*, 2881–2890. [CrossRef]

Journal of
Clinical Medicine

MDPI

Article

Angle-Adjustable Dynamic Hip Screw Plate for Unstable Trochanteric Fractures in Middle-Aged Patients: Mid-Term Outcomes and Return to Sport

Luca Andriollo [1,2], Giorgio Fravolini [1,2], Rudy Sangaletti [1], Loris Perticarini [1], Francesco Benazzo [1,3] and Stefano Marco Paolo Rossi [1,*]

1 Robotic Prosthetic Surgery Unit—Sports Traumatology Unit, Fondazione Poliambulanza Istituto Ospedaliero, 25124 Brescia, Italy; luca.andriollo@poliambulanza.it (L.A.); giorgio.fravolini01@icatt.it (G.F.); rudy.sangaletti@poliambulanza.it (R.S.); loris.perticarini@poliambulanza.it (L.P.); francesco.benazzo@poliambulanza.it (F.B.)

2 Department of Orthopedics, Catholic University of the Sacred Heart, 00168 Rome, Italy

3 Biomedical Sciences Area, IUSS University School for Advanced Studies, 27100 Pavia, Italy

* Correspondence: rossi.smp@gmail.com

Abstract: Background: There are conflicting results in the literature regarding the superiority of proximal femoral nails over dynamic hip screw (DHS) plates. The primary aim of this study is to evaluate mid-term post-injury patient-reported outcome measures (PROMs) and return to sport (RTS) in middle-aged patients treated with the DHS plate for unstable trochanteric fractures. Methods: Fifty-seven middle-aged patients (35–64 years) treated for proximal femoral fractures of type 31-A2 and 31-A3 according to the AO/OTA classification with the DMS Dynamic Martin Screw (KLS Martin Group, Jacksonville, FL, USA) between January 2017 and December 2019 were enrolled. Results: Forty-nine patients were included in this retrospective study, and the average age was 54.1 years (SD 8.4). The average follow-up duration at final follow-up was 60.5 months (SD 8.6). Post-operative complications included only one case of aseptic loosening of the implant, with a complication rate of 2%. There were no infections, peri-implant fractures, or other complications reported. Two out of the forty-nine patients (4.1%) required treatment with a total hip arthroplasty due to post-traumatic arthritis. The Harris Hip Score at final follow-up was 77.1 (SD 20.1), and the Western Ontario and McMaster Universities Osteoarthritis Index was 21.6 (SD 13.7). The overall rate of RTS was 57.7%. Conclusions: Treatment with DHS for unstable trochanteric fractures is a safe option in middle-aged patients, ensuring a good functional recovery.

Keywords: angle-adjustable dynamic hip screw; unstable trochanteric fracture; proximal femoral fracture; middle-aged; DHS

1. Introduction

Hip fractures are associated with high mortality and morbidity and are among the most common injuries worldwide [1]. Of these, almost 50% are accounted for by trochanteric fractures of the femur, which can be classified as either stable or unstable [2].

Specifically, the Arbeitsgemeinschaft für Osteosynthesefragen/Orthopedic Trauma Association (AO/OTA) classification divides trochanteric fractures into three groups: 31A1 simple pertrochanteric fractures, with two fragments, considered stable after anatomical reduction; 31A2 multifragmentary pertrochanteric fractures with disruption of the medial cortex, considered unstable; and 31A3 intertrochanteric fractures with reverse obliquity. Subtrochanteric fractures, where the fracture line extends distally to the lesser trochanter, are classified as 32A [3].

Treatment includes intramedullary fixation with proximal femoral nails (PFNs) and extramedullary fixation with dynamic hip screw (DHS) plates with or without a trochanteric stabilization plate (TSP), fixed-angle blade plates, and proximal femoral locking plates [4].

The DHS plate was once considered the benchmark for treating trochanteric fractures, particularly those that are stable [5,6]. PFNs have become an increasingly popular fixation technique for these fractures since their introduction in the 1980s [7,8]. PFNs represent a more recent innovation, featuring funnel-shaped intramedullary nails that are slightly curved to match the shape of the proximal femoral diaphyseal trochanteric region. The primary benefit of PFNs lies in their ability to minimize surgical damage to both bone and soft tissue [9].

Nowadays, there are conflicting results in the literature regarding the superiority of PFNs over DHS plates [2,10,11]. In particular, in unstable trochanteric fractures with lateral wall damage, DHS plates in conjunction with the TSP play a critical role in providing a buttressing effect and preventing excessive fracture collapse, excessive medialization, limb shortening, and varus malalignment [4,12,13]. PFNs have been shown to have advantages such as improved patient return to pre-operative status, reduced intraoperative blood loss, and a lower incidence of complications [14,15]. In addition, PFNs can also be used in the treatment of unstable fractures and subtrochanteric fractures [16].

Hip fractures in young adults (<65 years) are generally the result of high-energy trauma, often associated with high-impact injuries such as car accidents, sports injuries, or falls. In contrast, the highest peak in the older population is due to low-energy secondary injuries [17].

The majority of the international literature focuses on the outcomes of trochanteric fractures in older patients, despite the fact that younger patients have a higher risk of mortality than older patients who suffer a hip fracture [1]. In addition, the existing literature focuses on the most common intracapsular hip fractures, with very few publications on outcomes following extracapsular hip fractures [18]. Moreover, considering young patients, there is a lack of data on returning to sports activities.

Aim of this study is to evaluate mid-term post-injury patient-reported outcome measures (PROMs) and return to sport (RTS) in middle-aged (<65 years) patients treated with the DHS plate for unstable trochanteric fractures. The secondary objective is to assess peri-operative and post-operative complications, including the rate of surgical reintervention.

2. Materials and Methods

Patients treated with an angle-adjustable DHS plate system between January 2017 and December 2019 were retrospectively evaluated. All procedures were performed at a single center by experienced trauma surgeons.

In this study, middle-aged patients who had been treated with the DMS Dynamic Martin Screw (KLS Martin Group, Jacksonville, FL, USA) for proximal femoral fractures of type 31-A2 and 31-A3 according to the AO/OTA classification were enrolled.

The inclusion criteria comprised individuals aged between 35 and 64 years (as per the definition of early and late middle-aged), a follow-up of at least 48 months (more than 4 years), and the availability of radiographic documentation (X-rays or CT scans) for both the trauma and post-operative follow-up. Exclusion criteria included pathological fractures, polytraumatized patients, open fractures, and loss of follow-up data.

Demographic and peri-operative data were collected, including the time from trauma to surgery, American Society of Anesthesiologists (ASA) classification, in-hospital complications, length of hospital stay, hemoglobin levels, blood transfusions, surgical duration, and the type of anesthesia administered.

The assessment also included the evaluation of acute complications, such as post-surgical local hematoma, vascular injury, or nerve injury, as well as follow-up complications, including readmission or reoperation rates and their respective causes, such as infection, screw cut-out, aseptic mobilization, non-union, and peri-implant fracture.

At the final follow-up, all patients underwent a clinical examination which included patient-reported outcome measures (PROMs) such as the Western Ontario and McMaster Universities Osteoarthritis Index (WOMAC) and Harris Hip Score (HHS). Additionally, RTS was assessed, both in terms of participation and performance, and associations were evaluated between peri-operative characteristics and RTS as well as documenting the types of sports that patients resumed at the final follow-up.

Radiographic assessment was also performed during the final follow-up to evaluate the presence of device mobilization or any progression of osteoarthritis (Figure 1).

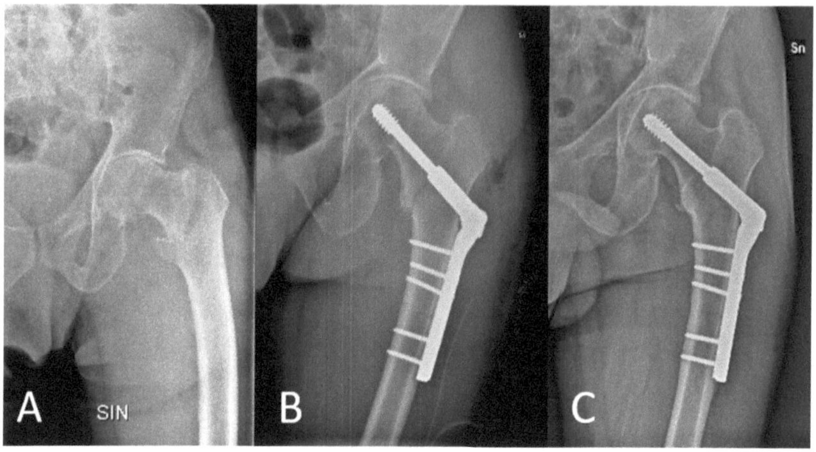

Figure 1. X-ray assessments at the time of trauma (**A**), immediately post-operatively (**B**), and at the final follow-up (**C**).

Patients received routine venous thromboembolism prevention with low-molecular-weight heparin until full weight-bearing was resumed. Alternatively, chronic anticoagulant therapy was administered as an option. Furthermore, cefazolin was used as a routine peri-operative prophylactic antibiotic. In detail, cefazolin 2 g was administered intravenously 30 min before the surgical procedure and cefazolin 1 g intravenously every 12 h for 36 h following the surgery. The post-operative rehabilitation protocol was not consistent for all patients, with variations in weight-bearing and joint mobilization recommendations.

2.1. Surgical Technique

The patient is placed in the dorsal decubitus position on a radiolucent operating table. A 15 cm long straight, lateral skin incision is made two finger widths proximally to the tip of the trochanter major. To countersink the femoral cortex, a 4.5 mm drill bit is used. The aiming device, which can be adjusted between 135° and 150°, is used to position the guide wire. The guide wire is then inserted under image intensifier control, ensuring that it is centrally located in the femoral head's mid-axis.

Once the guide wire is properly positioned, its length can be read off the scale of the measuring sleeve. After setting it to the measured value (−10 mm), the DMS combo reamer is drilled into the bone along the guide wire while being monitored by an image intensifier until the cone of the third stage has fully entered the lateral cortex. The tap is now screwed into a point 10 mm away from the cortex, optionally using the centering sleeve and the T-handle. The thread depth can be read directly from the mark on the centering sleeve. The length of the lag screw corresponds to the set drilling depth. To insert the lag screw, first attach it to the screwdriver and the connector before screwing it in with the safety inserter, 11 mm centering sleeve, and T-handle. After the lag screw has been properly positioned, the handle, safety inserter, and centering sleeve can be removed.

A plate of the proper length can now be passed over the screwdriver and onto the lag screw. Once the plate is in the proper position relative to the femoral axis, it is adjusted with the worm gear to correct any valgus or varus.

The worm gear is turned with a screwdriver until the plate is perfectly attached to the femur. The plate impactor is used to precisely adjust the DMS plate on the femur to ensure a secure seat. To secure the DMS plate to the femur, 4.5 mm cortical screws are used. A 6.5 mm cancellous screw can also be used for fixing the lesser trochanter in the plate hole directly underneath the worm gear. The fracture is finally compressed by inserting the DMS compression screw. Compression paths of up to 6 mm can occur in osteoporotic bone. The compression screw is removed after compression.

2.2. Statistical Analysis

Statistical analysis was performed using SPSS v18.0 (Chicago, IL, USA) by an independent statistician. Continuous variables were reported using averages and standard deviations (SD), while categorical variables were presented using frequency distributions and percentages. Biserial correlations were performed using a two-tailed test. The level of significance was set to $p < 0.05$.

3. Results

From January 2017 to December 2019, 57 patients were treated with the DMS Dynamic Martin Screw (KLS Martin Group, Jacksonville, FL, USA) for proximal femoral fractures of type 31-A2 and 31-A3 according to the AO/OTA classification. By the final follow-up, one patient (1.8%) had died from causes unrelated to the treatment, five patients (8.8%) met the exclusion criteria, and two patients (3.5%) were excluded due to a lack of data.

As a result, a total of 49 patients were included in this retrospective study; of these, 29 were male (59.2%) and 20 were female (40.8%). Nineteen cases (38.8%) involved the right hip and thirty (61.2%) involved the left hip. At the time of surgery, the average age was 54.1 years (SD 8.4).

Table 1 contains specifics about the baseline demographics at the time of surgery.

Table 1. Baseline demographic data at time of surgery.

Patient Population	Number	%
Total no.	57	100
Died	1	1.8
Non-traceable	2	3.5
Exclusion criteria	5	8.8
Available	49	85.9
Indication	**Number**	**%**
31 A2	39	79.6
31 A3	10	20.4
Sex	**Number**	**%**
Male	29	59.2
Female	20	40.8
Age	**Average (Y)**	**SD**
	54.1	8.4
Side	**Number**	**%**
Left	30	61.2
Right	19	38.8

Data on pre-traumatic health conditions are reported in Table 2.

The average time from trauma to surgery was 1.18 ± 0.7 days. Thirty-one (63.3%) patients received spinal anesthesia. Surgical procedures had an average duration of 110.8 ± 29.7 min. Cerclage wires were used in 18 patients (36.7%). Pre-operative hemoglobin levels averaged at 13.53 ± 1.29 g/L, while first-day post-operative hemoglobin was 9.83 ± 2.3 g/L and discharge hemoglobin was 9.74 ± 2.5 g/L. Packed red cells were transfused in 27 patients (55.1%).

Table 2. Data on pre-traumatic health conditions.

ASA	Average	SD
	1.7	0.6
ASA	**Number**	**%**
1	17	34.7
2	28	57.1
3	4	
BMI	**Average (kg/m^2)**	**SD**
	24.3	3.7
Osteoporosis	**Number**	**%**
	9	18.4

On the first or second day, 16 patients (32.7%) were mobilized into a vertical position with partial weight-bearing. The average duration of hospital stay was 6.5 ± 3.1 days. One patient experienced a post-surgical hematoma, which was surgically drained, and another patient had prolonged diffuse paresthesia in the surgically treated limb. No further complications, such as deep vein thrombosis or pulmonary embolism, urinary tract infection, heart failure, pneumonia, acute kidney injury, and vascular injury, arose during hospitalization in the analyzed patient cohort.

Complete intraoperative data, including in-hospital complications, are reported in Table 3.

Table 3. Peri-operative and in-hospital data.

Time from Trauma to Surgery	Average (Day)	SD
	1.18	0.7
Time from trauma to surgery	**Number**	**%**
Day 0	8	16.3
Day 1	24	49
Day 2	17	34.7
Surgical time	**Average (min)**	**SD**
	110.8	29.7
Cerclage	**No. of patients**	**%**
	18	36.7
Type of anesthesia	**Number**	**%**
Spinal	31	63.3
General	17	34.7
Hemoglobin (g/L)	**Average**	**SD**
Pre-operative	13.53	1.29
Day 1	9.83	2.3
At discharge	9.74	2.5
Transfusion of packed red cells	**No. of patients**	**%**
	27	55.1
Assisted verticalization with weight-bearing	**Number**	**%**
1st day	5	10.2
2nd day	11	22.5
By discharge	10	20.4
No verticalization at discharge	23	46.9

Table 3. *Cont.*

Days of hospitalization	Average (day)	SD
	6.5	3.1
In-hospital complications	**Number**	**%**
	2	4.1

The final evaluation was conducted on 49 patients, taking into consideration factors such as death and exclusion criteria. The average follow-up duration at final follow-up was 60.5 months (SD 8.6). During follow-up, no complications such as local infection or peri-implant fracture were observed. Seven patients (14.3%) underwent the removal of the synthesis devices, including one case due to aseptic mobilization despite osseous healing. Two of the patients (aged 58 and 61 years, 4.1%) who underwent synthesis device removal were subsequently treated with total hip replacement for post-traumatic arthritis (Figure 2).

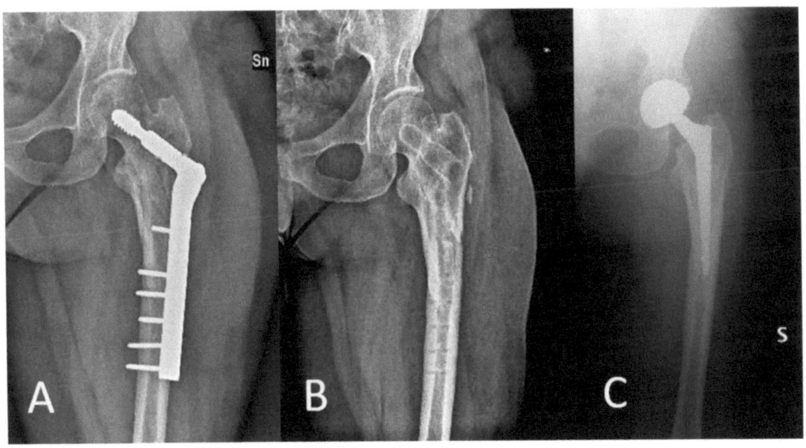

Figure 2. Patient underwent removal of synthesis devices and total hip replacement ((**A**): X-ray after treatment with DHS; (**B**): X-ray after removal of synthesis devices; (**C**): X-ray after total hip replacement surgery).

During radiographic assessment at the final follow-up, no further mobilizations or cut-outs were observed (Figure 3). In a single case, there was a presence of non-union of the greater trochanter, which remains clinically asymptomatic.

Of the patients enrolled in the study, 26 (53%) had been engaged in sports activities before the traumatic event. The overall rate of RTS was 57.7% (15 patients), defined as a return to participation, while the return to the same performance level occurred in 34.6% (nine patients). The average time for RTS for all sports was 34.3 weeks (SD 11.3).

The average HHS at final follow-up was 77.1 (SD 20.1). The average WOMAC score at final follow-up was 21.6 (SD 13.7). At the final follow-up, 15 (30.6%) showed excellent outcomes (HHS > 90), 14 (28.6%) good outcomes (HHS: 80–89), 13 (26.5%) fair outcomes (HHS: 70–79), and 7 (14.2%) poor outcomes (HHS < 70). Data related to PROMs and RTS are reported in Table 4.

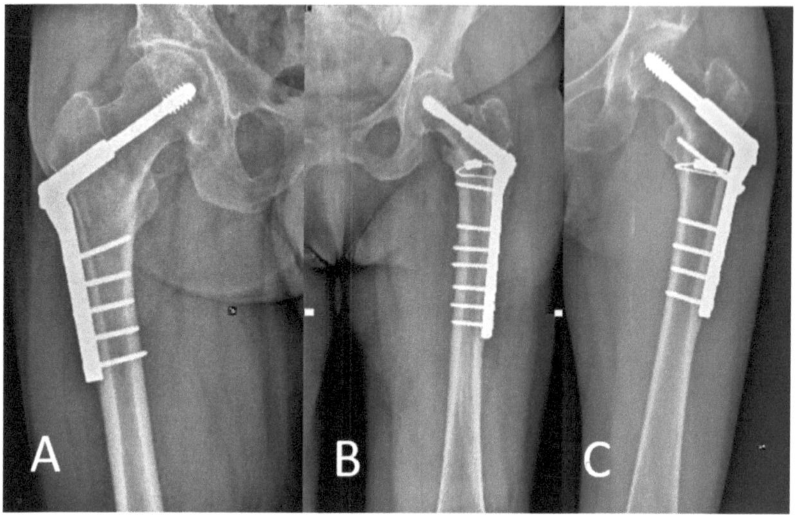

Figure 3. Three cases at follow-up: right hip with DHS (**A**) and left hip with DHS and cerclage (**B**,**C**); DHS = dynamic hip screw.

Table 4. Outcome data at final follow-up.

Final Follow-Up	Average (mos)	SD
	60.5	8.6
Return to sport	**Number**	**%**
Participation	15	53
Performance	9	34.6
Return to sport	**Average (w)**	**SD**
	34.3	11.3
Clinical outcome	**Average (pts)**	**SD**
HHS	77.1	20.1
WOMAC	21.6	13.7
Quality score HHS	**Number**	**%**
Excellent > 90	15	30.6
Good 80–89	14	28.6
Fair 70–79	13	26.5
Poor < 70	7	14.2

The correlation between patient characteristics in the peri-operative period, PROMs at final follow-up, and correlation with RTS, intended as participation, was evaluated. As documented in Table 5, no statistically significant correlations emerged, except with PROMs at final follow-up.

Of the fifteen patients who resumed sports activities, seven (47%) practiced cycling, two (13%) football, four (27%) swimming, and two (13%) running. All the patients participated in sports at a non-competitive level.

Table 5. Correlation between patient characteristics and return to sport.

	Return to Sport (N = 26)		
	Yes (N = 15)	**No (N = 11)**	***p* Value**
Age	55.54(SD 9.47)	55.45 (SD 4.95)	0.805
BMI	23.65 (SD 3.12)	23.63 (SD 3.5)	0.644
ASA	1.76 (SD 0.6)	1.72 (SD 0.47)	0.787
Time from trauma to surgery	1 (SD 1.15)	1.63 (SD 0.67)	0.142
Surgical time	105.6 (SD 31.5)	119.6 (SD 24.25)	0.229
Days of hospitalization	5.61 (SD 1.8)	5.4 (SD 2.4)	0.917
Harris Hip Score	90.15 (SD 13.7)	67.54 (SD 13.23)	<0.05
WOMAC	13.76 (9.9)	27.1 (SD 10.4)	<0.05

4. Discussion

To the best of our knowledge, this is the first study that evaluates the use of the DHS plate in a cohort of middle-aged patients treated for unstable trochanteric fractures. Specifically, the type of DHS used is angle-adjustable, enhancing anatomical fit and respect for the femoral phenotype being treated.

The optimal treatment for unstable trochanteric and intertrochanteric fractures, whether to use a DHS plate or a PFN, remains a topic of debate in the literature. Specifically, unstable trochanteric fractures, especially intertrochanteric fractures, continue to pose a challenge to the orthopedic surgeon. These fractures are linked with increased rates of failure and the need for subsequent surgical revisions, regardless of the method of fixation employed. Moreover, the literature does not clarify the role of DHS treatment in middle-aged patients (<65 years old), who are underrepresented in studies that predominantly focus on an older population. This older group, however, has different types of issues and functional demands.

The cohort enrolled in this study exhibits characteristics that are distinct from those of other studies in the literature. Specifically, the average age is 54.1 (SD 8.4) years, and patients underwent surgery within the first 48 h following trauma, with an average time from arrival at the emergency department to surgery of 1.18 (SD 0.7) days. The discussion, which aims to assess the role of DHS in the treatment of unstable trochanteric fractures in middle-aged patients, is based on studies in the literature with the closest matching average age and demographic characteristics to the cohort evaluated in this study.

The surgical time was 110.8 (SD 29.7) minutes. In the literature, shorter operative times are reported. Sharma et al., in their study involving 29 patients with an average age of 62.3 years treated with DHS, reported an average time of 69.7 min [19]. Adeel et al. reported an average time of 58.7 (SD 7.8) minutes in 34 patients with an average age of 60.9 (SD 12.5) years [20]. Even shorter durations are reported in treatments using PFNs, with Xu et al., in a meta-analysis of 1889 patients, highlighting a statistically significant difference in the duration of surgery, with an average of 9.5 min less for treatments using PFNs [21]. Furthermore, if there is a need for an antirotation screw in addition to the DHS, the time increases further, as found by Mueller et al. in a study of 375 patients [22].

The DHS carries the drawback of requiring significant exposure and soft tissue stripping, which may lead to significant blood loss [23,24]. The patients evaluated in this study experienced an average decrease in hemoglobin of 3.8 g/L from their arrival at the emergency department to discharge, with 55% of the patients requiring at least one transfusion of packed red cells. In the literature, there is heterogeneity in this aspect, with some studies reporting a transfusion rate of up to 67.9%, while another study reported only 3.4% [9,19,21,25].

A meta-analysis published by Xu et al. reports data indicating less blood loss in patients treated with PFN [26]. A meta-analysis by Hao et al. compared different surgical techniques for intertrochanteric femoral fractures, focusing on intraoperative blood loss [27]. Their results highlighted the notable advantage of proximal femoral nail antirotation (PFNA), which had the lowest blood loss and the shortest operative time of the five treatments considered. After PFNA, the order of blood loss for each method was observed in ascending order: proximal cortical contouring plate, gamma nail, femoral head resection, and DHS. Strategically reducing blood loss during surgery not only minimizes the need for allogeneic blood transfusions, but also reduces the potential risks associated with transfusion reactions, disease transmission, and immunomodulation [28,29]. The reduced duration of surgery and lower incidence of blood loss may be attributed to the smaller incision and lesser muscle trauma. The PFN implant is placed using a minimally invasive technique that does not involve exposing the fracture site, in contrast to the DHS, which requires a larger incision [9,26].

Although not assessed in this study, several studies in the literature have evaluated the use of intraoperative fluoroscopy. DHS typically requires less fluoroscopic exposure compared to PFN [11,25,30,31]. Given that PFN procedures are performed through a minimally invasive approach, it can be expected that more fluoroscopic guidance would be necessary to ensure correct implant placement, achieve good stability, and reduce the risk of implant failure. For this reason, some authors suggest that DHS might be the preferable option for patients who must limit their exposure to radiation, such as younger individuals or those with multiple chronic conditions [26].

The cohort of patients presented in this study showed a shorter length of hospital stay compared to the data reported in the literature, with an average stay of 6.5 (SD 3.1) days. This early discharge was made possible due to meticulous pharmacological management of peri-operative pain, immediate rehabilitation, and a reduced rate of peri-operative complications. In fact, during hospitalization, only one patient developed a post-operative hematoma that required surgical drainage, and another patient experienced diffuse paresthesia in the operated lower limb. No other intraoperative complications were reported. The literature reports lengths of stay ranging from 10 to 14 days on average, with no statistically significant difference between patients treated with DHS and those treated with PFNs [19,22,25,32].

In the patient cohort featured in this study, at the final follow-up, post-operative complications only included one case of aseptic loosening of the implant, with a complication rate of 2%. There were no infections, peri-implant fractures, or other complications reported. The reoperation rate was 14.3%, with six out of seven patients undergoing removal of the fixation devices for reasons not associated with treatment failure.

Failures in cases treated with DHS alone have often been linked to excessive sliding of the compression screw, which can lead to the collapse or medial shift of the distal fracture fragment. This can occur even if the compression screw is ideally placed within the femoral head. Such failures are typically due to the loss of support from the calcar or to a deficiency in the lateral femoral wall, resulting in fracture collapse under load [33–35]. In the literature, non-union and implant failure are common complications associated with compromised fixation stability [36]. Sharma et al., in a study of twenty-nine patients treated with DHS, reported one case of loss of reduction and one case of implant failure, with a total complication rate of 7% [19]. Huang et al., in a study of thirty patients, reported two cases of fixation failure (6.7%) [9]. Yu et al., in a study of 110 patients, reported a non-union rate of 1.8% [35]. The incidence of post-operative complications such as fracture non-union, implant failure, revision of fixation failure, or arthroplasty did not show a significant difference between the use of PFNs and DHS. This finding is highlighted by the comprehensive meta-analysis published by Xu et al., conducted on 1889 patients, which reported a non-union rate of 1.7% in patients treated with PFNs and 2% in patients treated with DHS, and an implant failure rate of 2.5% with PFNs and 3.5% with DHS, with no statistically significant differences [26].

In the cohort in this study, two out of forty-nine patients (4.1%) required treatment with a total hip arthroplasty due to post-traumatic arthritis. Saudan et al. reported a prosthetic implantation rate at the final follow-up of 2.2%, while Parker et al. reported a rate of 4.3%, with both studies having a minimum follow-up of one year [25,30]. Acute arthroplasty treatment is a trending topic in the current literature, with some authors suggesting immediate replacement treatment, especially in cases of existing osteoarthritis or poor bone quality [37–39].

There are limited studies in the literature that have evaluated modern PROMs, such as HHS and WOMAC. In our study, the functional outcomes at follow-up were satisfactory, with an HHS of 77.1 (SD 20.1) and a WOMAC score of 21.6 (SD 13.7). Memon et al., in a study of 122 patients treated for unstable pertrochanteric fractures, reported an average HHS of 69.3 (SD 10) at 2 years' follow-up [40]. In a study of 34 patients, Kassem et al. reported an HHS of 77.9 (SD 8.4) at 1 year follow-up [41]. The use of DHS in femoral neck fractures in adults aged between 18 and 69 years showed superior results, with an average HHS of 88 [42]. Watson et al. reported an average WOMAC score of 41 in a study involving 62 patients [43].

No study in the literature has evaluated RTS after proximal femur fractures. It can be hypothesized that the treatment we employed is less invasive on the gluteal muscles, which are necessary for sporting activity, when compared to PFNs. The findings of this study are thus capable of shedding light on the feasibility and success of resuming sporting activities after this type of surgery. This knowledge is crucial for both physicians and patients to understand the potential impact on an active lifestyle. However, the reported data are lower compared to the rates of RTS after elective hip arthroplasty in a middle-aged population [44].

This study has several limitations, including the lack of a control group, the limited number of patients assessed, the retrospective nature of the study, and the relatively brief duration of the follow-up period.

5. Conclusions

Treatment with angle-adjustable DHS plates for unstable trochanteric fractures is a safe option in middle-aged patients, ensuring good functional recovery comparable to outcomes achieved with intramedullary fixation or other extramedullary fixation systems.

Furthermore, this study represents the first publication on a cohort of patients treated with this device. Additional studies are required to assess complication rates and functional outcomes in comparison to patients treated with intramedullary nailing or with acute arthroplasty.

Author Contributions: Conceptualization, L.A. and F.B.; methodology, L.A. and S.M.P.R.; investigation, L.A. and G.F.; data curation, L.A. and G.F.; writing—original draft preparation, L.A. and G.F.; writing—review and editing, R.S., L.P. and S.M.P.R.; supervision, F.B. All authors have read and agreed to the published version of the manuscript.

Funding: This research received no external funding.

Institutional Review Board Statement: This study was conducted in accordance with the ethical standards of the 1964 Declaration of Helsinki and in compliance with HIPAA regulation. The Institutional Review Board (IRB) of the authors' institution defined this study as exempt from IRB approval (retrospective study on a well-established surgical procedure and commercialized device).

Informed Consent Statement: All patients involved in this study provided written, informed consent for the management of personal data.

Data Availability Statement: The data presented in this study are available on request from the corresponding author (privacy).

Conflicts of Interest: The authors declare no conflicts of interest.

References

1. Richmond, J.; Aharonoff, G.B.; Zuckerman, J.D.; Koval, K.J. Mortality Risk after Hip Fracture. *J. Orthop. Trauma* **2003**, *17*, 53–56. [CrossRef]
2. Selim, A.; Ponugoti, N.; Naqvi, A.Z.; Magill, H. Cephalo-Medullary Nailing versus Dynamic Hip Screw with Trochanteric Stabilisation Plate for the Treatment of Unstable per-Trochanteric Hip Fractures: A Meta-Analysis. *J. Orthop. Surg. Res.* **2021**, *16*, 47. [CrossRef] [PubMed]

3. Meinberg, E.G.; Agel, J.; Roberts, C.S.; Karam, M.D.; Kellam, J.F. Fracture and Dislocation Classification Compendium—2018. *J. Orthop. Trauma* **2018**, *320* (Suppl. 1), S1–S170. [CrossRef] [PubMed]
4. Selim, A.A.H.A.; Beder, F.K.; Algeaidy, I.T.; Farhat, A.S.; Diab, N.M.; Barakat, A.S. Management of Unstable Pertrochanteric Fractures, Evaluation of Forgotten Treatment Options. *SICOT J.* **2020**, *6*, 21. [CrossRef] [PubMed]
5. Parker, M.J.; Handoll, H.H. Gamma and Other Cephalocondylic Intramedullary Nails versus Extramedullary Implants for Extracapsular Hip Fractures in Adults. *Cochrane Database Syst. Rev.* **2010**, *9*, CD000093. [CrossRef]
6. Kaplan, K.; Miyamoto, R.; Levine, B.R.; Egol, K.A.; Zuckerman, J.D. Surgical Management of Hip Fractures: An Evidence-Based Review of the Literature. II: Intertrochanteric Fractures. *J. Am. Acad. Orthop. Surg.* **2008**, *16*, 665–673. [CrossRef] [PubMed]
7. Forte, M.L.; Virnig, B.A.; Kane, R.L.; Durham, S.; Bhandari, M.; Feldman, R.; Swiontkowski, M.F. Geographic Variation in Device Use for Intertrochanteric Hip Fractures. *J. Bone Jt. Surg. Am.* **2008**, *90*, 691–699. [CrossRef] [PubMed]
8. Anglen, J.O.; Weinstein, J.N.; American Board of Orthopaedic Surgery Research Committee. Nail or Plate Fixation of Intertrochanteric Hip Fractures: Changing Pattern of Practice. A Review of the American Board of Orthopaedic Surgery Database. *J. Bone Jt. Surg. Am.* **2008**, *90*, 700–707. [CrossRef] [PubMed]
9. Huang, S.-G.; Chen, B.; Zhang, Y.; Nie, F.-F.; Ju, L.; Li, M.; Zhang, Y.-H. Comparison of the Clinical Effectiveness of PFNA, PFLCP, and DHS in Treatment of Unstable Intertrochanteric Femoral Fracture. *Am. J. Ther.* **2017**, *24*, e659–e666. [CrossRef]
10. Chehade, M.J.; Carbone, T.; Awwad, D.; Taylor, A.; Wildenauer, C.; Ramasamy, B.; McGee, M. Influence of Fracture Stability on Early Patient Mortality and Reoperation After Pertrochanteric and Intertrochanteric Hip Fractures. *J. Orthop. Trauma* **2015**, *29*, 538–543. [CrossRef]
11. Zehir, S.; Zehir, R.; Zehir, S.; Azboy, İ.; Haykir, N. Proximal Femoral Nail Antirotation against Dynamic Hip Screw for Unstable Trochanteric Fractures; a Prospective Randomized Comparison. *Eur. J. Trauma Emerg. Surg.* **2015**, *41*, 393–400. [CrossRef]
12. Fu, C.-W.; Chen, J.-Y.; Liu, Y.-C.; Liao, K.-W.; Lu, Y.-C. Dynamic Hip Screw with Trochanter-Stabilizing Plate Compared with Proximal Femoral Nail Antirotation as a Treatment for Unstable AO/OTA 31-A2 and 31-A3 Intertrochanteric Fractures. *BioMed Res. Int.* **2020**, *2020*, 1896935. [CrossRef] [PubMed]
13. Gotfried, Y. The Lateral Trochanteric Wall: A Key Element in the Reconstruction of Unstable Pertrochanteric Hip Fractures. *Clin Orthop. Relat. Res.* **2004**, *425*, 82. [CrossRef]
14. Aktselis, I.; Kokoroghiannis, C.; Fragkomichalos, E.; Koundis, G.; Deligeorgis, A.; Daskalakis, E.; Vlamis, J.; Papaioannou, N. Prospective Randomised Controlled Trial of an Intramedullary Nail versus a Sliding Hip Screw for Intertrochanteric Fractures of the Femur. *Int. Orthop.* **2014**, *38*, 155–161. [CrossRef]
15. Shen, L.; Zhang, Y.; Shen, Y.; Cui, Z. Antirotation Proximal Femoral Nail versus Dynamic Hip Screw for Intertrochanteric Fractures: A Meta-Analysis of Randomized Controlled Studies. *Orthop. Traumatol. Surg. Res.* **2013**, *99*, 377–383. [CrossRef] [PubMed]
16. Mereddy, P.; Kamath, S.; Ramakrishnan, M.; Malik, H.; Donnachie, N. The AO/ASIF Proximal Femoral Nail Antirotation (PFNA): A New Design for the Treatment of Unstable Proximal Femoral Fractures. *Injury* **2009**, *40*, 428–432. [CrossRef]
17. Singer, B.; Mclauchlan, G.; Robinson, C.; Christie, J. Epidemiology of Fractures in 15 000 Adults: The Influence of Age and Gender. *J. Bone Jt. Surg.* **1998**, *80*, 243–248. [CrossRef]
18. Coughlin, T.A.; Nightingale, J.M.; Myint, Y.; Forward, D.P.; Norrish, A.R.; Ollivere, B.J. Patient-Reported Outcomes in Young Patients with Isolated Fracture of the Hip. *Bone Jt. J.* **2020**, *102*, 766–771. [CrossRef]
19. Sharma, A.; Sethi, A.; Sharma, S. Treatment of Stable Intertrochanteric Fractures of the Femur with Proximal Femoral Nail versus Dynamic Hip Screw: A Comparative Study. *Rev. Bras. Ortop.* **2017**, *53*, 477–481. [CrossRef]
20. Adeel, K.; Nadeem, R.D.; Akhtar, M.; Sah, R.K.; Mohy-Ud-Din, I. Comparison of Proximal Femoral Nail (PFN) and Dynamic Hip Screw (DHS) for the Treatment of AO Type A2 and A3 Pertrochanteric Fractures of Femur. *J. Pak. Med. Assoc.* **2020**, *70*, 815–819. [CrossRef]
21. Xu, K.; Chen, Q.; Yan, Q.; Wang, Q.; Sun, J. Comparison of Computer-Assisted Navigated Technology and Conventional Technology in Unicompartmental Knee Arthroplasty: A Meta-Analysis. *J. Orthop. Surg. Res.* **2022**, *17*, 123. [CrossRef]
22. Müller, F.; Doblinger, M.; Kottmann, T.; Füchtmeier, B. PFNA and DHS for AO/OTA 31-A2 Fractures: Radiographic Measurements, Morbidity and Mortality. *Eur. J. Trauma Emerg. Surg.* **2020**, *46*, 947–953. [CrossRef]
23. Verettas, D.-A.J.; Ifantidis, P.; Chatzipapas, C.N.; Drosos, G.I.; Xarchas, K.C.; Chloropoulou, P.; Kazakos, K.I.; Trypsianis, G.; Ververidis, A. Systematic Effects of Surgical Treatment of Hip Fractures: Gliding Screw-Plating vs Intramedullary Nailing. *Injury* **2010**, *41*, 279–284. [CrossRef]
24. Wandel, S.; Jüni, P.; Tendal, B.; Nüesch, E.; Villiger, P.M.; Welton, N.J.; Reichenbach, S.; Trelle, S. Effects of Glucosamine, Chondroitin, or Placebo in Patients with Osteoarthritis of Hip or Knee: Network Meta-Analysis. *BMJ* **2010**, *341*, c4675. [CrossRef] [PubMed]
25. Saudan, M.; Lübbeke, A.; Sadowski, C.; Riand, N.; Stern, R.; Hoffmeyer, P. Pertrochanteric Fractures: Is There an Advantage to an Intramedullary Nail?: A Randomized, Prospective Study of 206 Patients Comparing the Dynamic Hip Screw and Proximal Femoral Nail. *J. Orthop. Trauma* **2002**, *16*, 386–393. [CrossRef]
26. Xu, H.; Liu, Y.; Sezgin, E.A.; Tarasevičius, Š.; Christensen, R.; Raina, D.B.; Tägil, M.; Lidgren, L. Comparative Effectiveness Research on Proximal Femoral Nail versus Dynamic Hip Screw in Patients with Trochanteric Fractures: A Systematic Review and Meta-Analysis of Randomized Trials. *J. Orthop. Surg. Res.* **2022**, *17*, 292. [CrossRef] [PubMed]

27. Hao, Z.; Wang, X.; Zhang, X. Comparing Surgical Interventions for Intertrochanteric Hip Fracture by Blood Loss and Operation Time: A Network Meta-Analysis. *J. Orthop. Surg. Res.* **2018**, *13*, 157. [CrossRef] [PubMed]
28. White, J.J.E.; Khan, W.S.; Smitham, P.J. Perioperative Implications of Surgery in Elderly Patients with Hip Fractures: An Evidence-Based Review. *J. Perioper. Pract.* **2011**, *21*, 192–197. [CrossRef] [PubMed]
29. Xu, Y.Z.; Geng, D.C.; Mao, H.Q.; Zhu, X.S.; Yang, H.L. A Comparison of the Proximal Femoral Nail Antirotation Device and Dynamic Hip Screw in the Treatment of Unstable Pertrochanteric Fracture. *J. Int. Med. Res.* **2010**, *38*, 1266–1275. [CrossRef] [PubMed]
30. Parker, M.J.; Bowers, T.R.; Pryor, G.A. Sliding Hip Screw versus the Targon PF Nail in the Treatment of Trochanteric Fractures of the Hip: A Randomised Trial of 600 Fractures. *J. Bone Jt. Surg. Br.* **2012**, *94*, 391–397. [CrossRef]
31. Singh, N.K.; Sharma, V.; Trikha, V.; Gamanagatti, S.; Roy, A.; Balawat, A.S.; Aravindh, P.; Diwakar, A.R. Is PFNA-II a Better Implant for Stable Intertrochanteric Fractures in Elderly Population ? A Prospective Randomized Study. *J. Clin. Orthop. Trauma* **2019**, *10*, S71–S76. [CrossRef]
32. Madsen, J.E.; Naess, L.; Aune, A.K.; Alho, A.; Ekeland, A.; Strømsøe, K. Dynamic Hip Screw with Trochanteric Stabilizing Plate in the Treatment of Unstable Proximal Femoral Fractures: A Comparative Study with the Gamma Nail and Compression Hip Screw. *J. Orthop. Trauma* **1998**, *12*, 241–248. [CrossRef]
33. Sun, D.; Wang, C.; Chen, Y.; Liu, X.; Zhao, P.; Zhang, H.; Zhou, H.; Qin, C. A Meta-Analysis Comparing Intramedullary with Extramedullary Fixations for Unstable Femoral Intertrochanteric Fractures. *Medicine* **2019**, *98*, e17010. [CrossRef]
34. Zhang, W.-Q.; Sun, J.; Liu, C.-Y.; Zhao, H.-Y.; Sun, Y.-F. Comparing the Intramedullary Nail and Extramedullary Fixation in Treatment of Unstable Intertrochanteric Fractures. *Sci. Rep.* **2018**, *8*, 2321. [CrossRef]
35. Yu, X.; Wang, H.; Duan, X.; Liu, M.; Xiang, Z. Intramedullary versus Extramedullary Internal Fixation for Unstable Intertrochanteric Fracture, a Meta-Analysis. *Acta Orthop. Traumatol. Turc.* **2018**, *52*, 299–307. [CrossRef] [PubMed]
36. Ekinci, Y.; Gürbüz, K.; Batın, S.; Kahraman, M.; Doğar, F.; Kaya Erten, Z. A Multicenter Intertrochanteric Fracture Study in the Elderly: Hemiarthroplasty versus Proximal Femoral Nailing. *Jt. Dis. Relat. Surg.* **2020**, *31*, 209–217. [CrossRef] [PubMed]
37. Liu, L.; Sun, Y.; Wang, L.; Gao, Q.; Li, A.; Wang, J.; Gao, Y. Total Hip Arthroplasty for Intertrochanteric Fracture Fixation Failure. *Eur. J. Med. Res.* **2019**, *24*, 39. [CrossRef] [PubMed]
38. Chaudhry, H. Total Hip Arthroplasty after Hip Fracture. *BMJ* **2016**, *353*, i2217. [CrossRef]
39. Andriollo, L.; Sangaletti, R.; Are, L.; Perticarini, L.; Benazzo, F.; Rossi, S.M.P. Uncemented Hemiarthroplasty May Have a Role in the Treatment of Unstable Intertrochanteric Fractures in Elderly Patient. A Survival Complications and Functional Outcomes Analysis. *Int. J. Burns Trauma* **2023**, *13*, 126–135. [PubMed]
40. Memon, K.; Siddiqui, A.M.; Khan, Z.A.; Zahoor, A. Dynamic Hip Screw Fixation Vs. Proximal Femur Nail For Unstable Per-Trochanteric Fractures: A Comparative Analysis Of Outcomes And Complications. *J. Ayub Med. Coll. Abbottabad* **2021**, *33*, 34–38.
41. Kassem, E.; Younan, R.; Abaskhron, M.; Abo-Elsoud, M. Functional and Radiological Outcomes of Dynamic Hip Screw with Trochanteric Stabilizing Plate versus Short Proximal Femoral Nail in Management of Unstable Trochanteric Fractures: A Randomized-Controlled Trial. *Jt. Dis. Relat. Surg.* **2022**, *33*, 531–537. [CrossRef]
42. Fjeld, A.; Fülling, T.; Bula, P.; Bonnaire, F. Functional Outcomes and Perceived Quality of Life Following Fixation of Femoral Neck Fractures in Adults from 18 to 69 Years Using Dynamic Hip Screw (DHS) and an Additional Anti-Rotation Screw- a Retrospective Analysis of 53 Patients after a Mean Follow-up Time of 4 Years. *Eur. J. Trauma Emerg. Surg.* **2022**, *48*, 1893–1903. [CrossRef] [PubMed]
43. Watson, A.; Zhang, Y.; Beattie, S.; Page, R.S. Prospective Randomized Controlled Trial Comparing Dynamic Hip Screw and Screw Fixation for Undisplaced Subcapital Hip Fractures. *ANZ J. Surg.* **2013**, *83*, 679–683. [CrossRef] [PubMed]
44. Magan, A.A.; Radhakrishnan, G.T.; Kayani, B.; Ronca, F.; Khanduja, V.; Meek, R.M.D.; Haddad, F.S. Time for Return to Sport Following Total Hip Arthroplasty: A Meta-Analysis. *Hip Int.* **2023**, *33*, 221–230. [CrossRef] [PubMed]

Journal of
Clinical Medicine

MDPI

Article

Evaluation of Outcome after Total Hip Arthroplasty for Femoral Neck Fracture: Which Factors Are Relevant for Better Results?

Paolo Schiavi *, Francesco Pogliacomi, Matteo Bergamaschi, Francesco Ceccarelli and Enrico Vaienti

Orthopedic Clinic, Department of Medicine and Surgery, University Hospital of Parma, 43126 Parma, Italy; francesco.pogliacomi@unipr.it (F.P.); matteo.bergamaschi1@studenti.unipr.it (M.B.); francesco.ceccarelli@unipr.it (F.C.); enrico.vaienti@unipr.it (E.V.)

* Correspondence: pschiavi@ao.pr.it or ppschiav@gmail.com

Abstract: Background: Femoral neck fractures (FNFs) are frequent orthopedic injuries in elderly patients. Despite improvements in clinical monitoring and advances in surgical procedures, 1-year mortality remains between 15% and 30%. The aim of this study is to identify variables that lead to better outcomes in patients treated with total hip arthroplasty (THA) for FNFs. **Methods:** All patients who underwent cementless THA for FNF from January 2018 to December 2022 were identified. Patients aged more than 80 years old and with other post-traumatic lesions were excluded. Patient data and demographic characteristics were collected. The following data were also registered: time trauma/surgery, surgical approach, operative time, intraoperative complications, surgeon arthroplasty-trained or not, and anesthesia type. In order to search for any predictive factors of better short- and long-term outcomes, we performed different logistic regression analyses. **Results:** A total of 92 patients were included. From multivariable logistic regression models, we derived that a direct anterior surgical approach and an American Society of Anesthesiologists (ASA) classification < 3 can predict improved short-term outcomes. Moreover, THAs performed by surgeons with specific training in arthroplasty have a lower probability of revision at 1 year. Mortality at 1 year was ultimately influenced by the ASA classification. **Conclusions:** A direct anterior approach and specific arthroplasty training of the surgeon appear to be able to improve the short- and long-term follow-up of THA after FNF.

Keywords: femoral neck fracture; total hip arthroplasty; direct anterior approach; outcome

1. Introduction

Femoral neck fractures (FNFs) are very common injuries in the elderly population. Recent studies have reported that the prevalence of FNFs is expected to show a strong increase worldwide by 2035 to 2050 [1–6].

Hip fractures have an important impact on the US healthcare system, with an annual incidence of 1000 per 100,000 beneficiaries [7,8]. It is estimated that the incidence of FNFs will increase from 1.66 million in 1990 to 6.26 million by 2050 [9]. In terms of type of treatment, the anatomic site of fracture plays an important role in determining the procedure needed. Intracapsular injuries consist of subcapital and transcervical groups, with arthroplasty being the common surgical treatment. In contrast, extracapsular fractures occur distal to the joint capsule insertion and can be distinguished into basicervical, intertrochanteric, and pertrochanteric groups, with osteosynthesis being the best recognized treatment [9].

Despite improvements in clinical monitoring and advances in surgical treatment, the 1-year mortality rates in patients who reported an FNF remain considerable, being 15% to 30% [7,10].

Currently, the common treatment of FNFs is internal fixation in 60% of cases, hemiarthroplasty in 30% of cases, and total hip arthroplasty (THA) in the remaining percentage of cases [11,12].

However, we have to consider that the use of THA as the primary treatment of FNFs continues to increase annually [13].

These changes in the application of the different surgical options depend on the results reported in several randomized trials and have been confirmed by meta-analyses that compared THA to hemiarthroplasty and internal fixation for displaced FNFs, showing that THA is associated with better outcomes and a lower incidence of re-operations [14,15].

Many factors can play a significant role in determining the outcome after THA for FNF. Recently, many studies have investigated the consequence of a surgical approach (direct anterior [DA], posterolateral [PL], and lateral direct [LD]) for total hip arthroplasty on short- and long-term follow-ups. Reported benefits of the DA approach are as follows: minor dislocation risk [16–18], lesser pain, and higher functional recovery in the early postoperative days (first 2 weeks after surgery) compared to the PL approach [19,20] and higher self-reported scores for functional recovery at 2 weeks after surgery compared to the LD approach [21]. However, these postoperative advantages often were absent at 3-month and 1-year follow-up evaluations [20,22].

Functional status in the first postoperative days after THA may play a role of higher importance in FNF patients considering their generally increased age and reduced level of activity compared to their elective counterparts [23].

Furthermore, growing evidence has suggested that early postoperative deambulation in the group of patients who suffered an FNF could influence mortality at follow up [24–28].

The aim of this study is to identify the factors that lead to better outcomes in the early period and at 1-year follow-up in patients who underwent a THA operation after FNF.

2. Materials and Methods

2.1. Study Design and Patients

All patients who underwent cementless total hip arthroplasty for FNF from 1 January 2018 to 31 December 2022 were preliminarily identified. Patients who underwent THA for pathologic fracture, osteonecrosis, or lateral femoral fractures (trochanteric fractures) were excluded. Additionally, we considered exclusion criteria cases of bilateral FNF and the presence of ipsilateral acetabular injuries. Finally, patients aged more than 80 years old and subjects with a reported non-independent deambulatory capability at baseline were excluded.

The study was regularly approved by the North Aemilia Ethical Committee with number 631/2023 on 12 December 2023.

All procedures were performed after collecting written informed consent from each patient and in accordance with the ethical standards of the institutional and national committees of research and the 1964 Declaration of Helsinki and its subsequent amendments.

Patient data and demographic characteristics were collected, including age, gender, BMI, Garden classification of fracture, and ASA classification. Furthermore, we registered the following operative data: time between trauma and surgery (days), surgical approach (DA or LD), operative time, reported intraoperative complications (periprosthetic femoral fracture or surgical acetabular protrusion), and anesthesia type (spinal or general).

We verified, as previously reported, if the surgical procedure was performed by an arthroplasty-trained surgeon (AR-trained) or by a non-arthroplasty-trained surgeon (non-AR-trained).

2.2. Surgical Technique

In all patients, the THA was completed through an LD approach or a DA approach under spinal or general anesthesia. Both surgical approaches were performed in the supine position.

For DA, a regular operating room table was used, and the patient was positioned with the hip over the table break junction, thus allowing table reflexion and hyperextension of the hip joint. The contralateral leg was typically inserted in the sterilization procedure before incision in order to make possible a correct check of limb length during surgery and a correct figure-four adduction during the femoral exposure. In obese patients, we conducted a pannus retraction with adhesive tape to avoid any possible related difficulties during stem broaching and positioning. An oblique incision was made originating 2–4 cm distal and lateral to the ASIS. Dissection was taken deep to expose the overlying thin fascia of the tensor fascia lata, which was then incised with the same axis as the cutaneous incision. Blunt finger dissection was utilized afterward, and the interval was developed between the sartorius and the TFL. Two wound protectors were positioned at this point in order to reach the minimization of soft tissue, muscle, and skin damage caused by retraction. The ascending branch of the lateral circumflex femoral artery and vein was identified and tied before cauterization, and the anterior hip capsule was exposed. The femoral neck osteotomy was then completed either with a single cut or sometimes with a napkin-ring-type parallel two-cut technique to facilitate the removal of the femoral head. Femoral exposure on our regular operating room table started with external rotation of the femur typically over 90°. A proximal femoral hook was useful in this phase to elevate the proximal femur and facilitate better exposure. The leg was extended by lowering the leg to the floor followed by adduction of the extremity. The femoral exposure was accomplished by reflexing the table to extend the extremity and placing the leg figure-four under the opposite leg with flexion of the knee of the operated leg lower to 45°. A retractor was then placed on the femur medial to the neck cut and a double-pronged retractor was placed under the greater trochanter. Soft tissue releases were performed identifying the piriformis fossa and proceeding along the greater trochanter while elevating the proximal femur with the hook device. The visualization of the osteotomy plane enabled the broaching and placement of a femoral trial component to commence. Closure of the wound was initiated with repair of the TFL fascia with either a running or interrupted suture. In all cases, a drain was correctly positioned.

For the direct lateral approach, we proceeded with releases of the anterior third of the gluteus medius and minimus while preserving the posterior femoral attachment of the major part of these muscles. The proximal part of the incision was limited by the superior gluteal nerve and vessels, crossing 3–5 cm proximal to the tip of the greater trochanter. Distally, the anterior fibers of the vastus lateralis were elevated from the anterior femur. Next, the anterior attachment of the hip capsule was released from the anterior base of the femoral neck, and an anterior longitudinal capsulotomy was opened as necessary with a proximal transverse T-shaped incision. Femoral exposure was completed with careful release of the postero-lateral capsule and positioning of the leg in figure-four under the opposite leg with a flexion of the knee over 90°. Closure of the wound started from the muscular fibers of the gluteus medius and minimus and then with fascia repair with an interrupted suture. In all cases, a drain was correctly positioned.

During all surgeries, intraoperative fluoroscopic imaging was used in order to exclude possible complications. The DA approaches were performed by two different surgeons, whereas the LD approaches were performed by five different surgeons. The arthroplasty-trained surgeons were the two surgeons able to implant THA with both the LD and DA approaches.

Perioperative and postoperative institutional protocols were adhered to with minor variations depending on surgeon preference. All patients received preoperative antibiotics before incision.

If no surgical contraindications were present, then, in all patients, walking in the first 2 postoperative days was attempted with dedicated physiotherapy personnel. All included patients have a minimum of 1-year follow-up.

2.3. Radiographic Evaluation

Postoperative X-rays were checked by two orthopedic surgeons in order to verify correct component positioning: acetabular shell inclination and anteversion, as well as femoral subsidence and varus, were measured as previously reported in the literature [29,30].

Rotation of the proximal femur was verified by measuring the width of the lesser trochanter. Further fine adjustments were made using the ratio of the projection of the distal tip of the stem that was verified by known stem size. The inclination of the acetabular component referenced the interteardrop line and anteversion, following the previously reported method published by Haddad et al. [31]. The valgus/varus alignment of the stem was recorded using the method described by Khalily and Lester [32]. Subsidence was evaluated from the immediate postoperative radiographs and those at final follow-up as a vertical movement of the femoral component, as validated in previous study.

The postoperative radiographs from the first ten patients were separately analyzed and evaluated by two independent observers to assess interobserver reliability through the single measures and with a two-way mixed effect intra-class correlation coefficient. The registered inter-observer reliability coefficient was in the correct range of tolerance for each radiographic assessment.

2.4. Outcome Measurement

In order to search for any predictive factors of outcome in the early period and at 1-year follow-up, we performed different multivariable logistic regression analyses.

Early outcome was evaluated using two different parameters: early deambulation (ED) and capability to reach autonomy in deambulation (AD) without crutches in the first month after surgical procedure.

ED was attempted in all included cases where the patients in the first 2 postoperative days were able to complete a supported deambulation of at least 20 meters. The results of this attempt were independently registered by four physiotherapists blinded to the design and scope of the study.

The level of autonomy in deambulation (AD) was evaluated by an orthopedic surgeon during one-month follow-up visit registering whether it was possible for deambulation without crutches and with a correct muscular response to weightbearing. The results in terms of AD were independently registered by surgeons blinded to the design and the scope of the study.

Outcome at 1-year follow-up was evaluated using two different parameters: 1-year mortality and 1-year revision for any cause.

2.5. Statistical Analysis

All variables were checked in order to verify distribution, mean, median, interquartile range, and standard deviation.

A preliminary Kolmogorov–Smirnov test was performed for all variables in order to verify the normality distribution of the variable.

The variance inflation factor was used in order to verify the absence of multicollinearity inside each multivariate analysis.

The insertion of any variable in the multivariate analysis was followed by calculation of the derived adjusted R-squared to proceed to a correct adjustment of the models.

A multivariable logistic regression analysis was performed for the two short-term outcome parameters including the data reported above. These two multivariate analyses were performed in order to identify predictive factors for failure in achieving early deambulation and an inability to reach deambulation without crutches at one-month follow-up.

A multivariable logistic regression analysis was then performed searching predictive factors for 1-year mortality and 1-year revision for any cause including the data reported above and including measurements of short-term outcomes.

The significance level was set at $p < 0.05$.

Data elaboration and statistical analysis were performed using SPSS® statistics software 20.0 (IBM®, Armonk, New York, NY, USA).

3. Results

A total of 108 patients were preliminarily included in the study. After the final collection of data at follow-up, a total of 16 patients were excluded for unavailable complete information (Figure 1).

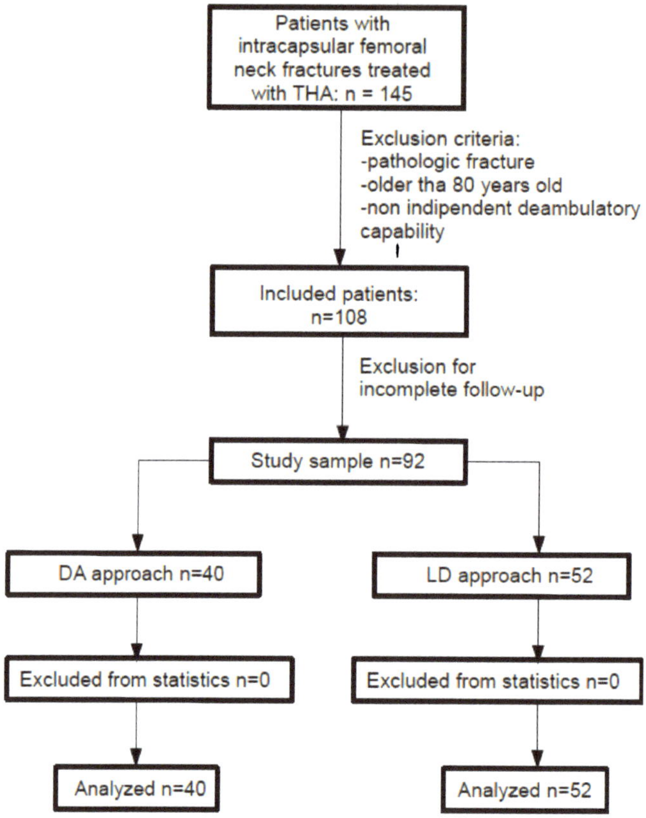

Figure 1. Flowchart of the studied population.

Thus, 92 patients constituted the pool of analysis of our study.

Demographic data are reported in Table 1.

An ED was registered as successful in 31 cases, and in 25 cases a successful AD at one month without crutches was possible with adequate muscular response to weightbearing.

The multivariable analysis for short-term outcomes is reported in Tables 2 and 3.

The logistic regression models showed the statistically significant predictive power of the surgical approach to influence ED. Specifically, the DA surgical approach could be considered a parameter able to predict the capability of reaching ED from our data (Figure 2). The second analysis performed for AD at one month showed the statistically significant predictive power of the surgical approach and ASA classification. Thus, the DA surgical approach and ASA classification < 3 were able to have a favorable influence on AD at one month.

The multivariable analysis for outcome at 1-year follow-up is reported in Tables 4 and 5.

Table 1. Patient characteristics and demographic data.

	N = 92
Age (mean ± std dev)	72.6 ± 7.3
Gender	
Male	38
Female	54
BMI	25.8 ± 3.1
ASA	
1	8
2	29
3	51
4	4
Garden fracture	
2	5
3	56
4	31
Time trauma/surgery (hours)	57.1 ± 13.5
Operative time (min)	118 ± 14.9
Intraoperative complications	
Surg acetabular protrusion	4
Femoral fracture	2
Surgical approach	
DA	40
LD	52
Surgical training	
AR	43
non-AR	49
Anesthesia type	
General	34
Spinal	58
Component positioning	
Correct	75
Incorrect	
Stem	
Varus	3
Acetabular	
Inclination	7
Anteversion	5

Table 2. Multivariable logistic regression analysis for failure in early deambulation.

	OR	95% Confidence Interval	p
Age	0.781	0.314–0.827	0.083
Female	1.026	0.526–1.331	0.645
BMI	0.890	0.673–0.995	0.286
ASA < 3	0.762	0.540–0.913	0.109
Time trauma/surgery	1.153	0.732–1.385	0.622
Operative time	0.807	0.691–1.469	0.581
No intraoperative complications	0.996	0.503–1.542	0.875
DA surgical approach	0.291	0.106–0.374	**<u>0.026</u>**
AR-trained surgeon	0.467	0.238–0.782	0.171
Spinal anesthesia	0.957	0.580–1.463	0.602
Correct component positioning	0.554	0.296–0.831	0.185

DA: direct anterior; AR: arthroplasty. Bolded and underlined values identify variable with statistical significance.

Table 3. Multivariable logistic regression analysis for inability of deambulation without crutches at one-month follow-up.

	OR	95% Confidence Interval	p
Age	0.862	0.764–1.351	0.098
Female	0.615	0.391–1.227	0.189
BMI	0.928	0.732–1.416	0.352
ASA < 3	0.349	0.206–0.518	**<u>0.034</u>**
Time trauma/surgery	0.786	0.365–1.191	0.432
Operative time	0.883	0.475–1.364	0.502
No intraoperative complications	0.512	0.256–0.729	0.091
DA surgical approach	0.447	0.315–0.580	**<u>0.026</u>**
AR-trained surgeon	0.546	0.129–0.866	0.312
Spinal anesthesia	0.904	0.563–1.672	0.633
Correct component positioning	0.735	0.306–1.147	0.567

DA: direct anterior; AR: arthroplasty. Bolded and underlined values identify variable with statistical significance.

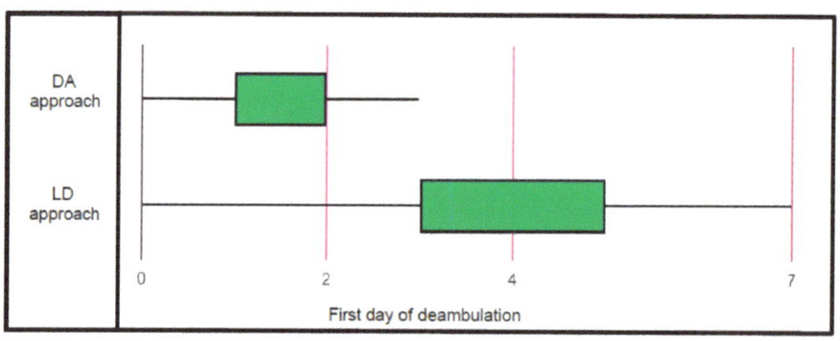

Figure 2. Graphical distribution of the first day of deambulation in Patients treated with direct anterior approach and lateral direct approach.

Table 4. Multivariable logistic regression analysis for revision surgery at one-year follow-up.

	OR	95% Confidence Interval	*p*
Age	0.741	0.489–1.266	0.659
Female	0.562	0.273–0.984	0.416
BMI	0.397	0.137–0.558	0.083
ASA < 3	0.604	0.218–1.165	0.687
Time trauma/surgery	0.856	0.649–1.453	0.705
Operative time	0.915	0.807–1.511	0.842
No intraoperative complications	0.789	0.625–1.139	0.821
DA surgical approach	0.423	0.156–0.727	0.234
AR-trained surgeon	0.258	0.114–0.392	**0.003**
Spinal anesthesia	0.891	0.565–1.376	0.908
Correct component positioning	0.672	0.496–0.978	0.536
Early deambulation completed	0.218	0.129–0.564	0.095

DA: direct anterior; AR: arthroplasty. Bolded and underlined values identify variable with statistical significance.

Table 5. Multivariable logistic regression analysis for mortality at one-year follow-up.

	OR	95% Confidence Interval	*p*
Age	0.471	0.206–0.872	0.247
Female	0.692	0.491–0.958	0.535
BMI	0.543	0.387–0.824	0.394
ASA < 3	0.367	0.194–0.525	**0.021**
Time trauma/surgery	0.825	0.657–1.237	0.780
Operative time	0.904	0.722–1.369	0.829
No intraoperative complications	0.786	0.315–1.196	0.452
DA surgical approach	0.217	0.108–0.313	0.096
AR-trained surgeon	0.338	0.239–0.482	0.081
Spinal anesthesia	1.026	0.524–1.361	0.755
Correct component positioning	0.487	0.280–0.712	0.274
Early deambulation completed	0.259	0.148–0.306	0.053

DA: direct anterior; AR: arthroplasty. Bolded and underlined values identify variable with statistical significance.

The analysis for 1-year mortality identified statistical significance in the ASA classification. In particular, we documented a higher mortality risk at 1 year for ASA classification > 3. Furthermore, we considered, of particular interest, the strong near-significance value of ED in relation to 1-year mortality; in fact, even if it were not really significant, the value of ED in this model could witness the existence of the relationship between early mobilization and better survival in our data, as already reported in the literature (Figure 3).

Revision surgery was performed in four cases: three cases for atraumatic dislocation, and one case for early periprosthetic joint infection.

The analysis for 1-year revision risk showed statistical significance for the training of the surgeons. This logistic regression analysis documented a higher risk for revision when the surgical procedure was performed by a non-AR-trained surgeon.

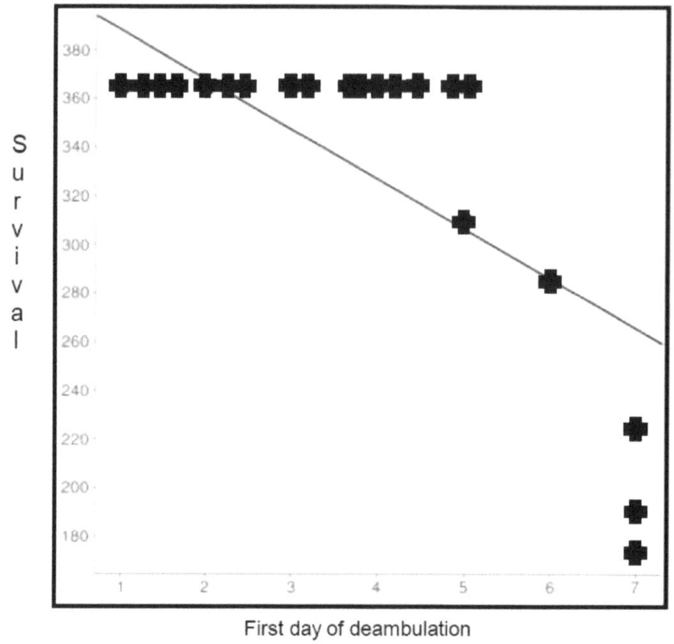

Figure 3. Survival of patients in relation to first day of registered deambulation.

4. Discussion

In this study, we present a case series of patients treated with THA after femoral neck fracture. After statistical processing of the data, we performed multivariate analyses in order to identify predictive factors of better outcomes in the first month and at 1-year follow-up.

From our data, it emerged that patients treated with THA through the DA surgical approach have a higher probability of reaching deambulation in the first days after surgery and to walk without crutches at one month. This could be derived from the minor muscular damage of this surgical approach, as is widely recognized in the literature.

Furthermore, we performed a multivariate analysis for revision risk at one year, which documented a higher risk of re-operation for patients operated on by a surgeon without specific arthroplasty training.

In our opinion, it is also of particular interest that the near-significance value resulted in ED predicting 1-year mortality. We suggest further studies to investigate this issue in this specific population of fractured patients.

Fractures of the femoral neck have important economic implications due to their direct and indirect medical costs. Total hip arthroplasty is a surgical procedure with a documented increase in number and extension year-by-year for clinical and epidemiological reasons. A recent study of the National Database documented, in the last 22 years (from 2001 to 2022), a growth rate of hip replacement surgery of +8.19% [33]. In the same study, the increase in THAs remains significant, especially when considering the progressive aging of the population in the last 22 years [33]. A previous study published by Pabinger and Geissler [34] similarly reported that hip arthroplasty is increasing exponentially in the OECD (Organization for Economic Cooperation and Development) with different rates across the countries: USA, +12.87%; Australia, +7.77%; United Kingdom, +6.95%; Germany, +6.07%; and Spain, +6.73%.

There is growing evidence that total hip arthroplasty may result in improved outcomes over hemiarthroplasty and internal fixation [13,14]. Furthermore, recent studies have also reported that THA could be more cost-effective in these patients when compared to other surgical treatments [13,14].

Recently, some authors have demonstrated that hospitals in which there is management of a high proportion of hip fracture patients may be unfairly penalized with the current models of payment [35–37]. In fact, it is recognized that there are pronounced differences between patients who underwent THA for osteoarthritis and those for hip fractures. Patients with an FNF tend to be older and with more significant clinical associated problems, frequently experience an increased length of hospitalization, more often need to be discharged to a rehabilitation facility, and show a higher readmission rate after surgery [35–37].

In our study, we performed an analysis that demonstrated a better short-term outcome in patients who underwent THA with the DA surgical approach and a better long-term outcome in terms of 1-year revision in patients operated on by an AR-trained surgeon. Furthermore, we consider the influence of ED on 1-year mortality, which could be desumed from the logistic regression analysis, to be of particular interest. In our opinion, this relationship needs to be clarified in a larger cohort of patients.

While the surgical approach for THA in elective cases is still a topic of debate with recognized difficulties in comparing the large number of reported papers [38,39], few studies to date have compared different surgical approaches in performing THA after FNF [40,41]. The results of a recent study by Cichos et al. showed that THA performed with the DA approach is associated with a lower risk of dislocation and mechanical revision at both 3 month and 1-year follow-ups when compared to the PL approach. Similarly, those authors reported that the DA approach was associated with an improvement in mortality rates compared to the PL approach at both 3-month and 1-year registered follow-ups [41].

Furthermore, the same study reported that utilization of the DA approach determined a higher overall survival at follow-up when compared to other surgical approaches [41].

In the first systematic review and meta-analysis investigating surgical approaches for arthroplasty after FNF [42], nine eligible studies were included with publication dates between 2012 and 2016. Data from this meta-analysis showed that the DA approach provided better early functional mobility in four studies according to other data reported in the literature.

Bucs et al., in a study that evaluated the efficacy of the DA approach in HHA for FNFs compared to the DL approach, demonstrated that patients operated on with the DA approach reported less postoperative pain, resulting in patients more frequently being able to complete earlier mobilization [43].

Nogler et al. confirmed these data and showed in a different study that patients operated on with the DA approach had less postoperative pain, minor blood loss, and an inferior length of hospital stay when compared to those treated with the PL or DL approaches [44].

Multiple prior studies on elective total hip arthroplasty showed an improvement in early functional scores, deambulation, and mobilization in DA-approach patients for the first few weeks after surgery [18,19]. While the consequences of these early improved capabilities in mobilization and deambulation for long-term outcomes in elective patients have still not yet been completely clarified, the FNF population is generally in a worse position compared to their elective counterparts [22,36], given the potential major benefits of these early small differences. A previous study reported that the level of deambulation at 2 weeks after surgery could be considered as a significant predictor of survivorship at 1 year in the FNF population [23]. Therefore, in our opinion, we have to give particular importance to reaching early deambulation after THA for FNFs, and surgery through the DA approach has a demonstrated positive influence in achieving this result.

Several studies have recently investigated the role of surgeon training in the treatment of FNF. Padilla et al. recently reported an interesting study in which the direct medical costs of THA performed for FNFs between orthopedic surgeons trained in different subspecialties were compared [45]. These authors demonstrated that in the FNF population, surgeons with specific training in arthroplasty achieve lower total costs for the THA episode of care, whereas surgeons without specific training in arthroplasty often exceed the bundled payment target. Similar results were also reported by Thomas et al. [46].

Prior studies have mainly sought to elucidate the relationship between the volume and outcome of the surgical procedures, and have demonstrated that an increase in the number of patients operated on leads to an improved outcome [47–50]. Maceroli et al. [50] analyzed the New York State System database to determine if patient outcomes following THA performed for FNF differed between hospitals with a significant volume of completed procedures. Those authors reported that patients treated with total hip arthroplasty at the highest volume hospitals had significantly lower 30-day and 1-year mortality rates and a minor complication rate at 3-month follow-up.

Browne et al. [49], in their analysis of a nationwide database, identified 97,894 patients affected by FNF surgically treated in different hospitals with different surgeon volumes. They found that in-hospital mortality and complication rates were significantly higher in subjects treated by lower-volume surgeons than higher-volume surgeons, and that complication rates were higher in hospitals with a lower volume of performed procedures. We have to consider that their study cohort included patients who underwent internal fixation, hemiarthroplasty, and total hip arthroplasty, potentially limiting the generalizability of the results to a THA-only population.

Few studies have investigated the relationship between surgeon specialization training and outcomes [51,52]. Previous articles have encompassed a limited number of surgical specialties, and few have been published investigating this item in Orthopedics and Traumatology. Hagen et al. [53] identified patients who underwent primary or revision hip and knee arthroplasty in the United States to study the relationship between hospital specialization and outcomes. They found an inversely proportional relationship between a hospital's degree of orthopedic specialization and the rates of adverse outcomes.

In fact, with an increase in orthopedic specialization, Hagen et al. [53] reported a progressive decrease in mortality, deep vein thrombosis, postoperative hemorrhage, and infection.

The results of our analysis on THA performed after FNF appear to be in accordance with the previous literature, underlining the importance of a surgical approach in determining a better outcome in the short term, leading to a better long-term outcome. Furthermore, our data confirm, as reported by other authors, that surgery for THA after FNF has significant advantages when performed by arthroplasty-trained surgeons.

This study should be interpreted considering its limitations. First of all, it has a retrospective design with the potential for transfer bias and the absence of randomization for surgical approaches. Additionally, the short- and long-term results at follow-up were collected by four different physiotherapists and by two different orthopedic surgeons. We followed previously published methods to verify correct femoral and acetabular positioning; however, all evaluations were performed by X-ray and not by CT imaging, with possible bias of underestimation. All people were blinded to the design of the study; however, possible bias could derive from excessive heterogeneity in participants in the data collection. Finally, this analysis was conducted on a limited number of patients at a single center and, thus, must be considered as only a preliminary indication to guide future multicenter prospective trials in order to reach definitive conclusions.

5. Conclusions

In our analysis, a direct anterior surgical approach and an ASA classification < 3 can predict improved results in the first month after THA for FNF. Furthermore, our results suggest that THAs performed by AR-trained surgeons have a lower probability of revision at 1 year. Mortality at 1 year was influenced by the ASA classification.

However, due to the results of our logistic regression models, we consider that the influence of early deambulation on 1-year mortality after THA for FNF is deserving of more clinical study.

Author Contributions: Conceptualization, P.S. and E.V.; Methodology, P.S. and F.P.; Investigation, F.P. and M.B.; Data curation, F.P., M.B. and E.V.; Writing—review & editing, P.S. and F.C.; Supervision, F.C. and E.V. All authors have read and agreed to the published version of the manuscript.

Funding: This research received no external funding.

Institutional Review Board Statement: The study was conducted in accordance with the Declaration of Helsinki, and approved by the Institutional Ethics Committee "North Emilia Ethical Commitee" protocol code 631/2023 date 12 December 2023.

Informed Consent Statement: Informed consent was obtained from all subjects involved in the study.

Data Availability Statement: Data are contained within the article.

Conflicts of Interest: The authors declare no conflicts of interest.

References

1. Brown, C.A.; Starr, A.Z.; Nunley, J.A. Analysis of past secular trends of hip fractures and predicted number in the future 2010–2050. *J. Orthop. Trauma.* **2012**, *26*, 117–122. [CrossRef]
2. Swayambunathan, J.; Dasgupta, A.; Rosenberg, P.S.; Hannan, M.T.; Kiel, D.P.; Bhattacharyya, T. Incidence of hip fracture over 4 decades in the Framingham Heart study. *JAMA Intern. Med.* **2020**, *180*, 1225–1231. [CrossRef]
3. Lewiecki, E.M.; Wright, N.C.; Curtis, J.R.; Siris, E.; Gagel, R.F.; Saag, K.G.; Singer, A.J.; Steven, P.M.; Adler, R.A. Hip fracture trends in the United States, 2002 to 2015. *Osteoporos. Int.* **2018**, *29*, 717–722. [CrossRef]
4. Chen, I.J.; Chiang, C.Y.; Li, Y.H.; Chang, C.H.; Hu, C.C.; Chen, D.W.; Chang, Y.; Yang, W.E.; Shih, H.-N.; Ueng, S.W.-N.; et al. Nationwide cohort study of hip fractures: Time trends in the incidence rates and projections up to 2035. *Osteoporos. Int.* **2015**, *26*, 681–688. [CrossRef]
5. Konnopka, A.; Jerusel, N.; Konig, H.H. The health and economic consequences of osteopenia- and osteoporosis-attributable hip fractures in Germany: Estimation for 2002 and projection until 2050. *Osteoporos. Int.* **2009**, *20*, 1117–1129. [CrossRef]
6. Rosengren, B.E.; Karlsson, M.K. The annual number of hip fractures in Sweden will double from year 2002 to 2050, projections based on local and nationwide data. *Acta Orthop.* **2014**, *85*, 234–237. [CrossRef]
7. Brauer, C.A.; Coca-Perraillon, M.; Cutler, D.M.; Rosen, A.B. Incidence and mortality of hip fractures in the United States. *JAMA* **2009**, *302*, 1573–1579. [CrossRef] [PubMed]
8. Schairer, W.W.; Lane, J.M.; Halsey, D.A.; Iorio, R.; Padgett, D.E.; McLawhorn, A.S. The Frank Stinchfield Award: Total hip arthroplasty for femoral neck fracture is not a typical DRG 470, a propensity-matched cohort study. *Clin. Orthop. Relat. Res.* **2017**, *475*, 353–360. [CrossRef] [PubMed]
9. Moldovan, F.; Ivanescu, A.D.; Fodor, P.; Moldovan, L.; Bataga, T. Correlation between Inflammatory Systemic Biomarkers and Surgical Trauma in Elderly Patients with Hip Fractures. *J. Clin. Med.* **2023**, *12*, 5147. [CrossRef] [PubMed]
10. Mundi, S.; Pindiprolu, B.; Simunovic, N.; Bhandari, M. Similar mortality rates in hip fracture patients over the past 31 years. *Acta Orthop.* **2014**, *85*, 54–59. [CrossRef] [PubMed]
11. Miller, B.J.; Callaghan, J.J.; Cram, P.; Karam, M.; Marsh, J.L.; Noiseux, N.O. Changing trends in the treatment of femoral neck fractures: A review of the American Board of Orthopaedic Surgery Database. *J. Bone Jt. Surg. Am.* **2014**, *96*, e149. [CrossRef]
12. Schiavi, P.; Pogliacomi, F.; Colombo, M.; Amarossi, A.; Ceccarelli, F.; Vaienti, E. Acetabular erosion following bipolar hemiarthroplasty: A Role for the size of femoral head? *Injury* **2019**, *50* (Suppl. S4), S21–S25. [CrossRef]
13. Stronach, B.M.; Bergin, P.F.; Perez, J.L.; Watson, S.; Jones, L.C.; McGwin, G.; Ponce, B.A. The rising use of total hip arthroplasty for femoral neck fractures in the United States. *Hip Int.* **2020**, *30*, 107–113. [CrossRef] [PubMed]
14. Goh, S.-K.; Samuel, M.; Su, D.H.C.; Chan, E.S.-Y.; Yeo, S.-J. Meta-analysis comparing total hip arthroplasty with hemiarthroplasty in the treatment of displaced neck of femur fracture. *J. Arthroplast.* **2009**, *24*, 400–406. [CrossRef]
15. Yu, L.; Wang, Y.; Chen, J. Total hip arthroplasty versus hemiarthroplasty for displaced femoral neck fractures: Meta-analysis of randomized trials. *Clin. Orthop. Relat. Res.* **2012**, *470*, 2235–2243. [CrossRef] [PubMed]
16. Awad, M.E.; Farley, B.J.; Mostafa, G.; Saleh, K.J. Direct anterior approach has short term functional benefit and higher resource requirements compared with the posterior approach in primary total hip arthroplasty: A meta-analysis of functional outcomes and cost. *Bone Jt. J.* **2021**, *103-B*, 1078–1087. [CrossRef] [PubMed]
17. Bergin, P.F.; Doppelt, J.D.; Kephart, C.J.; Benke, M.T.; Graeter, J.H.; Holmes, A.S.; Haleem-Smith, H.; Tuan, R.S.; Unger, A.S. Comparison of minimally invasive direct anterior versus posterior total hip arthroplasty based on inflammation and muscle damage markers. *J. Bone Jt. Surg. Am.* **2011**, *93*, 1392–1398. [CrossRef]
18. Miller, L.E.; Gondusky, J.S.; Kamath, A.F.; Boettner, F.; Wright, J.; Bhattacharyya, S. Influence of surgical approach on complication risk in primary total hip arthroplasty. *Acta Orthop.* **2018**, *89*, 289–294. [CrossRef]
19. Taunton, M.J.; Mason, J.B.; Odum, S.M.; Springer, B.D. Direct anterior total hip arthroplasty yields more rapid voluntary cessation of all walking aids: A prospective, randomized clinical trial. *J. Arthroplast.* **2014**, *29* (Suppl. S9), 169–172. [CrossRef]

20. Taunton, M.J.; Trousdale, R.T.; Sierra, R.J.; Kaufman, K.; Pagnano, M.W. John Charnley Award: Randomized clinical trial of direc anterior and miniposterior approach THA: Which provides better functional recovery? *Clin. Orthop. Relat. Res.* **2018**, *476*, 216–22 [CrossRef]
21. Peters, R.M.; van Beers, L.; van Steenbergen, L.N.; Wolkenfelt, J.; Ettema, H.B.; Ten Have, B.; Rijk, P.C.; Stevens, M.; Bulstra, S.K Poolman, R.W.; et al. Similar superior patient-reported outcome measures for anterior and posterolateral approaches after tota hip arthroplasty: Postoperative patient- reported outcome measure improvement after 3 months in 12,774 primary total hi arthroplasties using the anterior, anterolateral, straight lateral, or posterolateral approach. *J. Arthroplast.* **2018**, *33*, 1786–1793.
22. Sibia, U.S.; Turner, T.R.; MacDonald, J.H.; King, P.J. The impact of surgical technique on patient reported outcome measures an early complications after total hip arthroplasty. *J. Arthroplast.* **2017**, *32*, 1171–1175. [CrossRef]
23. Le Manach, Y.; Collins, G.; Bhandari, M.; Bessissow, A.; Boddaert, J.; Khiami, F.; Chaudhry, H.; De Beer, J.; Riou, B.; Landais, P et al. Outcomes after hip fracture surgery compared with elective total hip replacement. *JAMA* **2015**, *314*, 1159–1166. [CrossRef
24. Heinonen, M.; Karppi, P.; Huusko, T.; Kautiainen, H.; Sulkava, R. Post-operative degree of mobilization at two weeks predict one-year mortality after hip fracture. *Aging Clin. Exp. Res.* **2004**, *16*, 476–480. [CrossRef] [PubMed]
25. Imura, K.; Ishii, Y.; Yagisawa, K.; Matsueda, M. Postoperative ambulatory level after hip fracture in the elderly predicts surviva rate. *Arch. Orthop. Trauma. Surg.* **2000**, *120*, 369–371. [CrossRef] [PubMed]
26. Iosifidis, M.; Iliopoulos, E.; Panagiotou, A.; Apostolidis, K.; Traios, S.; Giantsis, G. Walking ability before and after a hip fracture in elderly predict greater longterm survivorship. *J. Orthop. Sci.* **2016**, *21*, 48–52. [CrossRef] [PubMed]
27. Cichos, K.H.; Mabry, S.E.; Spitler, C.A.; McGwin, J.r.G.; Quade, J.H.; Ghanem, E.S. Comparison between the direct anterior and posterior approaches for total hip arthroplasty performed for femoral neck fracture. *J. Orthop. Trauma.* **2021**, *35*, 41–48. [CrossRef] [PubMed]
28. Heiden, J.J.; Goodin, S.R.; Mormino, M.A.; Siebler, J.C.; Putnam, S.M.; Lyden, E.R.; Tao, M.A. Early ambulation after hip fracture surgery is associated with decreased 30-day mortality. *J. Am. Acad. Orthop. Surg.* **2021**, *29*, e238–e242. [CrossRef] [PubMed]
29. Pogliacomi, F.; Schiavi, P.; Grappiolo, G.; Ceccarelli, F.; Vaienti, E. Outcome of short versus conventional stem for total hip arthroplasty in the femur with a high cortical index: A five year follow-up prospective multicentre comparative study. *Int. Orthop* **2020**, *44*, 61–68. [CrossRef]
30. Loppini, M.; Schiavi, P.; Rocca, A.D.; Traverso, F.; Rocca, F.D.; Mazziotta, G.; Astore, F.; Grappiolo, G. Double-trabecular metal cup technique for the management of Paprosky type III defects without pelvic discontinuity. *Hip Int.* **2018**, *28* (Suppl. S2), 66–72 [CrossRef]
31. Hossain, F.; Konan, S.; Volpin, A.; Haddad, F.S. Early performance-based and patient-reported outcomes of a contemporary taper fit bone-conserving short stem femoral component in total hip arthroplasty. *Bone Jt. J.* **2017**, *99-B*, 49–55. [CrossRef]
32. Khalily, C.; Lester, D.K. Results of a tapered cementless femoral stem implanted in varus. *J. Arthroplast.* **2002**, *17*, 463–466 [CrossRef] [PubMed]
33. Moldovan, F.; Moldovan, L.; Bataga, T. A Comprehensive Research on the Prevalence and Evolution Trend of Orthopedic Surgeries in Romania. *Healthcare* **2023**, *11*, 1866. [CrossRef] [PubMed]
34. Pabinger, C.; Geissler, A. Utilization rates of hip arthroplasty in OECD countries. *Osteoarthr. Cartil.* **2014**, *22*, 734–741. [CrossRef]
35. Yoon, R.S.; Iorio, R.; Bosco, J.A.; Hutzler, L.H.; Mahure, S.A. Hip arthroplasty for fracture vs elective care. *J. Arthroplast.* **2017**, *32*, 2353–2358. [CrossRef] [PubMed]
36. Grace, T.R.; Patterson, J.T.; Tangtiphaiboontana, J.; Krogue, J.D.; Vail, T.P.; Ward, D.T. Hip fractures and the bundle: A cost analysis of patients undergoing hip arthroplasty for femoral neck fracture vs degenerative joint disease. *J. Arthroplast.* **2018**, *33*, 1681–1685 [CrossRef]
37. Kester, B.S.; Williams, J.; Bosco, J.A.; Slover, J.D.; Iorio, R.; Schwarzkopf, R. The association between hospital length of stay and 90-day readmission risk for femoral neck fracture patients: Within a total joint arthroplasty bundled payment initiative. *J. Arthroplast.* **2016**, *31*, 2741–2745. [CrossRef] [PubMed]
38. Miller, L.E.; Gondusky, J.S.; Bhattacharyya, S.; Kamath, A.F.; Boettner, F.; Wright, J. Does surgical approach affect outcomes in total hip arthroplasty through 90 days of follow-up? A systematic review with meta-analysis. *J. Arthroplast.* **2018**, *33*, 1296–1302. [CrossRef] [PubMed]
39. Malek, I.A.; Royce, G.; Bhatti, S.U.; Whittaker, J.P.; Phillips, S.P.; Wilson, I.R.; Wootton, J.R.; Starks, I. A comparison between the direct anterior and posterior approaches for total hip arthroplasty: The role of an 'enhanced recovery' pathway. *Bone Jt. J.* **2016**, *98-B*, 754–760. [CrossRef]
40. Haller, J.M.; Working, Z.M.; Ross, H.L.; Gililland, J.M.; Kubiak, E.N. Fewer hip dislocations with anterior total hip arthroplasty for displaced femoral neck fracture. *Orthopedics* **2021**, *44*, E248–E252. [CrossRef]
41. Cichos, K.H.; McGwin, G., Jr.; Boyd, B.; Arthroplasty for Hip Fracture Consortium; Ghanem, E.S. Direct Anterior Approach Total Hip Arthroplasty Is Associated with Reduced 1-Year Mortality and Surgical Complications After Femoral Neck Fracture. *J. Arthroplast.* **2023**, *38*, 2347–2354.e2. [CrossRef]
42. Kunkel, S.T.; Sabatino, M.J.; Kang, R.; Jevsevar, D.S.; Moschetti, W.E. A systematic review and meta-analysis of the direct anterior approach for hemiarthroplasty for femoral neck fracture. *Eur. J. Orthop. Surg. Traumatol.* **2018**, *28*, 217e2. [CrossRef] [PubMed]
43. Bucs, G.; Dande, A.; Patczai, B.; Sebestyen, A.; Almasi, R.; Not, L.G.; Wiegand, N. Bipolar hemiarthroplasty for the treatment of femoral neck fractures with minimally invasive anterior approach in elderly. *Injury* **2021**, *52* (Suppl. S1), S37–S43. [CrossRef] [PubMed]

44. Nogler, M.; Randelli, F.; Macheras, G.A.; Thaler, M. Hemiarthroplasty of the hip using the direct anterior approach. *Operat Orthop. Traumatol.* **2021**, *33*, 304–307. [CrossRef] [PubMed]
45. Padilla, J.A.; Gabor, J.A.; Ryan, S.P.; Long, W.J.; Seyler, T.M. Schwarzkopf RM Total Hip Arthroplasty for Femoral Neck Fracture: The Economic Implications of Orthopedic Subspecialty Training. *J. Arthroplast.* **2020**, *35*, S101–S106. [CrossRef] [PubMed]
46. Thomas, J.C.; Haidukewych , G.J. Total Hip Arthroplasty for Acute Femoral Neck Fractures: Who Should Perform the Operation-Adult Reconstructive or Trauma Surgeons? *J. Orthop. Trauma.* **2021**, *35*, 606–611. [CrossRef] [PubMed]
47. Katz, J.N.; Barrett, J.; Mahomed, N.N.; Baron, J.A.; Wright, R.J.; Losina, E. Association between hospital and surgeon procedure volume and the outcomes of total knee replacement. *J. Bone Jt. Surg. Ser. A* **2004**, *86*, 1909–1916. [CrossRef] [PubMed]
48. Katz, J.N.; Losina, E.; Barrett, J.; Phillips, C.; Mahomed, N.N.; Lew, R.A.; Guadagnoli, E.; Harris, W.H.; Poss, R.; Baron, J.A. Association between hospital and surgeon procedure volume with outcome of total hip replacement. *J. Bone Jt. Surg.* **2001**, *83*, 1622–1629. [CrossRef]
49. Shervin, N.; Rubash, H.E.; Katz, J.N. Orthopaedic procedure volume and patient outcomes. *Clin. Orthop. Relat. Res.* **2007**, *457*, 35–41. [CrossRef]
50. Maceroli, M.; Nikkel, L.E.; Mahmood, B.; Ketz, J.P.; Qiu, X.; Ciminelli, J.; Messing, S.M.; Elfar, J.C. Total hip arthroplasty for femoral neck fractures: Improved outcomes with higher hospital volumes. *J. Orthop. Trauma.* **2016**, *30*, 597–604. [CrossRef]
51. Sahni, N.R.; Dalton, M.; Cutler, D.M.; Birkmeyer, J.D.; Chandra, A. Surgeon specialization and operative mortality in United States: Retrospective analysis. *BMJ* **2016**, *354*, i3571. [CrossRef] [PubMed]
52. Hagen, T.P.; Vaughan-Sarrazin, M.S.; Cram, P. Relation between hospital orthopaedic specialisation and outcomes in patients aged 65 and older: Retrospective analysis of US Medicare data. *BMJ* **2010**, *340*, c165. [CrossRef] [PubMed]
53. Browne, J.A.; Pietrobon, R.; Olson, S.A. Hip fracture outcomes: Does surgeon or hospital volume really matter? *J. Trauma. Inj. Infect Crit. Care* **2009**, *66*, 809–814. [CrossRef] [PubMed]

Journal of
Clinical Medicine

MDPI

Article

Comparative Analysis of Complication Rates in Tibial Shaft Fractures: Intramedullary Nail vs. Ilizarov External Fixation Method

Danilo Jeremic [1,2,*], Nikola Grubor [3], Zoran Bascarevic [1,2], Nemanja Slavkovic [1,2], Branislav Krivokapic [1,2], Boris Vukomanovic [1,2], Kristina Davidovic [2,4], Zelimir Jovanovic [1] and Slavko Tomic [1,2]

1 Institute for Orthopeadics "Banjica", 11000 Belgrade, Serbia; zoran.bascarevic@iohbb.edu.rs (Z.B.); nemaslav@yahoo.com (N.S.); branislav.krivokapic@iohbb.edu.rs (B.K.); vukomanovicboris@gmail.com (B.V.); drzex@live.com (Z.J.); tomicslavko1956@gmail.com (S.T.)
2 Faculty of Medicine, University of Belgrade, 11000 Belgrade, Serbia; dr.kristina.davidovic@gmail.com
3 Institute for Medical Statistics and Informatics, Faculty of Medicine, University of Belgrade, 11000 Belgrade, Serbia; nickgrubor@gmail.com
4 Center for Radiology and Magnetic Resonance Imaging, University Clinical Center of Serbia, 11000 Belgrade, Serbia
* Correspondence: danilo.jeremic@iohbb.edu.rs

Abstract: Background: The external fixation (EF) Ilizarov method, shown to offer efficacy and relative safety, has unique biomechanical properties. Intramedullary nail fixation (IMN) is an advantageous alternative, offering biomechanical stability and a minimally invasive procedure. The aim of this study was to assess outcomes in patients undergoing tibia fracture fixation, comparing the Ilizarov EF and IMN methods in an early phase of IMN implementation in Serbia. **Methods:** This was a retrospective study including patients with radiologically confirmed closed and open (Gustilo and Anderson type I) tibial diaphysis fractures treated at the Institute for Orthopedic Surgery "Banjica" from January 2013 to June 2017. The following demographic and clinical data were retrieved: age, sex, chronic disease diagnoses, length of hospital stay, surgical wait times, surgery length, type of anesthesia used, fracture, prophylaxis, mechanism of injury, postsurgical complications, time to recovery, and pain reduction. Pain intensity was measured by the Visual Analog Scale (VAS), a self-reported scale ranging from 0 to 100 mm. **Results:** A total of 58 IMN patients were compared to 74 patients who underwent Ilizarov EF. Study groups differed in time to recovery ($p < 0.001$), length of hospitalization ($p = 0.007$), pain intensity at the fracture site ($p < 0.001$), and frequency of general anesthesia in favor of intramedullary fixation ($p < 0.001$). A shorter surgery time ($p < 0.001$) and less antibiotic use ($p < 0.001$) were observed when EF was used. Additionally, we identified that the intramedullary fixation was a significant predictor of pain intensity. **Conclusions:** The IMN method offers faster recovery and reduced pain intensity in comparison to EF, while the length of surgery predicted the occurrence of any complication.

Keywords: tibial shaft fracture; intramedullary fixation; external fixation; treatment strategies

1. Introduction

Fractures of the tibial diaphysis represent the most frequently encountered fractures of long bones [1]. With an incidence ranging from 8.1 to 37 per 100,000 individuals annually, these fractures pose a significant public health concern [1]. The vulnerability of these fractures to infection and nonunion is attributed to the absence of sufficient soft tissue coverage and the distinctive vascular supply to the affected region [2]. Furthermore, fractures of the tibial shaft are classified as injuries with severe quality-of-life impact with the potential for enduring disability [2,3].

Conservative management of stable tibial diaphyseal fractures, characterized by closed reduction and cast immobilization, is a common approach [4]. However, this method is not without complications, including an elevated risk of deep vein thrombosis, compartment syndrome, soft tissue damage, and chronic pain due to prolonged immobilization [5]. Despite the lower infection rate associated with conservative cast treatment, it concurrently exhibits the highest incidence of delayed union, nonunion, or inadequate union of fractures [6].

Intramedullary nail fixation is an advantageous alternative, offering biomechanical stability and a minimally invasive procedure [6]. Many experts consider intramedullary nails the treatment for tibial shaft fractures [7,8]. Comparative studies suggest the superiority of intramedullary nail fixation over external fixation in open tibial shaft fractures, mainly when wound closure is promptly executed following nail insertion [8]. The Ilizarov method is also discussed, emphasizing its efficacy and relative safety. This technique's unique biomechanical properties enable the application of tensioned wires to maintain stable fixation of bone fragments while facilitating fracture site dynamization [9–11]. Notable advantages of the Ilizarov method over closed fixation include closed reduction, minimal soft tissue damage, early mobilization, and simplified device removal [12].

The article delves into the controversy surrounding the choice of the most appropriate technique for stabilizing tibial fractures. With its ease of application and minimal impact on blood supply, the utility of external fixation is counterbalanced by a heightened pin tract infection rate, challenges in controlling soft tissue injuries, and a relatively elevated nonunion rate [13]. Conversely, reamed nails offer superior stability but entail a theoretical risk of increased infection and nonunion due to the compromise of endosteal blood supply [2]. Nevertheless, more evidence is required to substantiate this claim since several studies have shown conversely that reamed nails exhibit a higher incidence of union in comparison to non-reamed nails. Notably, the limited number of studies comparing complication rates, including compartment syndrome, poor union, nonunion, and delayed union, in tibial fractures treated with external and intramedullary fixation underscores the need for further research in this domain. Therefore, in this study, we aimed to assess outcomes in patients undergoing tibia fracture fixation, comparing the Ilizarov external fixation method (EF) and intramedullary nail placement (IMN) in an early phase of IMN implementation in Serbia.

2. Materials and Methods

This was a retrospective cohort study. Data about consecutive patients with radiologically confirmed closed and open (Gustilo and Anderson type I) tibial diaphysis fracture treated at the Institute for Orthopeadics "Banjica" from January 2013 to June 2017 were collected. The study was approved by the Ethical Committees of the Institute for Orthopedic Surgery "Banjica" (num: 16/2017) and Belgrade University, Faculty of Medicine (num: 2650/IV-16, date: 10 April 2018).

2.1. Eligibility Criteria

All consenting consecutive patients aged 18 or older with radiologically confirmed closed and open (Gustilo and Anderson type I) tibial diaphysis fractures, independent of fracture location, were included during the study period. The fractures were radiologically classified using The AO Foundation/Orthopaedic Trauma Association (AO/OTA) fracture classification system. The exclusion criteria were patients who had an open fracture above the Gustilo and Anderson type I classification, who had bone defects, injuries to nerves and blood vessels, and incomplete medical documentation, who were in an alcoholic state on admission, and who had a fracture of the diaphysis of the tibia as part of polytrauma.

2.2. Study Design and Data Collection

For patients who underwent external fixation (Ilizarov method) or reamed intramedullary nail fixation, the following demographic and clinical data were retrieved: age, sex, chronic disease diagnoses, length of hospital stay, surgical wait times, surgery length, type of anesthesia used, fracture, prophylaxis, mechanism of injury, postsurgical complications, time to recovery, and pain reduction. Pain intensity was measured by the Visual Analog Scale (VAS), a self-reported scale ranging from 0 to 100 mm [14]. The VAS scale was linguistically adapted to the local cultural area. Pain was evaluated on admission day (prior to surgery) and at last control, i.e., hospital discharge, in accordance with the protocol, at the fracture site and in two nearby joints (knee and ankle).

2.3. *Surgical Techniques*

The surgical choice in this study depended on the preference of the surgeon in charge. The indications for operative technique were the same for both groups, i.e., Gustilo and Anderson type I tibial diaphysis fractures, and surgery was performed independently of open or closed fracture types and fracture location. As IMN was introduced as a novel surgical technique, surgeries were performed by specialized surgeons with at least 5 years of experience performing multiple approaches to tibial diaphysis fractures.

2.3.1. Reamed Intramedullary Nail Fixation

Patients were positioned supine on the operating table to ensure radiolucency and facilitate access for tibial shaft surgery, with the knee flexed at an angle of 90–110°. Anesthesia was administered according to medical indications and the judgment of the anesthesiologist. The surgical area, namely the distal region of the upper leg, lower leg, and foot, was thoroughly sterilized. Prior to surgery, tourniquets were applied to the upper leg of all patients. After disinfecting and garnishing the operative field, we made an incision in the appropriate place on the skin above the tibial fracture (anterior approach to the knee, medial parapatellar approach). After access, we prepared the tibia to receive an intramedullary nail. The key is to precisely guide the intramedullary nail into the tibial canal. We did this under fluoroscopic (X-ray) control to ensure accurate positioning of the nails. After determining the starting point anterior to the articular plateau and medial to the lateral tibial spine and opening the canal, we placed a guide wire. Through the guide wire, we reamed the tibial canal 1.0 mm above the size of the final nail. The surgeon carefully pushed the nail over the guide wire through the tibial canal until it reached the desired position across the fracture. After proper placement of the nail, repositioning of the fracture, and obtaining a satisfactory position, we locked the nail through the guide with two proximal and two distal screws. Once the nail was securely placed and fixed, a final check of the nail's position was performed via fluoroscopy to ensure that everything was properly positioned. Once the nail was securely placed and fixed, the incision was carefully closed layer by layer. On the first postoperative day, all patients were verticalized with the help of crutches with a support on the operated leg, the wound was bandaged, and the neurovascular status was checked. All patients were included in the early physical rehabilitation program, with walking and support on the operated leg until discharge from the hospital. Regular bandages were applied on the second day.

2.3.2. External Fixation (Ilizarov Method)

Following the administration of anesthesia by the anesthesiologist, the patients were positioned on the operating table in the appropriate supine posture. Buttresses were positioned under the thigh and rear foot to elevate the lower leg to a sufficient height, creating space for the rings to move freely. Following disinfection and preparation of the surgical area (the lower portion of the upper leg and lower leg), we realigned the broken bone and began the process of attaching the Ilizarov external fixator. To achieve accurate positioning of the ring and maximum stability, we used X-ray guidance to attach the rings of the Ilizarov device to the bone using pins. The rings were affixed to the bone with the use of tensioned pins. Once the rings were connected, we inserted a spacer between them to create the outside structure of the Ilizarov external fixator. We affixed these spacers to the rings using screws or other fastening instruments. Once the device was positioned, a final assessment of the realignment of the fracture was conducted using X-rays. The construction of the devices was then carried out, and dressing was applied around the incisions where the pins penetrate the skin. On the first day after surgery, all patients were assisted in standing upright with assistance on the limb that was operated on. The neurovascular condition was assessed, and the wounds around the pins were dressed with bandages. As part of the early physical rehabilitation program, patients engaged in daily activities such as walking and receiving assistance on the leg that had surgery until discharge from the hospital.

2.4. Statistical Analysis

Measures of central tendency (mean and median) and variability (standard deviation and percentiles) were used to describe the study population. Categorical features were reported using absolute and relative frequencies. Data analysis used the null hypothesis significance testing paradigm, considering all p-values < 0.05 significant. We compared groups using the Student's t-test, Mann–Whitney U test, chi-square test, and generalized linear models. All statistical procedures used SPSS (SPSS for Windows, release 26.0, SPSS, Chicago, IL, USA).

3. Results

One hundred thirty-two patients with tibial diaphysis fractures were enrolled and followed in the study. Of the 132 patients, 62.9% were male, while 37.1% were female. The average age was 46.1 ± 16.4 years (range 18–73 years). In our cohort, 56.1% of patients underwent external fixation (Ilizarov method), while 43.9% underwent intramedullary nail fixation. Our samples were balanced concerning sociodemographic characteristics. The characteristics of the cohort are shown in Table 1.

Table 1. Characteristics of the cohort.

Variable	Intervention		p
	Intramedullary Nail Fixation (n = 58)	**External Fixation (n = 74)**	
Sex, n (%)			
Male	36 (62.1)	47 (63.5)	0.865
Female	22 (37.9)	27 (36.5)	
Age, x ± sd	43.28 ± 17.12	48.31 ± 15.58	0.082
Comorbidities			
Diabetes	4 (6.9)	9 (12.2)	0.314
Hypertension	11 (19.0)	21 (28.4)	0.210
Coronary Disease	1 (1.7)	2 (2.7)	0.708
Median Length of Hospitalization in Days (IQR)	20 (15–25)	23 (19–30)	0.007
Median Surgery Waiting Times in Days (IQR)	7 (3–8)	6 (3–8)	0.912
Mechanism of Injury, n (%)			
Fall onto a Flat Surface	33 (56.9)	50 (67.6)	0.386
Fall from Height	3 (5.2)	6 (8.1)	
Direct Trauma	9 (15.5)	8 (10.8)	
Motor Vehicle Accident	13 (22.4)	10 (13.5)	

Table 2 shows the types of fractures in total, as well as according to the type of intervention. There were 13 open Gustilo I fractures in the Ilizarov cohort (17.6%) and 9 open Gustilo I in the IMN cohort (15.5%). The 42-A type of fracture was the most common in our study sample (71.2%), followed by 42-B (19.0%). Comminuted fractures were more present in the EF group (20.3%); however, no statistical significance was found in the type of fracture according to the type of intervention (p = 0.079).

Table 2. Type of fractures in total, as well as according to type of intervention.

Type of Fracture, n (%)	Intervention	
	IMN (n = 58)	EF (n = 74)
42-A1	10 (17.2)	33 (44.6)
42-A2	26 (44.8)	12 (16.2)
42-A3	6 (10.3)	7 (9.4)
42-B1	1 (1.7)	2 (2.7)
42-B2	7 (12.1)	3 (4.0)
42-B3	3 (5.1)	2 (2.7)
42-C1	1 (1.7)	7 (9.4)
42-C2	3 (5.1)	3 (4.0)
42-C3	1 (1.7)	5 (6.7)

Type of Fracture, n (%)	Intervention	
	IMN (n = 58)	EF (n = 74)
42-A 94 (71.2)	42 (72.4)	52 (70.3)
42-B 18 (13.6)	11 (19.0)	7 (9.5)
42-C 20 (15.2)	5 (8.6)	15 (20.3)

Patients who underwent external fixation (Ilizarov method) had significantly longer hospital stays than patients who underwent intramedullary nail fixation, $p = 0.007$. No statistically significant difference was found when comparing groups by surgical wait times, mechanism of injury, or frequencies of different fracture types ($p > 0.05$). Patients who underwent intramedullary nail fixation had a significantly higher rate of procedural general anesthesia than patients who underwent external fixation (Ilizarov method), $p < 0.001$. We found a statistically significant difference in median surgical lengths among the two groups. Patients undergoing intramedullary nail fixation had significantly longer procedure lengths than those undergoing external fixation, $p < 0.001$. The two groups also differed in the rate of antibiotic usage, with those undergoing intramedullary nail fixation having higher frequencies of antibiotic use than those undergoing external fixation (Ilizarov method). These differences and their respective p-values are shown in Table 3.

Table 3. Characteristics of surgery in relation to the type of intervention for tibial fracture fixation in the study population.

Variable	Intervention		p
	Intramedullary Nail Fixation (n = 58)	External Fixation (n = 74)	
Anesthesia type, n (%)			
Spinal	26 (47.3)	56 (75.7)	
Block	8 (14.5)	12 (16.2)	<0.001
General	21 (38.2)	6 (8.1)	
Median Surgery Length in Minutes (IQR)	93 (75–130)	60 (50–80)	<0.001
Blood Transfusion, n (%)	1 (1.7)	0 (0.0)	0.257
Antibiotics, n (%)	38 (65.5)	18 (24.3)	<0.001
Low-Molecular-Weight Heparin (LMWH), n (%)	57 (98.3)	72 (97.3)	0.708

No statistically significant difference in frequencies of postoperative complications was found between the two study groups ($p > 0.05$). A statistically significant difference in recovery time was found favoring the intramedullary nail fixation group compared to the external fixation group ($p < 0.001$).

The average reported non-ambulatory knee pain before surgical intervention was 34.13 ± 18.45 in the group intended for external fixation (Ilizarov method) and 34.17 ± 18.26 in the group intended for intramedullary nail fixation. The average reported postsurgical non-ambulatory knee pain was 18.26 ± 18.17 and 16.67 ± 18.94 for both groups. Both groups experienced a statistically significant reduction in knee pain after surgery ($p < 0.001$). There was no statistically significant difference between groups in pre- and post-intervention knee pain measurement ($p = 0.619$) (Figure 1).

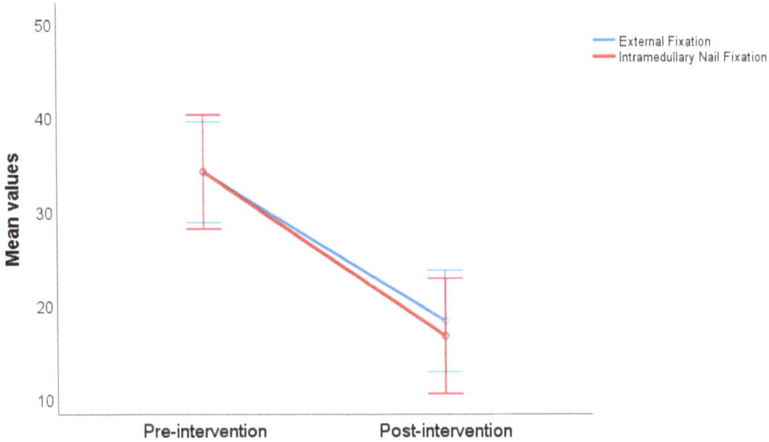

Figure 1. Non-ambulatory knee pain compared by pre- and post-treatment, stratified by intervention type.

The average reported non-ambulatory ankle pain before surgical intervention was 17.78 ± 19.53 in the group intended for external fixation (Ilizarov method) and 35.0 ± 18.90 in the group intended for intramedullary nail fixation. The average reported postsurgical non-ambulatory ankle pain was 8.22 ± 11.73 and 18.61 ± 17.91 for both groups. Both groups experienced a statistically significant reduction in ankle pain after surgery ($p < 0.001$). There was no statistically significant difference between groups pre- and post-intervention ankle pain measurement ($p = 0.056$) (Figure 2).

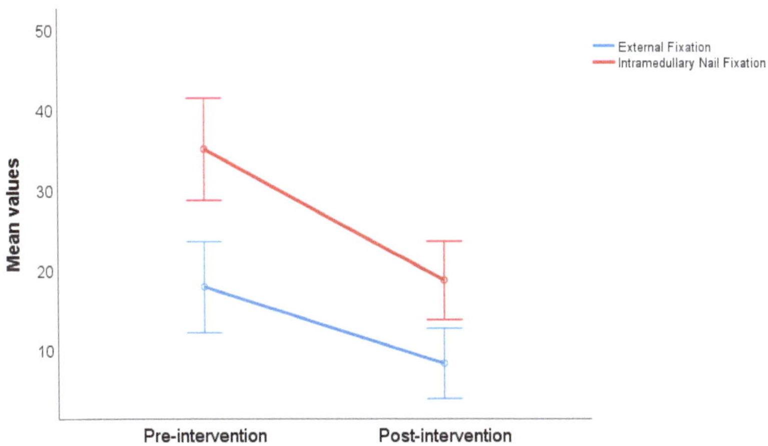

Figure 2. Non-ambulatory ankle pain compared by pre- and post-treatment, stratified by intervention type.

The average reported non-ambulatory pain at the fracture site before surgical intervention was 79.13 ± 10.92 in the group intended for external fixation (Ilizarov method) and 80.83 ± 9.06 in the group intended for intramedullary nail fixation. The average postsurgical non-ambulatory pain at the fracture site was 43.26 ± 20.88 and 13.47 ± 13.08 for both groups, respectively. Both groups experienced a statistically significant reduction in ankle pain after surgery ($p < 0.001$). Additionally, we found a statistically significant difference between pre- and post-intervention fracture site pain measurement ($p < 0.001$), with the group that underwent intramedullary nail fixation reporting significantly lower fracture site pain scores (Figure 3). There were no other significant predictors found for pain intensity after the surgical intervention in the logistic regression model ($p > 0.05$ for all assessed variables).

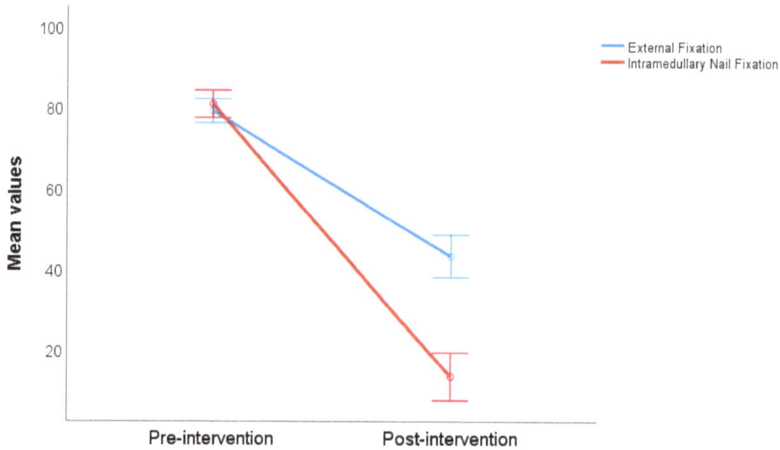

Figure 3. Non-ambulatory fracture site pain compared by pre- and post-treatment, stratified by intervention type.

We used univariant robust regression to assess variables, with time to recovery as the outcome. We found that intramedullary nail fixation was a significant predictor of recovery ($\beta = -1.08, p < 0.001$). Table 4 shows the β coefficients with their relevant *p*-values.

Table 4. Univariate robust regression model coefficients with recovery time treated as the outcome.

Variable	β Coefficient	*p*-Value
Sex (M/F)	0.016	0.955
Age (years)	0.014	0.063
Wait Time (min)	0.012	0.609
Intervention (nail vs. external)	−1.084	<0.001
Anesthesia		
Spinal (reference)		
Block	0.021	0.945
General	−0.095	0.792
Length of Surgery (min)	−0.001	0.889
Fracture Type		
42-A (reference)		
42-B	0.152	0.658
42-C	0.336	0.407
Mechanism of Injury		
Fall from a Flat Surface (reference)		
Fall from Height	0.650	0.297
Direct Trauma	−0.118	0.681
Motor Vehicle Accident	−0.019	0.961

We performed univariate screening for predictors of surgical complications with an exact logistic regression model. The statistically significant predictor of any surgical complication was the length of surgery ($\beta = 0.01, p = 0.015$). Table 5 shows the β coefficients with their relevant *p*-values.

Table 5. Univariate robust regression model coefficients with surgical complications as the outcome.

Variable	β Coefficient	p-Value	OR	95% Confidence Interval	
				Lower	Upper
Sex (M/F)	−0.466	0.532	0.63	0.11	2.57
Age (years)	0.023	0.273	1.02	0.98	1.07
Wait Time (min)	0.013	0.780	1.01	0.83	1.08
Intervention (nail vs. external)	0.257	0.710	1.29	0.32	5.23
Anesthesia					
Spinal (reference)					
Block	0.081	0.924	1.08	0.11	5.89
General	0.323		1.38	0.24	6.15
Length of Surgery (min)	0.011	0.015	1.011	1.002	1.021
Fracture Type					
42-A (reference)					
42-B	−0.821	0.204	0.44	0.003	4.16
42-C	1.180		3.26	0.70	13.47
Mechanism of Injury					
Fall from a Flat Surface (reference)					
Fall from Height	−0.073		0.93	0.007	9.86
Direct Trauma	1.450	0.330	4.26	0.87	19.49
Motor Vehicle Accident	0.164		1.18	0.11	6.81

4. Discussion

Our study aimed to assess outcomes in patients undergoing open and closed tibia fracture fixation, comparing the Ilizarov EF method and IMN in an early phase of IMN implementation in Serbia. We found no statistically significant difference in rates of postoperative complications between the two groups but noted longer hospitalization and recovery times in the Ilizarov group. Conversely, IMN patients experienced longer surgery durations and a higher frequency of antibiotic use. The study identified (EF) placement as a predictor for pain reduction at the fracture site and faster recovery, while longer surgery duration was associated with more frequent complications.

It remains uncertain whether surgical interventions, such as IMN or EF, result in better outcomes than conservative closed management with casting [15–18]. A meta-analysis of studies that compared cast treatment versus open reduction and internal fixation or intramedullary nailing of closed tibial shaft fractures found insufficient evidence to support the superiority of any approach [16]. Another review that pooled data from prospective studies of cast versus operative treatment in 895 fractures was also inconclusive [17]. Even if IMN is shown to be better than EF, there exists a lack of consensus regarding the best type of technique for IMN of the tibial shaft in adults [19]. A previous meta-analysis showed that IMN may be superior to other fixation strategies for open tibial shaft fractures. Using unreamed instead of reamed nails may be advantageous in setting open fractures. However, as with previous studies, confidence intervals around pooled malunion and infection risk estimates were extensive, and no recommendation could be given [20].

A recent updated meta-analysis pooling 16 randomized controlled trials found that IMN resulted in a lower rate of postoperative superficial infection and malunion rate but a higher hardware failure occurrence than EF. Additionally, the meta-analysis found no difference in union time, delayed union or nonunion rate, and postoperative deep infection rate between treatments [21]. Our study's findings agree with this meta-analysis regarding complication rate comparisons. It is still the case, though, that a small number of studies dominate effect sizes regarding certain quality-of-life and functional measures. Evidence synthesis in this field suffers from highly heterogeneous and uncertain data.

In our study, patients who underwent IMN fixation experienced a significantly longer surgery length and a higher frequency of antibiotic use. We identify the duration of surgery as a statistically significant predictor of postsurgical complications, with longer surgeries associated with higher complication rates. Though the effect of surgery length has not been directly compared for tibial shaft fractures, one study found that prolonged operative time increases the infection rate in tibial plateau fractures [22]. The method of fixation used does not seem to impact deep infection rates [23–25]. There is evidence that segmental tibial fractures might pose a greater deep infection risk with IMN than EF. However, these differences were minor (3% vs. 2.5%) [26]. Lower rates of superficial infection seem to favor IMN compared to EF [23,25]. Since surgery duration is related to case complexity and some studies indicate that surgical timing does not alter infection rates, other causes, such as expansive tissue injury due to more severe fractures, could be the unexplored etiology of this association [27]. Less antibiotic use found in our EF group might be attributed to hospital protocol recommendations for antibiotic use for all patients after the surgery at the start of this study. Intramedullary nailing was first introduced in Serbia in 2013 at the Institute for Orthopedic Surgery "Banjica", and the surgeons' lack of familiarity with a novel method might have resulted in prolonged surgical operations and a cautious approach that overestimated the necessity for antibiotics use. In contrast, surgeons were well experienced with the Ilizarov method, an external fixation technique that has been used in our country for the past 30 years. Thus, patients were given less antibiotics, but the study's hospitalization duration was significantly longer for patients treated with the Ilizarov external fixator than those treated with intramedullary nailing. This can be explained by the need for wound bandages around Ilizarov's external fixator, particularly around the pins. In addition, patients were hospitalized longer to facilitate rehabilitation and enable them to regain independent mobility via the assistance of physiotherapists. Due to this well-known concept of a learning curve influencing the outcomes of novel surgical techniques, in this study, we have presented the results of the first five years of IMN implementation in Serbia. This recognition of a measure of expertise might be beneficial to readers when assessing specific surgical techniques and their perioperative outcomes in other countries as well as for other surgical techniques. Some studies, such as the one conducted in Tanzania, showed that intramedullary fixation did not decrease treatment costs despite potentially shorter hospitalization periods [24]. In studies comparing IMN and EF in tibial fractures, recovery time is defined as the time to radiographic union [24,28], full weight-bearing [29], and unprotected weight-bearing. Recovery duration was significantly longer in Ilizarov patients in our study. However, there needs to be more consensus on the definition of recovery, which may have influenced different rates of recovery measurement, as some studies emphasize radiographic and others functional recovery [28]. It has been suggested that a composite measure, functional status combined with weight-bearing, could be used as an objective indicator of recovery. Some studies indicate that the type of fixation (IMN vs. EF) did not significantly differ in radiological healing outcomes after one year. In contrast, studies have reported differences in radiographic union scores and timing of visible fracture healing [24].

We continue to have low and uncertain data on functional outcomes and reoperations [16,19,21,25,30]. Our study observed that the IMN procedure predicted lower pain scores at the fracture site. The recent updated meta-analysis found that the composite pain score (from four RCTs) favored EF instead [10,21,28,29,31]. This apparent contrast appears to be only due to anterior knee pain, which had unexpectedly high rates after IMN procedures among patients in a subset of studies [23,29]. Therefore, intramedullary fixation could also be associated with higher rates of knee pain at one-year follow-up; all other pain measures were equal in both groups. One study showed that when functional outcomes were assessed, the differences usually disappeared by one year [24]. This equivalence in long-term outcomes emphasizes procedures that offer faster time to recovery, such as IMN, in our study. Another study observed that after one and a half years, there were no differences in knee motion, ankle motion, fracture site pain, or ankle pain [29]. It is still the case that functional outcomes, such as joint mobility, weight-bearing, rate of chronic pain, patient satisfaction, and quality of life, should be studied more rigorously [21].

Limitations

The limitations of this study are those familiar to single-center observational studies. It might not capture the variability seen in healthcare settings or populations, limiting external validity. The study relied on subjective measures, such as pain assessments, which can be influenced by individual patient perceptions. Variations in surgical techniques, anesthesia protocols, or postoperative care among health professionals and over the study period could introduce additional confounding. When interpreting the more frequent presence of general anesthesia in the IMN group, it should be noticed that the choice of anesthesia is, however, both anesthesiologist- and patient-dependent. In addition, as the choice of surgical technique in this study was surgeon-dependent, it should be noticed that possible selection bias might be present. However, although patients were not randomly assigned, groups were well balanced to the presence of open and closed fractures and other preoperative characteristics. As the study presents the results of early use of IMN in Serbia, the presence of a learning curve during the study period might have an effect on the duration of surgery and on the usage of antibiotics, particularly in more recent periods not presented in this study.

5. Conclusions

This study did not demonstrate a significant difference between postoperative complication rates and knee and ankle pain between intramedullary and external fixation. However, the two study groups differed in time to recovery, length of hospitalization, and pain intensity at the fracture site in favor of intramedullary fixation. Shorter surgery time and less antibiotic use were observed when external fixation was used. Additionally, we identified that intramedullary fixation was a significant predictor of pain intensity, and intramedullary fixation use predicted faster recovery. The length of surgery predicted the occurrence of any complication. Both methods should be compared more rigorously in multicentric randomized control trials.

Author Contributions: Conceptualization: D.J., N.G., Z.B., N.S., B.K., B.V., K.D., Z.J. and S.T.; methodology: D.J., N.G., Z.B., N.S., B.K., B.V., Z.J. and S.T.; software: D.J., N.G., K.D. and S.T.; validation: D.J., N.G., Z.B., N.S., B.K., B.V., K.D., Z.J. and S.T.; formal analysis: D.J., N.G. and S.T.; investigation: D.J., N.G., Z.B., N.S., B.K., B.V., K.D., Z.J. and S.T.; resources: D.J., N.G., Z.B., N.S., B.K., B.V., K.D., Z.J. and S.T.; data curation: D.J., Z.B., N.S., B.K., B.V., K.D., Z.J. and S.T.; writing—original draft preparation: D.J., N.G., Z.B., N.S., B.K., B.V., K.D., Z.J. and S.T.; writing—review and editing: D.J., N.G., Z.B., N.S., B.K., B.V., K.D., Z.J. and S.T.; visualization: D.J., N.G., K.D. and S.T.; supervision: D.J., Z.B., N.S., and S.T; project administration: D.J., Z.B. and S.T.; funding acquisition: D.J., Z.B., N.S. and S.T. All authors have read and agreed to the published version of the manuscript.

Funding: This research received no external funding.

Institutional Review Board Statement: The study was conducted in accordance with the Declaration of Helsinki and approved by the Institute for Orthopeadics "Banjica" (num: 16/2017) and Belgrade University Faculty of Medicine (Num: 2650/IV-16. date: 10 April 2018).

Informed Consent Statement: Informed consent was obtained from all subjects involved in the study.

Data Availability Statement: The data that support the findings of this study are available on request from the corresponding author.

Conflicts of Interest: The authors declare no conflicts of interest.

References

1. Metsemakers, W.-J.; Kortram, K.; Ferreira, N.; Morgenstern, M.; Joeris, A.; Pape, H.-C.; Kammerlander, C.; Konda, S.; Oh, J.-K.; Giannoudis, P.V.; et al. Fracture-Related Outcome Study for Operatively Treated Tibia Shaft Fractures (F.R.O.S.T.): Registry Rationale and Design. *BMC Musculoskelet. Disord.* **2021**, *22*, 57. [CrossRef] [PubMed]
2. Bode, G.; Strohm, P.C.; Südkamp, N.P.; Hammer, T.O. Tibial Shaft Fractures—Management and Treatment Options. A Review of the Current Literature. *Acta Chir. Orthop. Traumatol. Cech.* **2012**, *79*, 499–505. [CrossRef] [PubMed]

3. Grütter, R.; Cordey, J.; Bühler, M.; Johner, R.; Regazzoni, P. The Epidemiology of Diaphyseal Fractures of the Tibia. *Injury* **2000**, 3 (Suppl. S3), C64–C67. [CrossRef] [PubMed]
4. Sarmiento, A.; Gersten, L.M.; Sobol, P.A.; Shankwiler, J.A.; Vangsness, C.T. Tibial Shaft Fractures Treated with Functional Brace Experience with 780 Fractures. *J. Bone Jt. Surg. Br.* **1989**, *71*, 602–609. [CrossRef] [PubMed]
5. Mayr, E. Unterschenkelfrakturen. *Chirurg* **2002**, *73*, 642–663. [CrossRef] [PubMed]
6. Court-Brown, C.M.; Caesar, B. Epidemiology of Adult Fractures: A Review. *Injury* **2006**, *37*, 691–697. [CrossRef] [PubMed]
7. Bhandari, M.; Guyatt, G.H.; Tong, D.; Adili, A.; Shaughnessy, S.G. Reamed versus Nonreamed Intramedullary Nailing of Lowe Extremity Long Bone Fractures: A Systematic Overview and Meta-Analysis. *J. Orthop. Trauma* **2000**, *14*, 2–9. [CrossRef] [PubMed
8. Bhandari, M.; Guyatt, G.H.; Swiontkowski, M.F.; Schemitsch, E.H. Treatment of Open Fractures of the Shaft of the Tibia. *J. Bone J Surg. Br.* **2001**, *83*, 62–68. [CrossRef]
9. Jeremić, D.; Vitošević, F.; Glusčević, B.; Slavković, N.; Apostolović, M.; Lalošević, M.; Čolić, N.; Davidović, K. Single Cente Experience in Treatment of Tibial Shaft Fractures Using Ilizarov Technique. *Srp. Arh. Za Celok. Lek.* **2020**, *148*, 167–172. [CrossRef
10. Ramos, T.; Eriksson, B.I.; Karlsson, J.; Nistor, L. Ilizarov External Fixation or Locked Intramedullary Nailing in Diaphysea Tibial Fractures: A Randomized, Prospective Study of 58 Consecutive Patients. *Arch. Orthop. Trauma Surg.* **2014**, *134*, 793–802 [CrossRef]
11. Foster, P.a.L.; Barton, S.B.; Jones, S.C.E.; Morrison, R.J.M.; Britten, S. The Treatment of Complex Tibial Shaft Fractures by the Ilizarov Method. *J. Bone Jt. Surg. Br.* **2012**, *94*, 1678–1683. [CrossRef] [PubMed]
12. Reddy, R.S.; Kumar, C.Y.; Shah, H.M.; Golla, D.K.; Ganesh, D.J.N.; Kumar, P.A. Evaluation of Tibial Condyle Fractures Treated with Ilizarov Fixation, a Prospective Study. *J. Clin. Diagn. Res.* **2014**, *8*, LC05–LC07. [CrossRef]
13. Patzakis, M.J.; Wilkins, J.; Moore, T.M. Considerations in Reducing the Infection Rate in Open Tibial Fractures. *Clin. Orthop. Relat Res.* **1983**, *178*, 36–41. [CrossRef]
14. Downie, W.W.; Leatham, P.A.; Rhind, V.W.; Wright, V.; Branco, J.A.; Anderson, J.A. Studies with pain rating scales. *Ann. Rheum Dis.* **1978**, *37*, 378–381. [CrossRef] [PubMed]
15. Obremskey, W.T.; Cutrera, N.; Kidd, C.M. Southeastern Fracture Consortium A Prospective Multi-Center Study of Intramedullary Nailing vs Casting of Stable Tibial Shaft Fractures. *J. Orthop. Traumatol.* **2017**, *18*, 69–76. [CrossRef] [PubMed]
16. Littenberg, B.; Weinstein, L.P.; McCarren, M.; Mead, T.; Swiontkowski, M.F.; Rudicel, S.A.; Heck, D. Closed Fractures of the Tibial Shaft. A Meta-Analysis of Three Methods of Treatment. *J. Bone Jt. Surg. Am.* **1998**, *80*, 174–183. [CrossRef] [PubMed]
17. Coles, C.P.; Gross, M. Closed Tibial Shaft Fractures: Management and Treatment Complications. A Review of the Prospective Literature. *Can. J. Surg.* **2000**, *43*, 256–262. [PubMed]
18. Toivanen, J.A.; Honkonen, S.E.; Koivisto, A.M.; Järvinen, M.J. Treatment of Low-Energy Tibial Shaft Fractures: Plaster Cast Compared with Intramedullary Nailing. *Int. Orthop.* **2001**, *25*, 110–113. [CrossRef]
19. Duan, X.; Al-Qwbani, M.; Zeng, Y.; Zhang, W.; Xiang, Z. Intramedullary Nailing for Tibial Shaft Fractures in Adults. *Cochrane Database Syst. Rev.* **2012**, *1*, CD008241. [CrossRef] [PubMed]
20. Foote, C.J.; Guyatt, G.H.; Vignesh, N.K.; Mundi, R.; Chaudhry, H.; Heels-Ansdell, D.; Thabane, L.; Tornetta, P.I.; Bhandari, M Which Surgical Treatment for Open Tibial Shaft Fractures Results in the Fewest Reoperations? A Network Meta-Analysis. *Clin. Orthop. Relat. Res.* **2015**, *473*, 2179. [CrossRef] [PubMed]
21. Jeremić, D.; Rajovic, N.; Gluscevic, B.; Krivokapic, B.; Rajkovic, S.; Bogosavljevic, N.; Davidovic, K.; Tomic, S. Updated Meta-Analysis of Randomized Controlled Trials Comparing External Fixation to Intramedullary Nailing in the Treatment of Open Tibial Fractures. *Medicina* **2023**, *59*, 1301. [CrossRef] [PubMed]
22. Colman, M.; Wright, A.; Gruen, G.; Siska, P.; Pape, H.-C.; Tarkin, I. Prolonged Operative Time Increases Infection Rate in Tibial Plateau Fractures. *Injury* **2013**, *44*, 249–252. [CrossRef] [PubMed]
23. Zhuang, C.; Bin, Y. Unreamed Intramedullary Nailing Versus External Fixation for Type IIIA and IIIB Open Fractures of Tibial Shaft: A Subgroup Analysis of Randomized Trials. *J. Nov. Physiother.* **2013**, *3*, 144. [CrossRef]
24. Haonga, B.T.; Liu, M.; Albright, P.; Challa, S.T.; Ali, S.H.; Lazar, A.A.; Eliezer, E.N.; Shearer, D.W.; Morshed, S. Intramedullary Nailing Versus External Fixation in the Treatment of Open Tibial Fractures in Tanzania: Results of a Randomized Clinical Trial. *J. Bone Jt. Surg. Am.* **2020**, *102*, 896–905. [CrossRef] [PubMed]
25. Fu, Q.; Zhu, L.; Lu, J.; Ma, J.; Chen, A. External Fixation versus Unreamed Tibial Intramedullary Nailing for Open Tibial Fractures: A Meta-Analysis of Randomized Controlled Trials. *Sci. Rep.* **2018**, *8*, 12753. [CrossRef] [PubMed]
26. McMahon, S.E.; Little, Z.E.; Smith, T.O.; Trompeter, A.; Hing, C.B. The Management of Segmental Tibial Shaft Fractures: A Systematic Review. *Injury* **2016**, *47*, 568–573. [CrossRef] [PubMed]
27. Duyos, O.A.; Beaton-Comulada, D.; Davila-Parrilla, A.; Perez-Lopez, J.C.; Ortiz, K.; Foy-Parrilla, C.; Lopez-Gonzalez, F. Management of Open Tibial Shaft Fractures: Does the Timing of Surgery Affect Outcomes? *J. Am. Acad. Orthop. Surg.* **2017**, *25*, 230–238. [CrossRef] [PubMed]
28. Rohilla, R.; Arora, S.; Kundu, A.; Singh, R.; Govil, V.; Khokhar, A. Functional and Radiological Outcomes of Primary Ring Fixator versus Antibiotic Nail in Open Tibial Diaphyseal Fractures: A Prospective Study. *Injury* **2022**, *53*, 3464–3470. [CrossRef] [PubMed]
29. Bråten, M.; Helland, P.; Grøntvedt, T.; Aamodt, A.; Benum, P.; Mølster, A. External Fixation versus Locked Intramedullary Nailing in Tibial Shaft Fractures: A Prospective, Randomised Study of 78 Patients. *Arch. Orthop. Trauma Surg.* **2005**, *125*, 21–26. [CrossRef] [PubMed]

30. Alsharef, J.F.; Ghaddaf, A.A.; AlQuhaibi, M.S.; Shaheen, E.A.; AboAljadiel, L.H.; Alharbi, A.S.; AlHidri, B.Y.; Alamri, M.K.; Makhdom, A.M. External Fixation versus Intramedullary Nailing for the Management of Open Tibial Fracture: Meta-Analysis of Randomized Controlled Trials. *Int. Orthop.* **2023**, *47*, 3077–3097. [CrossRef] [PubMed]
31. Holbrook, J.L.; Swiontkowski, M.F.; Sanders, R. Treatment of Open Fractures of the Tibial Shaft: Ender Nailing versus External Fixation. A Randomized, Prospective Comparison. *J. Bone Jt. Surg. Am.* **1989**, *71*, 1231–1238. [CrossRef]

Journal of
Clinical Medicine

MDPI

Article

Periprosthetic Hip Fractures around the Stem: Can the Stem Design Affect Fracture Features?

Luca Costanzo Comba [1,*,†], Luca Gagliardi [2,†], Francesco Onorato [2] and Fabrizio Rivera [1]

1 Orthopedics and Trauma Department, SS Annunziata Hospital, ASL CN1, 12038 Savigliano, Italy
2 Orthopedics and Trauma Department, Univertità degli Studi di Torino, 10100 Turin, Italy
* Correspondence: lucacostanzo.comba@aslcn1.it
† These authors contributed equally to this work.

Abstract: Background: Total hip arthroplasty is one of the most successful orthopedic surgeries; nevertheless, many of these surgeries are the causes of failure, and among them, periprosthetic fractures are one of the major causes of revision. Our study focuses on periprosthetic hip fractures with two different stem designs. The aim of the study was to analyze the obtained results, focusing on the features of periprosthetic stem fractures observed. **Methods:** We retrospectively reviewed periprosthetic fractures occurring between 2010 and 2023, involving Alloclassic® or CLS® uncemented femoral stems. We analyzed demographic data, proximal femur morphology, and the fracture type. **Results:** We identified 97 patients. Considering the proximal femur morphology, we found that there was statistically significant prevalence of Dorr A proximal femur morphology in the CLS® group and of Dorr C in the Alloclassic® group. Considering the distribution of the fracture pattern, we reported a non-statistically significant prevalence of the fracture pattern with stable stems in the CLS® group. **Conclusions:** The choice of the prosthetic design of the femoral stem is a crucial element when planning total hip arthroplasty. However, we found a non-statistically significant difference between the two stems considered, raising questions about the real role of stem design as a primary determinant of periprosthetic hip fractures.

Keywords: cementless; periprosthetic femur fracture; stem design; total hip arthroplasty

1. Introduction

The ever-evolving field of orthopedics has experienced significant advancements in total hip arthroplasty (THA), including better materials, new prosthetic designs, and minimally invasive approaches. This development has allowed an improvement in functionality and quality of life for countless individuals [1]. The constantly growing number of implants suggests a potential increase in revision interventions in the future [2]. Periprosthetic femoral fractures (PFFs) remain one of the major causes of revision surgeries, with considerable implications for patients' functional outcomes, morbidity, and mortality [3]. Moreover, they contribute to increased healthcare costs due to prolonged hospital stays, extended rehabilitation periods, and high rates of hospital readmission [4].

Although the literature has already suggested several patient risk factors, including age, gender, and the presence of osteoporosis and rheumatoid arthritis, the contribution of implant design on PFF risk is less clear [5]. Recent studies have suggested that cemented femoral stem fixation could reduce the risk of intra-operative and post-operative PFFs following THA for femoral neck fractures (FNFs), as well as after elective THA [6–8].

A cemented femoral stem leads to a modification of the load transfer in the case of both taper slip and composite beam designs [6,7]. Notwithstanding, cementless fixation remains widely performed, such as in the United States, possibly due to shorter surgery times, concerns about potential embolization risks, and the challenges associated with revision surgeries. Despite the decades of research focused on optimizing load transfer at the prosthesis–bone interface, stress shielding is still considered one of the important factors in the long-term survival of femoral stem components. For this reason, the use of patient-specific stem designs considering individual characteristics to provide optimal implant solutions is rapidly increasing [9]. Nowadays, a wide range of stem designs is currently available on the market, allowing surgeons to optimize the stem choice based on patient femur characteristics [10]. Nevertheless, there is still an ongoing debate regarding the various factors influencing the incidence and type of fractures around the stem [11].

Even though numerous classifications have been proposed, the historical Vancouver classification [12] remains widely used and reliable, primarily due to its simplicity in guiding treatment decisions and reproducibility. Moreover, understanding the intricate interplay between patient factors, surgical variables, and implant characteristics necessitates thorough investigation and careful consideration to reduce the impact of periprosthetic hip fractures. Surprisingly few reports in the literature reported the clinical PFF rates among different cementless stem designs.

In our study, we retrospectively analyzed the observed PFFs at a single institution, comparing the two different stem designs implanted with a cementless fixation technique. Given the wide array of stem designs available, the endpoint of our investigation sought to determine whether specific stem designs may be correlated with a specific fracture pattern.

2. Material and Methods

We retrospectively reviewed the periprosthetic fractures of the proximal femur which occurred in the period between 2010 and 2023 and were surgically treated at SS Annunziata Hospital, Savigliano, Italy. Among them, we focused on periprosthetic fractures involving CLS® or Alloclassic® Zimmer (Woso, IN, USA) uncemented femoral stems. Patients were therefore divided into two distinct groups: Group A, comprising individuals with PFFs who previously underwent uncemented primary hip replacement with the Zweymuller Alloclassic® stems (Zimmer), and Group B, consisting of patients with PFFs on a Spotorno CLS® stem (Zimmer) [Figures 1 and 2].

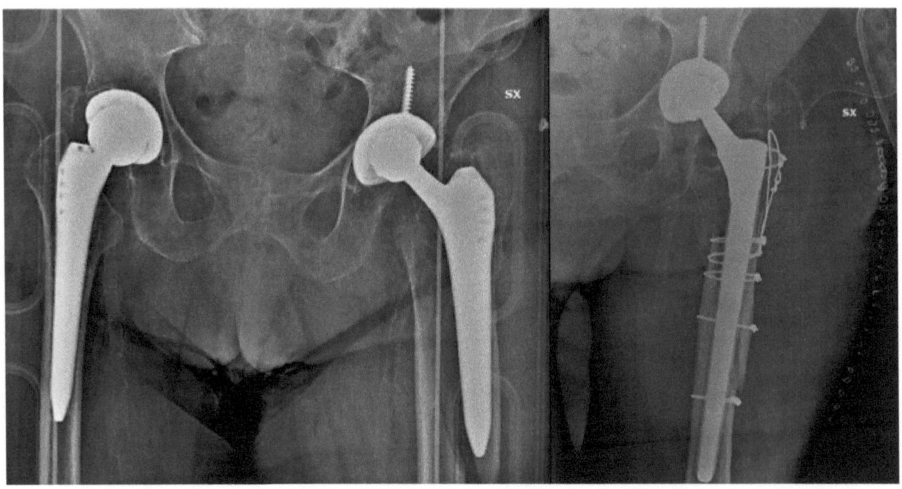

Figure 1. Periprosthetic fracture with unstable stem (Alloclassic), which underwent revision surgery.

We only considered PFFs following primary THAs originally implanted for hip osteoarthritis (OA). Only post-operative fractures occurring at least one month after the surgery were included, therefore excluding all intra-operative and early post-operative fractures within the first month after surgery (to minimize the risk of including intra-operative fractures not seen during surgery). Additionally, we excluded THAs on previous failed osteosynthesis and pathological fractures. We only selected patients who underwent a complete preoperative radiological study, including an antero-posterior (AP) and axial X-ray of the pelvis and hip as standardized in our institution; for the most complex cases where stem loosening was uncertain, a preoperative CT study was also performed.

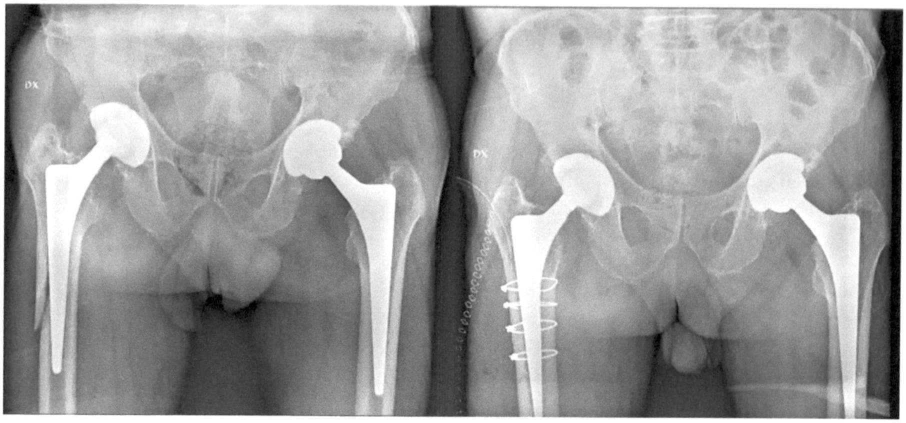

Figure 2. Periprosthetic fracture with stable stem (CLS), which underwent osteosynthesis surgery.

Cases were analyzed according to demographic data (gender and age), proximal femur morphology through the Dorr classification (due to the interobserver and intraobserver reliability) [13,14], and fracture type conforming to Vancouver classification (because of the reproducibility and the simple clinical application) [12]. In this regard, a re-evaluation of implant stability and osteointegration was always performed intraoperatively for definitive diagnosis before proceeding with the appropriate treatment, so that an eventual change in the initial assessment could then be reported in the surgical report and correctly retrieved by the authors.

Demographic data among the two groups, as well as proximal femur morphology and the fracture pattern distribution, were compared. Statistical analysis was performed using the Fisher's test to compare nominal variables. p values of <0.05 were considered to be significant.

3. Results

We identified 97 patients with periprosthetic fractures of the proximal femur in the examined period. Among them, 37 (38%) were male and 60 (62%) were female, with a mean age of 81 (range 51–96) years. In Group A, we reported 55 patients, of which 13 (24%) were male and 42 (76%) were female, with a mean age of 81 years (range 51–96). In Group B, we reported 42 patients, of which 24 (57%) were male and 18 (43%) were female, with a mean age of 81 years (range 65–96). No difference was found regarding the average age of patients; however, we reported a statistically significant prevalence of women in Group A ($p = 0.0014$), as depicted in Table 1.

Table 1. Patients' demographics.

Patients, n	Alloclassic (A)	CLS (B)	p Value
Patients, n	55	42	
Sex (male/female), n	13/42	24/18	$p = 0.0014$
Mean age	81 (51–96)	81 (65–96)	$p > 0.05$

Considering the distribution of proximal femur morphology with Dorr classification, we found 4 cases of Dorr A, 35 cases of Dorr B, and 16 cases of Dorr C in Group A;

conversely, we found 18 cases of Dorr A, 21 cases of Dorr B, and 3 cases of Dorr C in Group B [Table 2]. Comparing these results, we found that there was a statistically significant prevalence of the Dorr A proximal femur morphology in Group B ($p = 0.000095$) and a statistically significant prevalence of the Dorr C proximal femur morphology in Group A ($p = 0.009$).

Table 2. Proximal femur morphology (Dorr classification).

	Alloclassic (A)	CLS (B)	*p* Value
Dorr A	4	18	$p = 0.000095$
Dorr B	35	21	$p > 0.05$
Dorr C	16	3	$p = 0.009$

Considering the distribution of fracture patterns with Vancouver classification, we found 6 cases of type A fractures, 19 cases of B1, 17 cases of B2, 9 of B3, and 4 type C fractures in Group A. Conversely, we found 4 cases of type A fractures, 21 of B1, 12 of B2, 5 of B3, and no cases of type C PFFs in Group B, as reported in Table 3. It could be inferred that the femoral stem was assessed as stable in 54 cases (56%) and unstable in 43 cases (44%). Fracture patterns with stable stems had a higher incidence in Group B (60% vs. 53%); thus, the unstable pattern was more common in Group A. However, this difference was evaluated as not statistically significant ($p = 0.5415$).

Table 3. Fracture pattern (Vancouver classification). Green cells: stable stem. Red cells: unstable stem.

Vancouver	Alloclassic (A)	CLS (B)	*p* Value
A	6	4	$p > 0.05$
B1	19	21	$p > 0.05$
B2	17	12	$p > 0.05$
B3	9	5	$p > 0.05$
C	4	0	$p > 0.05$

4. Discussion

The main finding of the present study was a significant incidence of PFFs in Dorr A femoral phenotypes which underwent THA with the Spotorno CLS® (Zimmer) femoral stem. In contrast, patients with a Dorr C femoral bone were subjected to PFFs in a statistically higher proportion when implanted with the Zweymuller Alloclassic® stems (Zimmer). However, no significant difference in a specific fracture pattern occurrence or stem loosening was observed between the two stems.

The great success of THA and the large number of patients undergoing this procedure over the years clearly highlight the importance of managing complications as a priority. Among these complications, PFFs play an important role, and even more so within an audience of increasingly elderly patients [15]. In fact, periprosthetic fracture represents the fourth cause of failure of a THA, after aseptic loosening, hip dislocation, and the wear of materials [16].

The selection of the femoral stem design in hip arthroplasty represents a crucial decision involving considerations such as the material, geometry, fixation method, and modularity. No prosthetic stem can perfectly replicate the physiological load transmission; each stem is associated with a specific load pattern and consequently with a specific periprosthetic bone remodeling. In 2018, Rivière and colleagues [17] analyzed long-term bone remodeling in five widely used types of femoral stems, including those evaluated in our study. They observed a meta-diaphyseal grip in the Alloclassic stem, with proximal cortex atrophy as a primary sign of stress shielding, typically appearing approximately two years post-implantation, but stabilizing at around five years.

Conversely, the CLS stem's triple taper tended to achieve both metaphyseal and metaphyseal-diaphyseal grip, generating compressive forces with proximal load transfer, thereby partially mitigating bone remodeling secondary to stress shielding, especially in proximal femurs with a Dorr A type morphology. Conversely, in cases of Dorr C type morphology, the presence of signs of stress shielding indicated osteointegration at the inter-subtrochanteric level.

While the role of cementation in preventing PFFs (defined by the interplay of implant load and stiffness on one side, and bone or compound material resistance with bone cement on the other) seems clear in the literature, with stem fixation considered one of the most important revision risk factors in older patients [18,19], for younger patients preserving optimal bone stock, the influence of prosthetic stem design on the type of PFFs is less defined [5].

In the present study, the Zweymuller stem was implanted more often in Dorr type C "stovepipe" femoral shafts with a relative greater risk of PFF. This finding could be interpreted in two different ways. The underlying femoral osteopenia typical of Dorr type C, also confirmed by Dorr's original histological studies, could demand the use of a cemented stem, irrespective of the patient's age. On the other hand, the findings might be a selective bias related to surgeon stem choice at the time of surgery, where achieving a solid diaphyseal fixation in type C proximal femur diaphyseal-engaging stems was the preferred choice.

However, recent studies of modern femoral stem designs have demonstrated durable fixation with the use of cementless fixation in Dorr type C bone, although this was only performed by highly experienced surgeons [20,21]. A recent study by Jeong, Sang-Jin, et al. [22] found that a taper rectangular stem (i.e., an Alloclassic stem) was associated with a higher incidence of PFFs and femoral stem revision compared to flat taper and quadrangular taper stems. We know that in a non-cemented implant, femoral stems with different designs lead to different load transmission at the level of the prosthesis–bone interface, favoring phenomena such as stress shielding and bone resorption. Whenever an accidental fall occurs, this different stress distribution may thus influence a different location of the fractures [23]. This phenomenon has also been studied in cemented implants. In 2020, Windell and colleagues [24] compared three different polish tapered cemented stems by recreating periprosthetic fractures in sawbone models and observing their biomechanics, location and the energy needed to reach the breaking point.

Within our cohort, we reported a significantly higher prevalence of women with PFFs in Group A compared to Group B; this finding is consistent with several studies in the literature reporting a higher risk of PFFs in females. Konow, Tobias, et al. identified several PFF risk factors by analyzing over 200,000 cases from the German Arthroplasty Registry, including elderly patients, females, and uncemented and collarless stem designs [25]. Similarly, in 2021, Sershon and colleagues [26] attributed greater influence to the stem design in determining the risk of PFFs within three months post-surgery compared to other factors, such as the surgical approach choice, and reported a 2.6-fold and a 2.3-fold increased risk of PFFs with collarless or single-wedged stems compared to collared or fit-and-fill stems, respectively.

In a 2019 study [27], the incidence and pattern of periprosthetic fractures were analyzed based on anatomical or straight stem designs, and the authors reported a higher overall incidence of periprosthetic fractures with anatomical stems, which was also associated with a higher incidence of Clamshell-type fractures compared to Vancouver type B fractures. Matthias Luger et al. investigated the rate of PFFs within the first year post-surgery between cementless short and straight stem THA, concluding that short stem THA reduces Vancouver type A PFFs in the trochanteric region compared to straight stem THA, while Vancouver type B fractures are comparable [28].

In our study, we found that in cases of a periprosthetic hip fracture in the presence of an Alloclassic stem, there is a relative greater percentage of stem loosening compared to that found in the presence of a CLS stem; however, this difference was not statistically significant.

Although the choice of stem during the initial implantation seems to be influenced by achieving metaphyseal filling for an optimal press-fit, and therefore by the Dorr index, with a statistically significant prevalence of Dorr type C femurs in the Alloclassic group compared to a prevalence of type A in the CLS group, the larger dimensions of the metaphyseal portion of the Alloclassic stem could partly influence fracture biomechanics and bone integration loss. Considering the need for different surgical treatment in cases of prosthetic stem instability in a periprosthetic fracture (i.e., stem revision and reimplantation in the case of B2 and B3 Vancouver fractures), with the associated impact on patient outcomes, if this trend is confirmed with greater statistical power, it will introduce another factor to consider when choosing the initial implant prosthetic stem. This will be particularly important in Dorr B-type femoral canals, where both prosthetic models can ensure an adequate press-fit.

We encourage the use of preoperative templating to ensure a stem choice which fits the geometry of a patient's femoral canal to decrease the risk of iatrogenic fractures in patients who undergo THA. Lastly, we must consider the elderly age of this patient population and their associated comorbidities, which in some cases may have led the surgeon to opt for synthesis even if revision would have been indicated, in order to limit surgical time and associated intra- and post-operative complications [29].

Our study has several limitations. Firstly, the retrospective design and limited sample size. Moreover, the heterogeneity of the two groups in terms of the female ratio represents another confounding factor; we observed a greater presence of females in Group A, which was statistically significant, and therefore we cannot exclude that this may have influenced our results. Additionally, the exclusion of fractures occurring intraoperatively or within the first month post-surgery to minimize the risk of including intraoperative fractures not observed during surgery might bias the study. Despite the clear literature evidence regarding modifiable and unmodifiable PFFs risk factors that may already guide surgeon preferences [30–32], further studies are necessary to build evidence capable of deeply influencing our clinical practice.

5. Conclusions

Periprosthetic hip fractures represent a challenging complication in the realm of orthopedic surgery, particularly around the femoral stem, prompting a critical examination of the potential influence of stem design on fracture features. When approaching a first implant, the choice of prosthetic design of the femoral stem must be carefully taken into consideration to achieve a good press-fit in relation to the morphology of the proximal femur. In our study, the Alloclassic stem reported a relatively higher incidence of stem instability in cases of periprosthetic fracture compared to that detected for the CLS stem, although with a non-statistically significant difference. On the other hand, the lack of a significant difference in fracture patterns between the Alloclassic and CLS stems raises questions about the real role of stem design as a primary determinant of periprosthetic hip fractures. While the biomechanical characteristics of these stems differ, it appears that other factors, such as patient demographics, bone quality, and surgical technique may exert a more substantial influence on fracture outcomes. These findings highlight the need for a more comprehensive understanding of the multiple factors contributing to periprosthetic fractures, and call for further research to refine risk stratification and improve patient outcomes in hip arthroplasty.

Author Contributions: Conceptualization, L.C.C., L.G. and F.R.; methodology, L.C.C. and L.G.; data curation, F.O. and F.R.; writing—original draft, L.C.C. and L.G.; writing—review and editing, F.O. and F.R.; supervision, F.R. All authors have read and agreed to the published version of the manuscript.

Funding: This research received no external funding.

Institutional Review Board Statement: The study was conducted according to the guidelines of the Declaration of Helsinki. Considering the retrospective nature of the study, we assert that ethical approval is not necessary, as we solely analyzed pre-existing and anonymous data.

Informed Consent Statement: Informed consent was obtained from the subjects involved in the study.

Data Availability Statement: For full disclosure, a paper copy is available at SS Annunziata Hospital, Savigliano, Italy.

Conflicts of Interest: The authors declare no conflict of interest.

References

1. Learmonth, I.D.; Young, C.; Rorabeck, C. The operation of the century: Total hip replacement. *Lancet* **2007**, *370*, 1508–1519. [CrossRef]
2. Kurtz, S.; Ong, K.; Lau, E.; Mowat, F.; Halpern, M. Projections of primary and revision hip and knee arthroplasty in the United States from 2005 to 2030. *J. Bone Joint Surg. Am.* **2007**, *89-A*, 780–785.
3. Deng, Y.; Kieser, D.; Wyatt, M.; Stringer, M.; Frampton, C.; Hooper, G. Risk factors for periprosthetic femoral fractures around total hip arthroplasty: A systematic review and meta-analysis. *ANZ J. Surg.* **2020**, *90*, 441–447. [CrossRef]
4. Patsiogiannis, N.; Kanakaris, N.K.; Giannoudis, P.V. Periprosthetic hip fractures: An update into their management and clinical outcomes. *EFORT Open Rev.* **2021**, *6*, 75–92. [CrossRef]
5. Carli, A.V.; Negus, J.J.; Haddad, F.S. Periprosthetic femoral fractures and trying to avoid them. *Bone Jt. J.* **2017**, *99-B*, 50–59. [CrossRef]
6. Edelstein, A.I.; Hume, E.L.; Pezzin, L.E.; McGinley, E.L.; Dillingham, T.R. The impact of femoral component cementation on fracture and mortality risk in elective total hip arthroplasty: Analysis from a national Medicare sample. *J. Bone Jt. Surg. Am.* **2022**, *104*, 523–529. [CrossRef]
7. Kelly, M.P.; Chan, P.H.; Prentice, H.A.; Paxton, E.W.; Hinman, A.D.; Khatod, M. Cause-specific stem revision risk in primary total hip arthroplasty using cemented vs cementless femoral stem fixation in a US cohort. *J. Arthroplast.* **2022**, *37*, 89–96.e1. [CrossRef]
8. Song, J.S.A.; Dillman, D.; Wilson, D.; Dunbar, M.; Richardson, G. Higher periprosthetic fracture rate associated with use of modern uncemented stems compared to cemented stems in femoral neck fractures. *Hip Int.* **2019**, *29*, 177–183. [CrossRef] [PubMed]
9. Savio, D.; Bagno, A. When the Total Hip Replacement Fails: A Review on the Stress-Shielding Effect. *Processes* **2022**, *10*, 612. [CrossRef]
10. Noble, P.C.; Alexander, J.W.; Lindahl, L.J.; Yew, D.T.; Granberry, W.M.; Tullos, H.S. The anatomic basis of femoral component design. *Clin. Orthop. Relat. Res.* **1988**, *235*, 148–165. [CrossRef]
11. Weissinger, M.; Helmreich, C.; Pöll, G. Periprosthetic fractures of the hip. *Acta Chir. Orthop. Traumatol. Cech.* **2009**, *76*, 179–185. [CrossRef]
12. Duncan, C.P.; Masri, B.A. Fractures of the femur after hip replacement. *Instr. Course Lect.* **1995**, *44*, 293–304. [PubMed]
13. Dorr, L.D.; Faugere, M.C.; Mackel, A.M.; Gruen, T.A.; Bognar, B.; Malluche, H.H. Structural and cellular assessment of bone quality of proximal femur. *Bone* **1993**, *14*, 231–242. [CrossRef] [PubMed]
14. Wilkerson, J.; Fernando, N.D. Classifications in Brief: The Dorr Classification of Femoral Bone. *Clin. Orthop. Relat. Res.* **2020**, *478*, 1939–1944. [CrossRef] [PubMed]
15. Karachalios, T.S.; Koutalos, A.A.; Komnos, G.A. Total hip arthroplasty in patients with osteoporosis. *Hip Int.* **2020**, *30*, 370–379. [CrossRef] [PubMed]
16. Torre, M.; Leone, L.; Carrani, E.; Di Benedetto, C.; Manno, V.; Luzi, I.; Masciocchi, M. *Progetto Registro Italiano ArtroProtesi (RIAP): Risultati della Fase Pilota sugli Interventi di Protesi D'anca*; Rapporti ISTISAN; Istituto Superiore di Sanità: Rome, Italy, 2012; 12/32. Available online: https://www.yumpu.com/it/document/view/27991936/progetto-riap-risultati-della-fase-pilota-sugli-interventi-oer-puglia (accessed on 5 March 2024).
17. Rivière, C.; Grappiolo, G.; Engh, C.A., Jr.; Vidalain, J.P.; Chen, A.F.; Boehler, N.; Matta, J.; Vendittoli, P.A. Long-term bone remodelling around 'legendary' cementless femoral stems. *EFORT Open Rev.* **2018**, *3*, 45–57. [CrossRef] [PubMed]
18. Fernandez, M.A.; Achten, J.; Parsons, N.; Griffin, X.L.; Png, M.E.; Gould, J.; McGibbon, A.; Costa, M.L. Cemented or Uncemented Hemiarthroplasty for Intracapsular Hip Fracture. *N. Engl. J. Med.* **2022**, *386*, 521–530. [CrossRef] [PubMed]
19. Draenert, K.D.; Draenert, Y.I.; Krauspe, R.; Bettin, D. Strain adaptive bone remodelling in total joint replacement. *Clin. Orthop. Relat. Res.* **2005**, *430*, 12–27. [CrossRef] [PubMed]
20. Hatem, M.A.; Ferreira da Luz, B.; Nishi, R.N.; Cimbalista de Alencar, P.G. Evaluation of the results from proximal fixation of uncemented conical femoral components in Dorr type C femurs. *Rev. Bras. Ortop.* **2014**, *49*, 260–266.
21. Meding, J.B.; Galley, M.R.; Ritter, M.A. High survival of uncemented proximally porous-coated titanium alloy femoral stems in osteoporotic bone. *Clin. Orthop. Relat. Res.* **2010**, *468*, 441–447. [CrossRef]
22. Jeong, S.-J.; Park, C.-W.; Cho, K.; Jeong, J.; Lim, S.-J.; Park, Y.-S. Rectangular Taper Stem Designs Are Associated with a Higher Risk for Periprosthstic Femoral Fractures after Cementless Total Hip Arthroplasty. *J. Arthroplast.* **2023**, *38*, 2379–2385. [CrossRef]
23. Franceschini, M.; Barbera, L.; Anticonome, A.; Ottardi, C.; Tanaka, A.; Villa, T. Periprosthetic femoral fractures in sideways fall configuration: Comparative numerical analysis of the influence of femoral stem design. *Hip Int.* **2020**, *30*, 86–93. [CrossRef] [PubMed]
24. Windell, L.; Kulkarni, A.; Alabort, E.; Barba, D.; Reed, R.; Singh, H.P. Biomechanical Comparison of Periprosthetic Femoral Fracture Risk in Three Femoral Components in a Sawbone Model. *J. Arthroplasty* **2021**, *36*, 387–394. [CrossRef] [PubMed]

25. Konow, T.; Baetz, J.; Melsheimer, O.; Grimberg, A.; Morlock, M. Factors influencing periprosthetic femoral fracture risk: A German registry study. *Bone Jt. J.* **2021**, *103*, 650–658. [CrossRef] [PubMed]
26. Sershon, R.A.; McDonald, J.F., 3rd; Ho, H.; Hamilton, W.G. Periprosthetic Femur Fracture Risk: Influenced by Stem Choice, Not Surgical Approach. *J. Arthroplasty* **2021**, *36*, S363–S366. [CrossRef] [PubMed]
27. Cottino, U.; Dettoni, F.; Caputo, G.; Bonasia, D.E.; Rossi, P.; Rossi, R. Incidence and pattern of periprosthetic hip fractures around the stem in different stem geometry. *Int. Orthop.* **2020**, *44*, 53–59. [CrossRef] [PubMed]
28. Luger, M.; Feldler, S.; Pisecky, L.; Klasan, A.; Gotterbarm, T.; Schopper, C. Periprosthetic femoral fractures in cementless short versus straight stem total hip arthroplasty: A propensity score matched analysis. *J. Arthroplast.* **2023**, *38*, 751–756. [CrossRef] [PubMed]
29. González-Martín, D.; Hernández-Castillejo, L.E.; Herrera-Pérez, M.; Pais-Brito, J.L.; González-Casamayor, S.; Garrido-Miguel, M. Osteosynthesis versus revision arthroplasty in Vancouver B2 periprosthetic hip fractures: A systematic review and meta-analysis. *Eur. J. Trauma Emergy Surg.* **2023**, *49*, 87–106. [CrossRef] [PubMed]
30. Lindahl, H.; Malchau, H.; Herberts, P.; Garellick, G. Periprosthetic femoral fractures. *J. Arthroplast.* **2005**, *20*, 857–865. [CrossRef] [PubMed]
31. Sidler-Maier, C.C.; Waddell, J.P. Incidence and predisposing factors of periprosthetic proximal femoral fractures: A literature review. *Int. Orthop.* **2015**, *39*, 1673–1682. [CrossRef]
32. Learmonth, I.D. The management of periprosthetic fractures around the femoral stem. *J. Bone Jt. Surg. Br.* **2004**, *86*, 13–19. [CrossRef]

Journal of
Clinical Medicine

MDPI

Brief Report

Potential of Titanium Pins Coated with Fibroblast Growth Factor-2–Calcium Phosphate Composite Layers to Reduce the Risk of Impaired Bone–Pin Interface Strength in the External Fixation of Distal Radius Fractures

Hirotaka Mutsuzaki [1,2,*], Yohei Yanagisawa [3], Hiroshi Noguchi [4], Atsuo Ito [5] and Masashi Yamazaki [4]

1 Center for Medical Science, Ibaraki Prefectural University of Health Sciences, Ami 300-0394, Japan
2 Department of Orthopedic Surgery, Ibaraki Prefectural University of Health Sciences Hospital, Ami 300-0331, Japan
3 Department of Emergency Medicine, University of Tsukuba, 1-1-1 Tennodai, Tsukuba 305-8575, Japan; yanagisawa@tsukuba-seikei.jp
4 Department of Orthopaedic Surgery, University of Tsukuba, 1-1-1 Tennodai, Tsukuba 305-8575, Japan; noguhiro0164@tsukuba-seikei.jp (H.N.); masashiy@md.tsukuba.ac.jp (M.Y.)
5 Health and Medical Research Institute, National Institute of Advanced Industrial Science and Technology (AIST), AIST Tsukuba Central 6, 1-1-1 Higashi, Tsukuba 305-8566, Japan; atsuo-ito@aist.go.jp
* Correspondence: mutsuzaki@ipu.ac.jp; Tel.: +81-29-888-4000

Abstract: Background: The risk of impaired bone–pin interface strength in titanium (Ti) pins coated with fibroblast growth factor (FGF)–calcium phosphate (CP) composite layers is yet to be evaluated in a clinical study. This retrospective study used Weibull plot analysis to evaluate bone–pin interface strength in Ti pins coated with FGF-CP layers for external distal radius fracture fixation. **Methods**: The distal radial fractures were treated with external fixation. The FGF-CP group comprised five patients (all women, aged 70.4 ± 5.9 (range: 62–77) years), and the uncoated pin group comprised ten patients (eight women and two men, aged 64.4 ± 11.7 (range: 43–83) years). The pins were removed after six weeks. The insertion and extraction peak torques were measured. The extraction peak torque was evaluated using Weibull plot analysis. **Results**: We compared the extraction torque of the two groups at or below 506 Nmm for a fair comparison using Weibull plot analysis. The Weibull plots were linear for both the FGF-CP and uncoated pin groups. The slope of the regression line was significantly higher in the FGF-CP group (1.7343) than in the uncoated pin group (1.5670) (p = 0.011). The intercept of the regression line was significantly lower in the FGF-CP group (−9.847) than in the uncoated pin group (−8.708) (p = 0.002). Thus, the two regression lines significantly differed. **Conclusions**: Ti pins coated with FGF-CP layers exhibit the potential to reduce the risk of impaired bone–pin interface strength in the external fixation of distal radius fractures.

Keywords: fibroblast growth factor-2 (FGF-2); calcium phosphate; coating; external fixation; distal radius fractures; impaired bone fixation; Weibull plot analysis

1. Introduction

Screw loosening is a severe clinical problem in orthopedic surgery that leads to unfavorable clinical results, including incomplete healing of bone fractures and delayed union [1–3]. Plasma-sprayed apatite coating is known to increase the extraction torque of external fixation pins compared with that of uncoated pins [4,5]. Calcium titanate screws have an increased fixation index, which is the quotient of maximum extraction torque over maximum insertion torque for external fixation compared with uncoated pins [6]. Bisphosphonate coatings for external fixation in metaphyseal fixation strength are similar to hydroxyapatite coatings [7]. In these studies, average values of bone–pin interface strength were compared between treated pins and untreated pins. However, an average value does not necessarily reflect an incidence probability of an outlier, such as a very low value of bone–pin interface strength, since an outlier rather relates to dispersion.

We developed titanium (Ti) screws coated with human recombinant fibroblast growth factor (FGF)-2–calcium phosphate (CP) composite layers by immersing them in an infusion fluid-based supersaturated CP solution containing FGF-2 at 37 °C for 48 h [8]. The risk of impaired bone apposition to the screw was analyzed using Weibull plot analysis, a method commonly employed to analyze the lifetime, failure probability or risk, and reliability of industrial products [9]. As FGF-2 is a human recombinant protein, pedicle screws coated with an FGF-CP layer were implanted in cynomolgus monkey spines to simulate potential clinical use [8]. The pedicle screws coated with FGF-CP layers exhibited a significantly lower risk of impaired bone formation, as analyzed using Weibull plots [8]. In a clinical trial, Ti pins coated with FGF-CP layers in external fixation of distal radius fractures demonstrated safety and a tendency towards a reduced pin tract infection rate [10]. However, it is unclear whether the Ti pins coated with FGF-CP layers reduce the risk of impaired bone–pin interface strength in clinical studies. Using Weibull plot analysis, the purpose of this study was to retrospectively analyze the clinical trial data to evaluate the risk of impaired bone–pin interface strength in pins coated with FGF-CP layers. We hypothesized that Ti pins coated with FGF-CP layers would reduce the risk of impaired bone–pin interface strength that leads to pin loosening.

2. Materials and Methods

2.1. Participants

Fifteen patients who had fractures of the distal radius with unstable and displaced fragments were enrolled [10]. Fractures were treated using external fixation [10]. In the FGF-CP-coated pin group, five consecutive patients (all women, aged 70.4 ± 5.9 (range: 62–77) years) were enrolled between February 2013 and January 2015 [10]. In the uncoated pin group, ten consecutive patients (eight women and two men, aged 64.4 ± 11.7 (range: 43–83) years) were enrolled between January 2015 and August 2017 [10]. The exclusion criteria were as follows: patients with skin disease, a severe systemic disease (heart, lung, liver, or kidney disease, etc.), a malignant tumor within 5 years before the fracture, pregnant, and who were determined by the doctor as inappropriate [10].

2.2. Study Design

This study was a retrospective study that analyzed biomechanical data from the previous open-label controlled feasibility studies [10].

2.3. FGF-CP Coating Technique

Ti pins were immersed in a supersaturated calcium phosphate solution containing FGF-2 (4.0 μg/mL) at 37 °C for 48 h under air cleanliness condition class 5 using a clean bench in a clean room (class 6) [10] (Figure 1). The Ca/P molar ratio was 1.67 [10]. The layers retained their FGF-2 mitogenic activity, examined by fibroblastic NIH3T3 cell proliferation [10]. All the supersaturated CP solutions were aseptic, revealed by the bacteriologic and endotoxin tests [10].

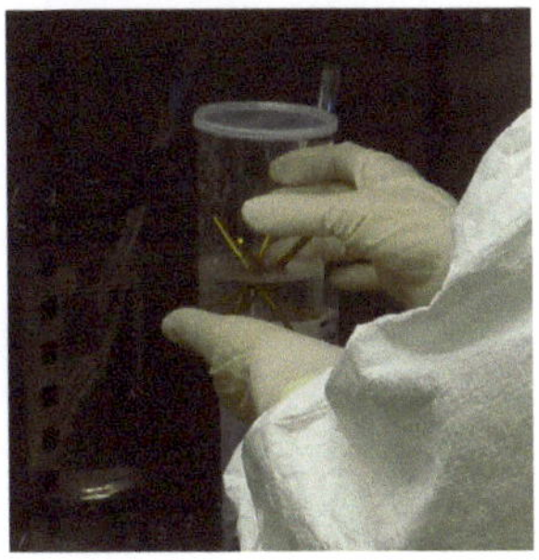

Figure 1. FGF-CP-coated pins.

2.4. Operation and Measurement Procedures

All operations were performed with external fixation using an external distal radius fixator (bridging and unilateral types: DePuy Synthes, Zuchwil, Switzerland), following the original operation manual to standardize pin insertion techniques [10]. Two pins were inserted into the radial shaft through a 10 mm incision, while the other two pins were inserted into the second metacarpal [10] (Figure 2). After six weeks, the pins were removed [10] (Figure 2). The insertion and extraction peak torques were measured using a digital torque wrench (HTG2-5G; IMADA, Toyohashi, Aichi, Japan) [10].

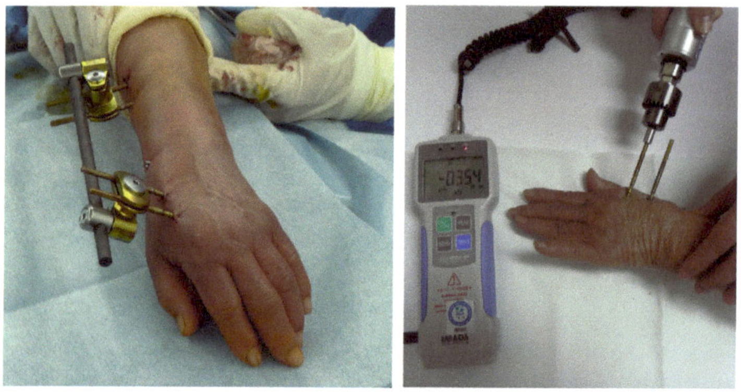

Figure 2. External fixation for fractures of the distal radius. Immediately after surgery (**left**) and extraction peak torque measurement (**right**).

2.5. Weibull Plot Analysis

The extraction peak torque was analyzed using Weibull plot analysis according to the following Weibull equation:

$$\ln\ln\,[1/(1-S)] = m\ln\sigma - m\ln\xi,$$

where ln, S, m, σ, and ξ indicate the natural log, failure probability, Weibull parameter, extraction peak torque, and scale parameter, respectively. Thus, the plot of "ln σ" against "lnln $[1/(1-S)]$" gives a straight line with a slope of "m". In this study, S is the probability of obtaining an extraction peak torque at or less than σ. The measured σ values were arranged in ascending order, such as σ_1, σ_2, σ_j, and σ_N, where j is the order of an individual σ value and N is the total number of measured σ values. S was derived from the median rank method using $S_j = (j - 0.3)/(N + 0.4)$.

2.6. Statistical Analysis

Student's t-test was used to evaluate statistically significant differences. The level of significance was set at $p < 0.05$.

3. Results

Figure 3 shows the relationship between insertion and extraction torques. The FGF-CP group had the highest value of 505 Nmm in extraction torque. The uncoated pin group showed a bimodal correlation between insertion and extraction torques, with a boundary at approximately 500 Nmm in extraction torque. Above the boundary, eight of the twelve points belonged to the three youngest patients (patients C1, C3, and C6 in [10]). The slope and intercept of the regression line above the boundary significantly differed from those below the boundary (slope: $p = 9.7 \times 10^{-6}$, intercept: $p = 1.3 \times 10^{-4}$) and those for the coated pin group (slope: $p = 1.1 \times 10^{-4}$, intercept: $p = 2.6 \times 10^{-4}$). Conversely, no significant difference was noted in the slope and intercept between the regression line below the boundary and those for the FGF-CP group (slope: $p = 0.46$, intercept: $p = 0.26$). Thus, we compared the extraction torques of the two groups at or below 506 Nmm for a fair comparison using Weibull plot analysis.

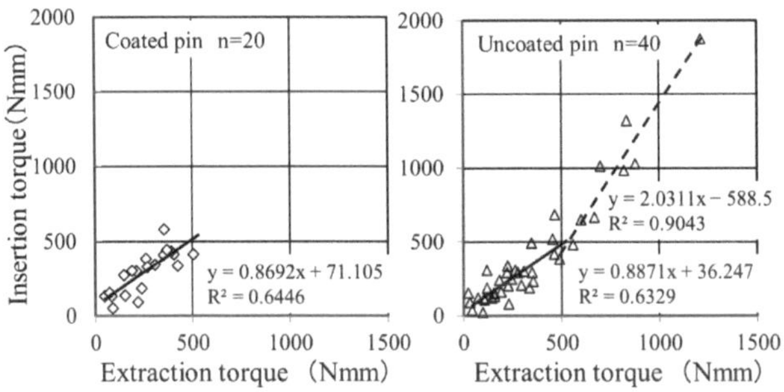

Figure 3. Relationship between the insertion and extraction torques. FGF-CP (**left**) and uncoated (**right**) pin groups.

The Weibull plots were linear for both the FGF-CP and uncoated pin groups (Figure 4). The slope of the regression line was significantly higher in the FGF-CP group (1.7343) than in the uncoated pin group (1.5670) ($p = 0.011$). The intercept of the regression line was significantly lower in the FGF-CP group (−9.847) than in the uncoated pin group (−8.708) ($p = 0.002$). Thus, the two regression lines exhibited a significant difference.

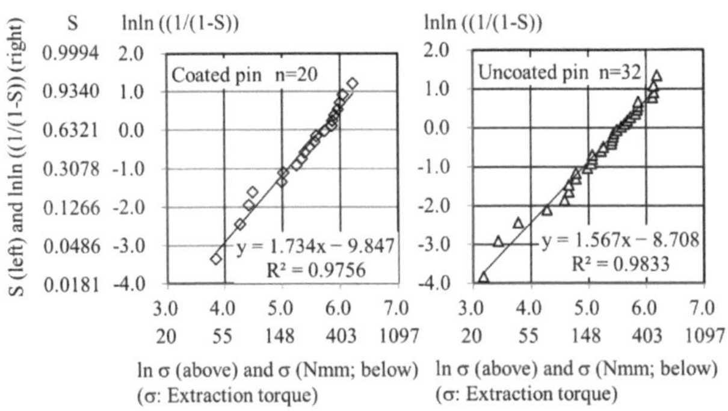

Figure 4. The Weibull plot of extraction torque for the FGF-CP (**left**) and uncoated pin (**right**) groups.

The regression lines enabled us to assess the risk of impaired bone–pin interface strength by calculating the probability of obtaining specific low values of the extraction torque, which were arbitrarily selected. For instance, if the impaired bone–pin interface strength was defined as an extraction torque (σ) at or less than 20 Nmm, then "ln σ" gives a value of 3.0 (Figure 4). Since "ln σ" is "x" of the linear regression function, "ln σ = 3.0" gives y values of −4.651 and −4.013 for FGF-CP and uncoated pin groups, respectively. Since "y" is "lnln ((1/(1 − *S*))", one can obtain the failure probabilities, *S*, of 0.9% and 1.8% in the FGF-CP and uncoated pin groups, respectively. Similarly, if the impaired bone–pin interface strength was defined as an extraction torque of ≤100 Nmm, the probabilities were 14% and 20% in the FGF-CP and uncoated pin groups, respectively. Thus, the risk of impaired bone–pin interface strength was lower in the FGF-CP group than in the uncoated pin group.

Similarly, the Weibull plots for all the 40 extraction torques in the uncoated pin group had a regression line with a slope that was significantly lower (1.340; $p = 1.2 \times 10^{-8}$) than that in the FGF-CP group (Figure S1). This again showed that the risk of impaired bone–pin interface strength was lower in the FGF-CP group than in the uncoated pin group.

4. Discussion

The risk of pin loosening is lower in the FGF-CP group than in the uncoated pin group, as shown by Weibull plot analysis. Stability of the bone–pin interface is achieved in the FGF-CP group. The Weibull plots are analyzed with the linear regression of plots (Figure 4). The greater the slope of the regression line is, the lower the probability of failure is, meaning that a more consistent treatment outcome is potentially obtained. When the slope is the same, a lower position of the regression line corresponds to a lower probability of failure. In the Weibull plot of extraction torque regression for the FGF-CP group, the line exhibits a greater slope and runs at a lower level compared to that of the uncoated pin group. This indicates that FGF-CP demonstrates a more consistent treatment outcome and a tendency to reduce the probability of impaired bone–pin interface strength in comparison to the uncoated pin group.

The mode of action on bone–pin interface strength is different between hydroxyapatite-coated and FGF-CP-coated pins. The average bone–pin interface strength for hydroxyapatite-coated pins is higher than that of uncoated pins [4,5,11–14]. In general, the higher bone–pin interface strength in average led to low incidence rates of impaired bone–pin interface strength [15,16]. In some reports, the incidence rates of impaired bone–pin interface strength, as low as 100 and 20 Nmm, in extraction torque that are associated with radiolucency, or as low as those that are manually extractable, are nearly the same between hydroxyapatite-coated and uncoated pins [11,14]. In contrast, FGF-CP-coated pins decrease the probability of impaired bone–pin interface strength without significant increases in average bone–pin interface strength. The average bone–pin interface strength for FGF-CP-coated pins (254 $\pm$ 132 Nmm (n = 20)) is not significantly higher than that of uncoated pins (227 $\pm$ 131 Nmm (n = 32) and 338 $\pm$ 269 Nmm (n = 40)). However, the probability of impaired bone–pin interface strength as low as 100 and 20 Nmm is lower in the FGF-CP pin group than in the un-coated pin group. It is suggested that Ti screws coated with FGF-CP layers are more reliable than uncoated pins for preventing impaired bone–pin interface strength that causes pin loosening.

5. Limitations

The current study is a retrospective study, and furthermore, a small number of patients were enrolled. In the future, prospective randomized controlled studies with increased enrollment of patients are needed. In addition, it may be necessary to show the relationship with bone mineral density in the future.

6. Conclusions

In the Weibull plot analysis of extraction torques, the slope of the regression line was higher in the FGF-CP group than in the uncoated pin group. Furthermore, the intercept of the regression line was significantly lower in the FGF-CP group than in the uncoated pin group. The two regression lines significantly differed. Therefore, Ti pins coated with FGF-CP layers have the potential to reduce the risk of impaired bone–pin interface strength in the external fixation of distal radius fractures.

Supplementary Materials: The following supporting information can be downloaded at: https://www.mdpi.com/article/10.3390/jcm13113040/s1, Figure S1: The Weibull plot of all the 40 extraction torques for uncoated pin groups.

Author Contributions: Conceptualization, H.M., Y.Y. and A.I.; Methodology, H.M., Y.Y. and A.I.; Software, H.M., Y.Y. and A.I.; Validation, H.M., Y.Y. and A.I.; Formal Analysis, Y.Y. and A.I.; Investigation, H.M., Y.Y. and A.I.; Resources, H.M., Y.Y. and A.I.; Data curation, Y.Y. and A.I.; Writing Original Draft Preparation, H.M. and Y.Y.; Writing Review and Editing, H.M., Y.Y., H.N., A.I. and M.Y.; Visualization, H.M., Y.Y. and A.I.; Supervision, H.M., Y.Y., H.N., A.I. and M.Y.; Project Administration, H.M., Y.Y., H.N., A.I. and M.Y.; Funding Acquisition, M.Y.; All authors have read and agreed to the published version of the manuscript.

Funding: This study was supported by a grant from the Initiative for Accelerating Regulatory Science in Innovative Drug, Medical Device, and Regenerative Medicine of the Ministry of Health, Labour and Welfare, Japan.

Institutional Review Board Statement: This study was conducted in accordance with the Declaration of Helsinki and approved by the ethics committees of the University of Tsukuba Hospital and Mito Kyodo Hospital (protocol code H23-37 and date of approval 18 March 2014, protocol code H25-124 and date of approval 4 March 2014, and protocol code H29-86 and date of approval 9 August 2017) and the National Institute of Advanced Industrial Science and Technology (protocol code I 2013-031 and date of approval 8 August 2013, protocol code I 2013-031A and date of approval 26 March 2014, protocol code I 2014-031 and date of approval 18 July 2014, protocol code I 2014-031ABC, and protocol code I 2017-041 and date of approval 6 December 2017).

Informed Consent Statement: Informed consent was obtained from all patients.

Data Availability Statement: The datasets generated and analyzed during the current study are available from the corresponding authors upon reasonable request.

Conflicts of Interest: The authors declare no conflicts of interest.

References

1. Galbusera, F.; Volkheimer, D.; Reitmaier, S.; Berger-Roscher, N.; Kienle, A.; Wilke, H.J. Pedicle screw loosening: A clinically relevant complication? *Eur. Spine J.* **2015**, *24*, 1005–1016. [CrossRef] [PubMed]
2. Wu, J.C.; Huang, W.C.; Tsai, H.W.; Ko, C.C.; Wu, C.L.; Tu, T.H.; Cheng, H. Pedicle screw loosening in dynamic stabilization: Incidence, risk, and outcome in 126 patients. *Neurosurg. Focus* **2011**, *31*, E9. [CrossRef] [PubMed]
3. Kocak, T.; Cakir, B.; Reichel, H.; Mattes, T. Screw loosening after posterior dynamic stabilization–review of the literature. *Acta Chir. Orthop. Traumatol. Cech.* **2010**, *77*, 134–139. [CrossRef] [PubMed]
4. Moroni, A.; Cadossi, M.; Romagnoli, M.; Faldini, C.; Giannini, S. A biomechanical and histological analysis of standard versus hydroxyApatite-coated pins for external fixation. *J. Biomed. Mater. Res. B Appl. Biomater.* **2008**, *86*, 417–421. [CrossRef] [PubMed]
5. Moroni, A.; Pegreffi, F.; Cadossi, M.; Hoang-Kim, A.; Lio, V.; Giannini, S. Hydroxyapatite-coated external fixation pins. *Expert Rev. Med. Devices.* **2005**, *2*, 465–471. [CrossRef]
6. Gathen, M.; Ploeger, M.M.; Jaenisch, M.; Koob, S.; Cucchi, D.; Kasapovic, A.; Randau, T.; Placzek, R. Outcome evaluation of new calcium titanate schanz-screws for external fixators. First clinical results and cadaver studies. *J. Mater. Sci. Mater. Med.* **2019**, *30*, 124. [CrossRef] [PubMed]
7. Toksvig-Larsen, S.; Aspenberg, P. Bisphosphonate-coated external fixation pins appear similar to hydroxyapatite-coated pins in the tibial metaphysis and to uncoated pins in the shaft. *Acta Orthop.* **2013**, *84*, 314–318. [CrossRef] [PubMed]
8. Matsumoto, Y.; Mutsuzaki, H.; Hara, Y.; Nagashima, K.; Okano, E.; Yanagisawa, Y.; Noguchi, H.; Sankai, T.; Yamazaki, M. Safety and osteointegration of titanium screws coated with a fibroblast growth factor-2-calcium phosphate composite layer in non-human primates: A pilot study. *J. Funct. Biomater.* **2023**, *14*, 261. [CrossRef] [PubMed]
9. Weibull, W. A statistical distribution function of wide applicability. *J. Appl. Mech.* **1951**, *18*, 293–297. [CrossRef]
10. Yanagisawa, Y.; Ito, A.; Hara, Y.; Mutsuzaki, H.; Murai, S.; Fujii, K.; Sogo, Y.; Hirose, M.; Oyane, A.; Kobayashi, F.; et al. Initial clinical trial of pins coated with fibroblast growth factor-2-apatite composite layer in external fixation of distal radius fractures. *J. Orthop.* **2019**, *16*, 69–73. [CrossRef] [PubMed]
11. Pieske, O.; Kaltenhauser, F.; Pichlmaier, L.; Schramm, N.; Trentzsch, H.; Löffler, T.; Greiner, A.; Piltz, S. Clinical benefit of hydroxyapatite-coated pins compared with stainless steel pins in external fixation at the wrist: A randomised prospective study. *Injury* **2010**, *41*, 1031–1036. [CrossRef] [PubMed]
12. Pieske, O.; Pichlmaier, L.; Kaltenhauser, F.; Schramm, N.; Rubenbauer, B.; Greiner, A.; Piltz, S. Hydroxyapatite-coated pins versus titanium alloy pins in external fixation at the wrist: A controlled cohort study. *J. Trauma.* **2011**, *70*, 845–851. [CrossRef]
13. Saithna, A. The influence of hydroxyapatite coating of external fixator pins on pin loosening and pin track infection: A systematic review. *Injury* **2010**, *41*, 128–132. [CrossRef] [PubMed]
14. Moroni, A.; Aspenberg, P.; Toksvig-Larsen, S.; Falzarano, G.; Giannini, S. Enhanced fixation with hydroxyapatite coated pins. *Clin. Orthop. Relat. Res.* **1998**, *346*, 171–177.
15. Moroni, A.; Faldini, C.; Marchetti, S.; Manca, M.; Consoli, V.; Giannini, S. Improvement of the bone-pin interface strength in osteoporotic bone with use of hydroxyapatite-coated tapered external-fixation pins. A prospective, randomized clinical study of wrist fracture. *J. Bone Joint Surg. Am.* **2001**, *83*, 717–721. [CrossRef]
16. Pizà, G.; Caja, V.L.; González-Viejo, M.A.; Navarro, A. Hydroxyapatite-coated external-fixation pins. The effect on pin loosening and pin-track infection in leg lengthening for short stature. *J. Bone Joint Surg. Br.* **2004**, *86*, 892–897. [CrossRef] [PubMed]

Journal of
Clinical Medicine

MDPI

Article

Early Postoperative Weight-Bearing Ability after Total Hip Arthroplasty versus Bipolar Hemiarthroplasty in Elderly Patients with Femoral Neck Fracture

Chiara Grabmann [1], Ibrahim Hussain [2], Anne Zeller [1], Sertac Kirnaz [2], Vincent Sullivan [3] and Fabian Sommer [2,*]

1 University Hospital of Munich, Ludwig Maximilian University, 81377 Munich, Germany
2 New York Presbyterian Hospital, Weill Cornell Medicine, New York, NY 10065, USA
3 Department of Biological Sciences, University of South Carolina, Columbia, SC 29208, USA
* Correspondence: publications@drsommer.net

Abstract: Background: Femoral neck fractures are among the most common types of fractures and particularly affect elderly patients. Two of the most common treatment strategies are total hip arthroplasty (THA) and bipolar hemiarthroplasty (BA). However, the role of the different treatment strategies in the postoperative weight-bearing ability in the early postoperative phase is still not entirely clear. **Methods:** Patients who underwent either THA or BA were consecutively included in our prospective cohort study. Gait analysis was performed during the early postoperative period. The gait analysis consisted of a walking distance of 40 m coupled with the turning movement in between. During the gait analysis, the duration of the measurement, the maximum peak force and the average peak force were recorded. **Results:** A total of 39 patients were included, 25 of whom underwent BA and 14 of whom underwent THA. The maximum peak force during the gait analysis was, on average, 80.6% ± 19.5 of the body weight in the BA group and 78.9% ± 21.6 in the THA group. The additionally determined average peak force during the entire gait analysis was 66.8% ± 15.8 of the body weight in the BA group and 60.5% ± 15.6 in the THA group. **Conclusions:** Patients with femoral neck fractures undergoing THA and BA can achieve sufficient weight bearing on the operated leg in the early postoperative period. In our study, BA did not allow for a significantly higher average and maximum loading capacity compared with THA.

Keywords: fracture; femoral neck; hip; arthroplasty; hemiarthroplasty; weight bearing; mobilization

1. Introduction

Hip fractures, especially the subgroup of femoral neck fractures, are among the most common types of fractures and particularly affect elderly patients [1]. This is a global health problem that is particularly prevalent in older women [2]. The region of the proximal femur is anatomically exposed and usually has a relatively low amount of protective soft tissue coverage, which increases the injury risk in case of a fall on the hip [3,4]. Contrarily, young people generally have better bone stability and femoral neck fractures rarely occur and are in most cases a consequence of high energy trauma, such as traffic accidents [5,6]. In elderly people, bone stability physiologically decreases with age, and the natural degradation of bones combined with osteoporosis can have a significant impact on bone quality [1]. Additionally, the soft tissue covering of the hip region decreases in elderly people, affording less protection against impacts from falling [4,7]. Therefore, in elderly patients, low impact trauma, such as a light fall on the hip, can lead to femoral neck fractures [8]. In addition to the cause of the injury, the treatment goals also differ between these two age groups. While younger people usually have a higher functional demand and can undergo more complex surgical procedures and post-treatment regimens, older people are often functionally limited and have more comorbidities that increase the risk of surgery [1,9,10]. Taking this into consideration, the treatment goal in geriatric patients is early mobilization with ideally postoperative full weight bearing to reduce the risk of postoperative complications due to immobilization [11,12]. Prolonged immobilization has been shown to increase both mortality and the risk of irreversible loss of mobility [13,14]. Thus, the earliest possible postoperative mobilization is one of the main treatment goals in elderly patients [11,12,15]. For this reason, surgical techniques that require postoperative weight-bearing restrictions and do not permit the patient to apply full weight bearing postoperatively should be avoided. For the evaluation of weight-bearing capacity, special devices have been available recently, which are not larger than a normal insole and can be inserted into the patient's shoes to evaluate the individual weight-bearing capacity of the affected leg. These devices have already been used in other studies for the scientific evaluation of postoperative weight-bearing capacity and demonstrated a simple applicability and relatively precise measurement results [16].

Early mobilization has a significant impact on the further course of rehabilitation and the final functional outcome for the patient [11,15]. To meet this therapeutic goal, the first treatment option for femoral neck fractures in geriatric patients in many cases is direct joint replacement [17,18]. Two of the most common procedures are total hip arthroplasty (THA) (Figure 1), which consists of a replacement of both the femoral head and acetabulum, and bipolar hemiarthroplasty (BA) (Figure 2), in which only the femoral head is replaced [17,19].

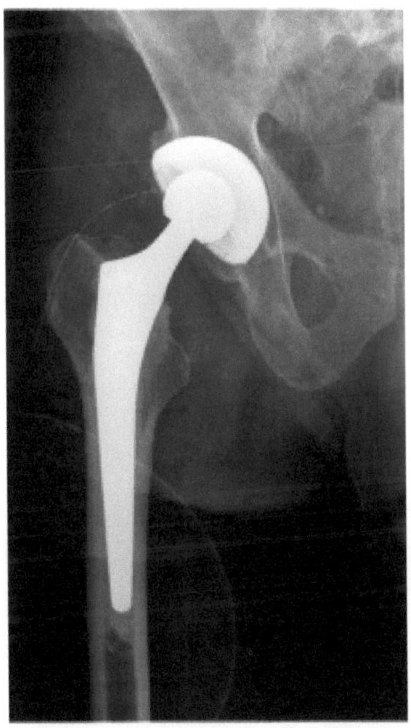

Figure 1. Early postoperative X-ray of the right hip joint in AP view of a male patient after femoral neck fracture who underwent total hip arthroplasty (THA).

BA is typically the shorter and less invasive surgery, since the procedure steps to prepare the acetabulum for an implant are not necessary [20,21]. On the other hand, THA could show a better outcome in patients with pre-existing coxarthrosis and a higher functional demand [17,22–24]. However, the role of the different treatment strategies in the postoperative weight-bearing ability in the early postoperative phase is still not entirely clear. In patients without a clear indication for either surgical procedure, the postoperative weight-bearing ability, and thus, the possibility of early mobilization, may be a crucial factor to consider when choosing the best surgical treatment. Furthermore, an evaluation of the postoperative weight-bearing ability could also help patients who have a clear indication for either procedure to more accurately adjust postoperative mobilization regimens and pain medication to achieve the best possible functional outcome.

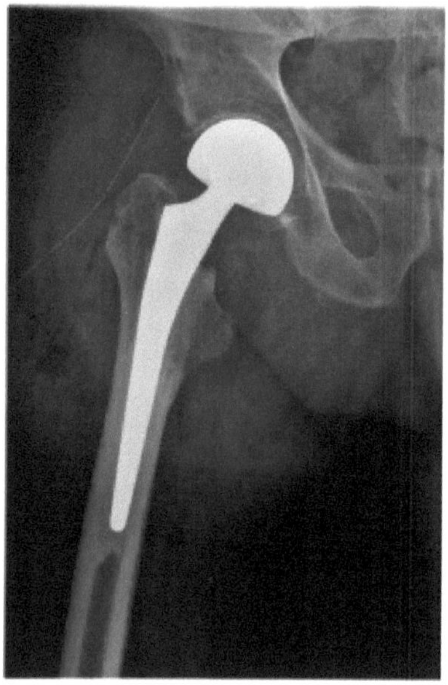

Figure 2. Early postoperative X-ray of the right hip joint in AP view of a male patient after femoral neck fracture who underwent bipolar hemiarthroplasty (BA).

For this reason, our group evaluated and compared the weight-bearing ability in the early postoperative period in elderly patients with femoral neck fracture who underwent THA or BA as part of a prospective cohort study.

2. Materials and Methods

To evaluate the early postoperative weight-bearing ability in elderly patients after hip replacement surgery, we conducted a prospective cohort study. The study was reviewed and approved by the Institutional Review Board (IRB) (Ethic Committee Name: Ethic Committee of the Ludwig Maximilian University of Munich (LMU), Approval Code: 214-16, Approval Date: 28 June 2016). Patients over the age of 60 years who underwent surgical treatment for a femoral neck fracture, either THA or BA, were consecutively included in the study. Our study focused exclusively on fractures in the femoral neck region that can be treated with THA or BA, following the recommendations of the AO Foundation. These include dislocated subcapital, transcervical and basicervical femoral neck fractures, according to AO classifications 31B1, 31B2 and 31B3 [25]. Patients who were not able to perform a postoperative gait analysis were excluded. These included patients with relevant cognitive impairment (for example, dementia, postoperative delirium), pre-existing immobility (for example, bedridden patients, musculoskeletal disorders) and other restricting comorbidities that were limiting postoperative mobilization.

Prior to the gait analysis, cognitive impairment, the presence of comorbidities and the mobility of patients before trauma were assessed using standardized questionnaires. The Mini-Mental State Examination was used to evaluate cognitive impairment [26]. Co-morbidities were assessed using the Charlson Index [27]. Patients' mobility and daily living ability were assessed using the Parker Mobility Score (PMS) and the Barthel Index (BI) [28,29]. These functional scores were assessed for the first time right after hospital admission to estimate the functional scores before the accident at the earliest possible time point and for the second time on the date of the postoperative gait analysis.

Postoperatively, all patients were treated according to the World Health Organization (WHO) standardized pain management guidelines [30]. During the whole study, all patients were mobilized by the same experienced physiotherapy team. All patients were allowed full weight bearing immediately following operation without weight-bearing restrictions, meaning the operated leg was allowed to be loaded with the full body weight. Prior to mobilization, patients were provided with an appropriate dose of analgesia, according to the WHO pain management guidelines, depending on their individual pain level, if necessary, in order to facilitate mobilization with minimum pain.

Postoperative gait analysis was performed using insoles with integrated force sensors (Figure 3). The insoles were matched to the patients' shoe size and placed in both shoes before the gait analysis. The insoles' force sensor measures the actual applied plantar force between the foot and the shoe and reflects the load on the leg with each step. The measuring range of the pressure sensors in the model used ranges from 20 N to 2500 N at a maximum sampling rate of 200 Hz, meaning 200 measurements per second. The electronic hardware for recording and transmitting was located in a small box connected to the soles by a cable and was attached to the outer shoe during the test (Figure 4). The weight of the box was only a few grams and did not cause the patients any impairment during the gait analysis. The data were transmitted via Bluetooth to a mobile tablet PC during the gait analysis and stored using a dedicated software application (loadsol version 1.4.72). Before each measurement, the sensor soles were calibrated. All measurements in the study were performed with the same test setup.

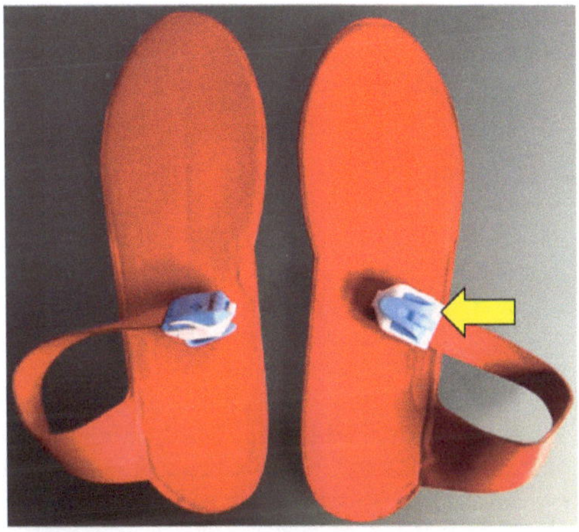

Figure 3. Example of a pair of insoles with integrated force sensors that were used for the gait analysis. The electronic hardware is located in a small box (yellow arrow) that is connected to the soles by a cable. The insoles are about 2–3 mm thick, so the soles do not significantly interfere with walking.

Gait analysis was performed during the hospital stay in the early postoperative period and was adapted to the individual patient's mobilization ability. During the gait analysis, the duration of the measurement in seconds [s], the maximum peak force and the average peak force in Newton [N] were recorded by the insoles. The maximum peak force is defined as the highest load that the patient is able to apply during the measurement period and usually occurs during walking in the phase when the foot hits the ground. This value depends on the walking speed and can exceed 100% of the body weight due to the kinetic energy acting in addition to the body weight. The average peak force is a parameter calculated by the software application that takes the measurements of the applied force during each step and calculates an average value for all steps during the measurement period. To avoid bias from inconsistent force application, at the beginning of walking, the first three steps from each recording period were excluded from the determination of the average peak force. In addition to the load, the walking speed in meters per second [m/s] was calculated. These parameters were determined for all patients in the BA group and the THA group and compared to determine whether one of the two treatment groups was able to show a higher postoperative weight-bearing capacity. Walking speed was measured to estimate the impact of the additional kinetic energy generated during walking on our measurements.

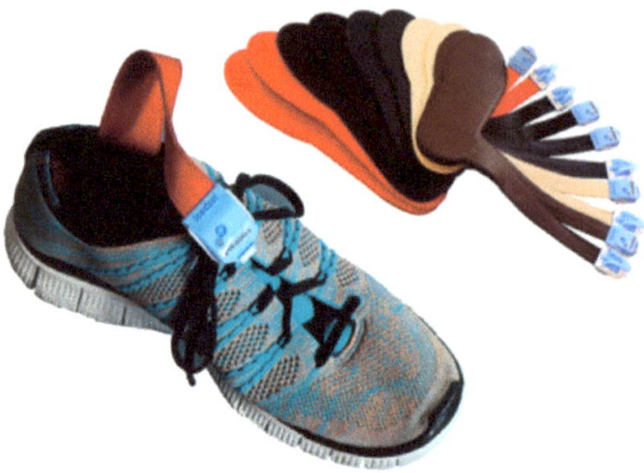

Figure 4. Examples of insoles with different sizes that were used for the gait analysis, each size being assigned a different color. The insoles were selected individually to match the patients' shoe size and placed in the patients' shoes before the gait analysis. The small box containing the hardware is attached to the outer shoe, where it does not interfere with walking.

For the gait analysis, patients were provided with a walking aid of their choice (crutches, walker or rollator). The decision regarding which type of walking aid was used depended on the individual patient's ability to bear weight and coordination. Crutches were used for patients with good coordination, and a walker or rollator was used for patients with impaired coordination. The walking aid was initially used in all patients and was then adjusted and reduced in further course based on the patient's individual load-bearing capacity and individual coordination ability. In our study, the walking aid served to reduce the load on the extremity and to prevent falls during mobilization. For this reason, the walking aid continued to be used in some patients who were already able to bear weight sufficiently but had an increased risk of falling due to impaired coordination. Because the use of the walker was not exclusively linked to weight-bearing capacity, this parameter was not included in our analysis due to its limited informative value. During mobilization, all patients were supported by a physiotherapist who ensured correct movement and was present for fall prevention. The sequence of the load measurement was the same for all patients and consisted of a walking distance of two 20 m stretches with a 180 degree turn in between. In total, the gait analysis consisted of a walking distance of 40 m coupled with the turning movement in between.

Statistical Analysis

A statistical analysis of the results was performed using the IBM SPSS software (Version 28.0, IBM corporation, Armonk, NY, USA). Before comparing the two groups, the parameters were tested for normal distribution using the Shapiro–Wilk test. For the comparison of maximum peak force and average peak force during walking, the unpaired *t*-test was used to identify significant differences between the two groups. Due to lack of normal distribution in the score values, the non-parametric Mann–Whitney-U-test was used for comparing the score values between the two groups. The significance level was set at $p < 0.05$.

3. Results

A total of 39 patients with femoral neck fracture met the inclusion criteria and were included in the study. Depending on the discretion of the operating surgeon, who was not directly involved in this study, 25 (14 male/11 female) patients underwent BA, and 14 (6 male/8 female) patients underwent THA. The mean age in the BA group was 82.5 ± 7.0 years and 74.0 ± 7.9 years in the THA group (Table 1). Age was normally distributed in both groups and presented no statistically significant difference between groups.

Table 1. Demographics of patients in the THA group and BA group.

	THA	BA
Number in total	14	25
Age, mean ± SD	74.0 ± 7.9 years	82.5 ± 6.9 years
Sex		
Male	6 (43%)	14 (56%)
Female	8 (57%)	11 (44%)
ASA, mean ± SD	2.6 ± 0.6	2.9 ± 0.5

ASA: American Society of Anesthesiologists physical status classification system.

3.1. Postoperative Weight Bearing

The evaluation of the gait analysis showed that both groups were able to achieve a maximum load of more than 75% of their own body weight, on average, during walking. The maximum peak force during the gait analysis was, on average, 80.6% ± 19.5 of the body weight in the BA group and 78.9% ± 21.6 in the THA group (Figure 5). The difference between the two groups was not statistically significant ($p = 0.799$). The additionally determined average peak force (average of maximum force for each step) during the entire gait analysis was 66.8% ± 15.8 of the body weight in the BA group and 60.5% ± 15.6 in the THA group (Figure 6). Although the average peak force was found to be around 6 points higher in the BA group, the difference between the two groups was not statistically significant ($p = 0.272$). Due to a connection loss between the soles and the mobile tablet PC during the recording of the average peak force, this value was not saved for two patients from the THA group and for four patients from the BA group; therefore, they could not be included in the evaluation. This referred only to the average peak force; all other parameters were transferred correctly by the software.

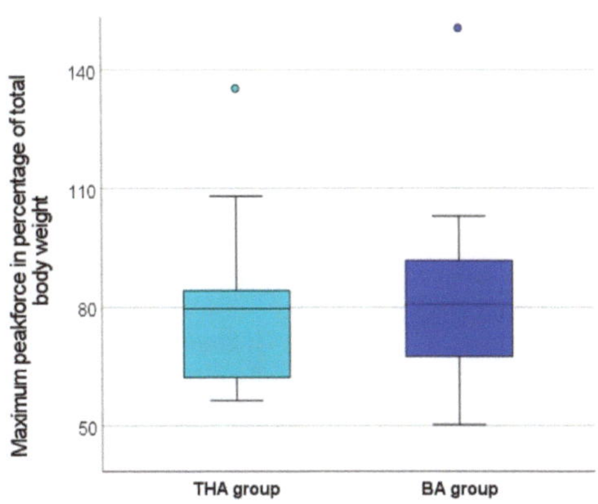

Figure 5. Box plot comparing the maximum peak force during the gait analysis between the BA group and the THA group. The maximum peak force is presented in relation to the body weight of the study participants. There was no significant difference ($p = 0.799$) between both groups.

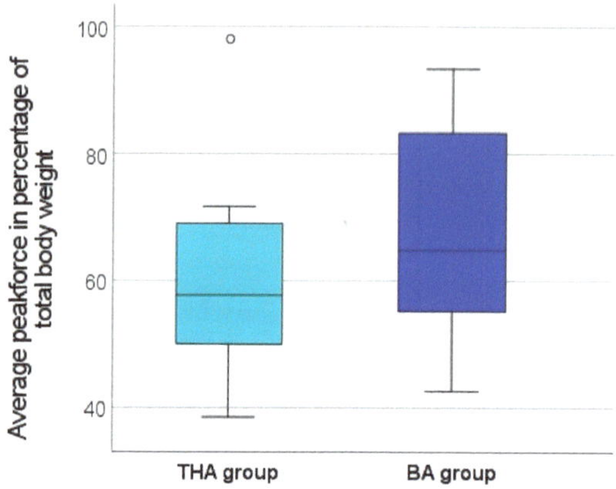

Figure 6. Box plot comparing the average peak force during the gait analysis between the BA group and the THA group. The average peak force is presented in relation to the body weight of the study participants. There was no significant difference ($p = 0.272$) between both groups.

Walking speed was, on average, 0.31 m/s ± 0.14 in the BA group and 0.32 m/s ± 0.19 in the THA group. Thus, no significant difference was found in walking speed between the two patient groups ($p = 0.890$). The difference in walking speed between the two groups was not statistically significant.

3.2. Mobility and Comorbidity

A comparison of the patients' mobility and health-related quality of life before trauma and after surgery, as assessed by the PMS and BI, revealed no significant difference between the two groups.

4. Discussion

Our study showed no significant difference in postoperative weight bearing in the early postoperative period in patients with femoral neck fracture, regardless of whether they underwent THA or BA. Both groups were able to achieve a maximum peak force of more than 75% of their own body weight, on average, on the operated leg during postoperative mobilization. A healthy person can statically load their leg with 100% of their body weight while standing. In the case of a dynamic load, such as walking or running, this value can also increase to more than 100% of the body weight, since, in addition to the body weight, the kinetic energy also puts force on the limb. In our study, however, postoperative mobilization was performed very slowly in all cases, since the physiotherapy team primarily focused on the correct execution of the movement sequence and not on the speed. Therefore, very low kinetic energies occurred when the leg touched the ground. In order to better quantify the influence of kinetic energy on our measurements, walking speed was additionally measured. In healthy subjects, the walking speed is about 1.5 m/s [31]. In our study, the walking speed in both groups was about 0.3 m/s, which is only about 20% of the normal walking speed. Since walking speed affects kinetic energy mathematically to the second power, a reduction in speed to 20% lowers the total corresponding kinetic energy to 4%. Due to this particular feature in the mobilization, the additional kinetic energy acting on the limb during walking is considered low and can be practically neglected for better comparability. This is also evident in the observation that the maximum peak load in our measurements, which usually occurs when the foot hits the ground, is above 100% in only a few cases (see Figure 5).

There is a consensus in the guidelines of several countries that the earliest possible postoperative mobilization should be a treatment goal in elderly trauma patients [32–35]. This treatment strategy showed a reduced complication rate and improved long-term outcome [11,12,15]. For these reasons, BA is often preferred in elderly patients with femoral neck fracture.

The choice of the surgical procedure depends on several additional factors, such as age, functional expectations, the amount of displacement of the fracture fragments or the patient's comorbidities [19,36]. BA typically represents the less invasive procedure of the two treatment strategies [20,21]. The average duration of surgery of a BA is shorter, and it has less average blood loss compared to a THA [20,21]. However, one of the disadvantages of BA is the high rate of painful acetabular erosions in the long term. In the literature, the rate of acetabular erosions in BA is described as being up to 36% [24,37]. This is another reason why the revision rate of BA within the first few years is higher compared to THA [22]. Therefore, the indication for BA is mainly given in elderly patients with a low functional demand and an increased operative risk. Even in this group, due to the growing life expectancy over the last decades, these implants may lead to complaints over the years [38].

Both surgical procedures have different advantages and disadvantages and their corresponding indications. Mobile and independent elderly patients with femoral neck fractures usually benefit more from THA. In the long term, THA has a better functional outcome and has fewer revisions than hemiarthroplasty [22–24]. A major disadvantage of the procedure is a higher risk of dislocation, particularly in the first period after surgery [22,23]. In addition, the operation takes longer and usually causes greater blood loss during the surgery, since the acetabular bone needs to be prepared for the hip cup implant [20,21]. Overall, THA represents the more invasive surgical procedure but is associated with better joint function in the long term than BA.

Which of the procedures, BA or THA, offers advantage for the actual postoperative weight-bearing ability of geriatric patients has not yet been investigated, and it is an important factor to consider when choosing the right treatment for a patient. Another study has already shown that hip replacement surgery allows effective loading in the early postoperative period [16]. However, the relatively small sample size in the described study specifically limits the findings related to the THA group. The extent of how much the postoperative weight bearing differs in detail between BA and THA could only be assessed to a limited extent due to the small number of cases, consisting of fewer than 10 cases in the THA group in the mentioned study.

There are clear indications for both surgical procedures where one procedure is more suitable and the patient is more likely to benefit from one particular procedure. In between, however, there are also patients without clear indications for one of the two procedures and who are suitable for both operative techniques. Patients without a clear indication for BA or THA are particularly challenging for the decision-making surgeon. Especially in older patients, where early postoperative mobilization is the therapeutic goal, Bhandari et al. were able to show that surgeons tend to prefer BA in case of doubt [18]. In this regard, some patients without a clear indication for either procedure could potentially benefit from the higher functionality of THA.

Our analysis showed no significant differences in weight bearing after either surgical procedure in the early postoperative period. Patients treated with both surgical techniques, THA and BA, were able to bear sufficient weight on the operated limb postoperatively. BA did not show a significant advantage for older patients to allow earlier full weight bearing compared to patients who underwent THA. This finding should be taken into consideration when planning the surgical treatment strategy.

Nevertheless, our study has a few limitations. It must be taken into account that the measurement took place at an early postoperative point of time and thus does not provide any information on the load-bearing ability in the long-term course. However, mobility in the early postoperative period during the hospital stay represents an important prognostic factor for the outcome of the patients [39]. Early mobilization, within 48 h of surgery, showed an increased functional recovery. Additionally, a higher rate of early mobilized patients were able to return directly back home after the surgery and showed lower rates of discharge to high-level care centers [39]. Several international guidelines recommend starting the postoperative mobilization on the first postoperative day for geriatric patients with femoral neck fracture if no contraindications exist [33,34]. Patients with femoral neck fracture lose, on average, more than 50% of their muscle strength within the first postoperative week in the affected leg compared to the non-affected leg, which affects the mobilization of elderly patients in particular [40–43]. For these reasons, we decided to conduct our evaluation in the early postoperative period.

Another limiting factor of our study is the sample size. In our study, only patients who were able to perform the gait analysis correctly were included, since this was the only way to obtain valid and comparable measurements. This resulted in a smaller sample size, but the group size of our study is comparable with other gait analysis studies that have used similar measurement procedures with sensor soles in determining the postoperative weight-bearing ability [44,45]. Due to the selection beforehand, all included patients were able to successfully perform gait analysis under appropriate guidance, and no patient needed to be excluded due to inability to follow the instructions during the gait analysis.

In addition, it is theoretically possible that our exclusion criteria might contribute to a selection bias. Since we did not include bedridden and severely mentally impaired patients in our analysis, we cannot draw any conclusions regarding this group of patients. For bedridden patients, this might be of limited significance, since weight bearing was already impossible before the injury. However, it could be that postoperative weight bearing differs between the two procedures in cognitively impaired patients and that this was not noticed due to the exclusion of this patient group. However, severely mentally impaired patients would not primarily be considered as ideal candidates for THA because of the higher postoperative dislocation and complication risk; therefore, this potential bias might be primarily of theoretical interest. Furthermore, the exclusion was made because we do not currently have a valid method to obtain reproducible and comparable data from patients who do not adhere exactly to the procedural instructions. As soon as we have the possibility to do so, we will include this patient group in future weight-bearing studies. In order to avoid selection bias and increase comparability, we limited our evaluation exclusively to patients with traumatic hip fractures and excluded patients who underwent elective THA due to advanced osteoarthritis of the hip joint, since mobilization of patients after traumatic injuries is typically more challenging than after elective surgery.

The second potential bias in our evaluation is a recall bias, since functional scores before the accident were determined based on the patient's memory. This can result in the subjectively perceived mobility before the accident being classified as too high or too low. For elective surgery, it is possible to obtain the functional scores directly before the operation or even to determine them directly. This is not possible in the case of accidents, since it is impossible to anticipate an accident, and therefore, it is not possible to collect data in advance. However, since our study only evaluates patients after an accident, this is the most accurate way to determine mobility before the accident. In addition, to minimize the risk of recall bias, patients were asked about their pre-accident mobility as soon as possible after hospital admission. In addition, we focused the evaluation on the objective data from our weight-bearing analysis and not on the subjective information provided by the patients.

The focus of our study was to determine and compare the actual weight-bearing ability of older patients with femoral neck fracture in the early postoperative period who underwent either THA or BA. Our study showed no significant difference between the two procedures regarding the weight-bearing ability. This might indicate that the effect of the comparatively more invasive procedure of THA on the postoperative weight-bearing ability of older patients may be overestimated. For a more accurate evaluation, future studies should investigate weight bearing after THA and BA in the medium- and long-term course and with an increased sample size.

5. Conclusions

Our study shows that older patients with femoral neck fracture undergoing THA and BA can achieve sufficient weight bearing on the operated leg in the early postoperative period. In our study, BA did not allow for a significantly higher average and maximum loading capacity in the early postoperative period compared with THA, meaning there were no relevant differences in terms of weight-bearing ability between the two groups. In our study, we were able to quantify the difference and objectify this hypothesis. This finding should be considered during the decision-making process of surgical treatment, especially in patients without a clear indication for one of the two surgical procedures. The extent to which the weight-bearing ability differs between the two surgical procedures in the long term must be shown in further studies.

Author Contributions: Methodology, C.G.; Formal analysis, C.G.; Investigation, C.G.; Data curation, C.G. and A.Z.; Writing—Original draft, C.G. and F.S.; Writing—Review and editing, C.G., I.H., S.K., V.S. and F.S.; Visualization, C.G. and F.S.; Supervision, F.S.; Project administration, C.G. and F.S. All authors have read and agreed to the published version of the manuscript.

Funding: This research received no external funding.

Institutional Review Board Statement: The study was conducted in accordance with the Declaration of Helsinki, and approved by the Institutional Review Board (IRB) (Ethic Committee Name: Ethic Committee of the Ludwig Maximilian University of Munich (LMU), Approval Code: 214-16, Approval Date: 28 June 2016)

Informed Consent Statement: Informed consent was obtained from all subjects involved in the study.

Data Availability Statement: Dataset available on request from the authors.

Acknowledgments: The authors would like to thank the research group for geriatric traumatology at the Ludwig Maximilian University of Munich for their friendly support. Furthermore, the authors would like to thank the entire team of the physiotherapy department at the Ludwig Maximilian University of Munich for their kind support in this project.

Conflicts of Interest: The authors declare no conflicts of interest.

References

1. Johnell, O.; Kanis, E.J. Epidemiology of osteoporotic fractures. *J. Clin. Orthop. Trauma* **2005**, *16* (Suppl. 2), S3–S7. [CrossRef] [PubMed]
2. Lorentzon, M.; Johansson, H.; Harvey, N.C.; Liu, E.; Vandenput, L.; McCloskey, E.V.; Kanis, J.A. Osteoporosis and fractures in women: The burden of disease. *Climacteric* **2022**, *25*, 4–10. [CrossRef] [PubMed]
3. Weyler, E.J.; Gandjour, A. Socioeconomic Burden of Hip Fractures in Germany. *Gesundheitswesen* **2007**, *69*, 601–606. [CrossRef] [PubMed]
4. Greenspan, S.L.; Myers, E.R.; Maitland, L.A.; Resnick, N.M.; Hayes, W.C. Fall Severity and Bone Mineral Density as Risk Factors for Hip Fracture in Ambulatory Elderly. *J. Am. Med. Assoc.* **1994**, *271*, 128–133. [CrossRef]
5. Broos, P.L.; Vecruyssee, R.; Fourneau, I.; Driesen, R.; Stappaerts, K.H. Unstable femoral neck fractures in young adults: Treatment with the AO 130-degree blade plate. *J. Orthop. Trauma* **1998**, *12*, 235–239. [CrossRef] [PubMed]
6. Zetterberg, C.H.; Irstam, L.; Andersson, B.J. Femoral Neck Fractures in Young Adults. *Acta Orthop.* **1982**, *53*, 427–435. [CrossRef] [PubMed]
7. Bales, C.W.; Ritchie, C.S. Sarcopenia, weight loss, and nutritional frailty in the elderly. *Annu. Rev. Nutr.* **2002**, *22*, 309–323. [CrossRef] [PubMed]
8. Karagas, M.R.; Lu-yao, G.L.; Barrett, J.A.; Beach, M.L.; Baron, J.A. Heterogeneity of Hip Fracture: Age, Rac, Sex, and Geographic Patterns of Femoral Neck and Trochanteric Fractures among the US Elderly. *Am. J. Epidemiol.* **1996**, *143*, 677–682. [CrossRef] [PubMed]
9. Girard, J.; Glorion, C. Risk Factors for Revision of Hip Arthroplasties in Patients Younger Than 30 Years. *Clin. Orthop. Relat. Res.* **2011**, *469*, 1141–1147. [CrossRef]
10. Sierra, T.P.; Martín, I.B.; Solís, J.R.; Goitiandia, L.B. Predictive factors of hospital stay, mortality and functional recovery after surgery for hip fracture in elderly patients. *Rev. Esp. Cir. Ortop. Traumatol.* **2017**, *61*, 427–435. [CrossRef]

11. Yoo, J.; Ha, Y.; Lim, J.; Kang, H.; Yoon, B.; Kim, H. Early Rehabilitation in Elderly after Arthroplasty versus Internal Fixation for Unstable Intertrochanteric Fractures of Femur: A Systematic Review and Meta-Analysis. *J. Korean Med. Sci.* **2017**, *32*, 858–867. [CrossRef] [PubMed]
12. Rapp, K.; Rothenbacher, D.; Magaziner, J.; Becker, C.; Benzinger, P.; König, H.-H.; Jaensch, A.; Büchele, G. Risk of Nursing Home Admission after Femoral Fracture Compared with Stroke, Myocardial Infarction, and Pneumonia. *J. Am. Med. Dir Assoc.* **2015**, *16*, e7–e715. [CrossRef]
13. Ariza-vega, P.; Kristensen, T.; Jime, J.; Martı, L. Predictors of Long-Term Mortality in Older People With Hip Fracture. *Arch. Phys. Med. Rehabil.* **2015**, *96*, 1215–1221. [CrossRef] [PubMed]
14. Friedman, S.M.; Mendelson, D.A. Epidemiology of Fragility Fractures. *Clin. Geriatr. Med.* **2014**, *30*, 175–181. [CrossRef]
15. Baer, M.; Neuhaus, V.; Pape, H.C.; Ciritsis, B. Influence of mobilization and weight bearing on in-hospital outcome in geriatric patients with hip fractures. *SICOT-J.* **2019**, *5*, 4. [CrossRef]
16. Pfeufer, D.; Grabmann, C.; Mehaffey, S.; Keppler, A.; Böcker, W.; Kammerlander, C.; Neuerburg, C. Weight bearing in patients with femoral neck fractures compared to pertrochanteric fractures: A postoperative gait analysis. *Injury* **2019**, *50*, 1324–1328. [CrossRef]
17. Blomfeldt, R.; Törnkvist, H.; Ericksson, K.; Söderqvist, A.; Ponzer, S.; Tidermark, J. A randomised controlled trial comparing bipolar hemiarthroplasty with total hip replacement for displaced intracapsular fractures of the femoral neck in elderly patients. *J. Bone Jt. Surg. Ser. B* **2007**, *89*, 160–165. [CrossRef] [PubMed]
18. Bhandari, M.; Devereaux, P.; TornettaIII, P.; Swiontkowski, M.F.; Berry, D.J.; Haidukewych, G.; Schemitsch, E.H.; Hanson, B.P.; Koval, K.; Dirschl, D.; et al. Operative Management of displaced femoral neck fractures in elderly patients: An international survey. *J. Bone Jt. Surg. Am.* **2005**, *87*, 2122–2131. [CrossRef] [PubMed]
19. Masson, M.; Parker, M.J.; Schoelzl, S. Internal fixation versus arthroplasty for intracapsular proximal femoral fractures in adults. *Cochrane Database Syst. Rev.* **2003**, CD001708. [CrossRef]
20. Schleicher, I.; Kordelle, J.; Jürgensen, I.; Haas, H.; Melzer, C. Die schenkelhalsfraktur beim alten menschen—Bipolare hemiendoprothese vs. total-endoprothese. *Unfallchirurg* **2003**, *106*, 467–471. [CrossRef]
21. Sharma, V.; Awasthi, B.; Kumar, K.; Kohli, N.; Katoch, P. Outcome analysis of hemiarthroplasty vs. Total hip replacement in displaced femoral neck fractures in the elderly. *J. Clin. Diagn. Res.* **2016**, *10*, RC11–RC13. [CrossRef] [PubMed]
22. Avery, P.P.; Baker, R.P.; Walton, M.J.; Rooker, J.C.; Squires, B.; Gargan, M.F.; Bannister, G.C. Total hip replacement and hemiarthroplasty in mobile, independent patients with a displaced intracapsular fracture of the femoral neck: A seven- to ten-year follow-up report of a prospective randomised controlled trial. *J. Bone Jt. Surg. Ser. B* **2011**, *93B*, 1045–1048. [CrossRef] [PubMed]
23. Baker, R.P.; Squires, B.; Gargan, M.F.; Bannister, G.C. Total Hip Arthroplasty and Hemiarthroplasty in Mobile, Independent Patients with a Displaced Intracapsular Fracture of the Femoral Neck. *J. Bone Jt. Surg. Am.* **2006**, *88*, 2583–2589. [CrossRef] [PubMed]
24. Squires, B.; Bannister, G. Displaced intracapsular neck of femur fractures in mobile independent patients: Total hip replacement or hemiarthroplasty? *Injury* **1999**, *30*, 345–348. [CrossRef] [PubMed]
25. Apivatthakakul, T.; Oh, J.-K. AO Surgery Reference, Proximal Femur. 2022. Available online: https://surgeryreference.aofoundation.org/orthopedic-trauma/adult-trauma/proximal-femur (accessed on 4 July 2022).
26. Tombaugh, T.N.; Mclntyre, N.J. The Mini-Mental State Examination. *J. Am. Geriatr. Soc.* **1992**, *40*, 922–935. [CrossRef] [PubMed]
27. D'Hoore, W.; Sicotte, C.; Tilquin, C. Risk adjustment in outcome assessment: The Charlson comorbidity index. *Methods Inf. Med.* **1993**, *32*, 382–387. [CrossRef]
28. Lübke, N.; Meinck, M.; Von Renteln-Kruse, W. Der Barthel-Index in der geriatrie. Eine kontextanalyse zum Hamburger Einstufungsmanual. *Z. Gerontol. Geriatr.* **2004**, *37*, 316–326. [CrossRef]
29. Parker, M.J.; Palmer, C.R. A new mobility score for predicting mortality after hip fracture. *J. Bone Jt. Surg. Ser. B* **1993**, *75*, 797–798. [CrossRef]
30. Anekar, A.A.; Cascella, M. WHO analgesic ladder. In *StatPearls [Internet]*; StatPearls Publishing: Treasure Island, FL, USA, 2021.
31. Samson, M.M.; Crowe, A.; de Vreede, P.L.; Dessens, J.A.G.; Duursma, S.A.; Verhaar, H.J.J. Differences in gait parameters at a preferred walking speed in healthy subjects due to age, height and body weight. *Aging Clin. Exp. Res.* **2001**, *13*, 16–21. [CrossRef] [PubMed]
32. Mak, J.C.S.; Cameron, I.D.; March, L.M. Evidence-based guidelines for the management of hip fractures in older persons: An update. *Med. J. Aust.* **2010**, *192*, 37–41. [CrossRef]
33. Ftouh, S.; Morga, A.; Swift, C. Management of hip fracture in adults: Summary of NICE guidance. *BMJ* **2011**, *342*, d3304. [CrossRef] [PubMed]
34. Mitchell, R. *Australian and New Zealand Hip Fracture Hospitalisation Trends: 2000–2001 to 2011–2012: Informing the Development of the Australian and New Zealand Hip Fracture Registry*; Australian & New Zealand Hip Fracture Registry: Sydney, Australia, 2014.
35. Bonnaire, F.; Weber, A. Schenkelhalsfraktur des Erwachsenen. *Leitlinien Unfallchirurgie* **2015**. Available online: https://www.awmf.org/uploads/tx_szleitlinien/012-001l_S2e_Schenkelhalsfraktur_2015-10-abgelaufen_02.pdf (accessed on 4 July 2022).
36. Tidermark, J. Quality of life and femoral neck fractures. *Acta Orthop.* **2003**, *74*, 1–42. [CrossRef]
37. Calder, S.J.; Anderson, G.H.; Jagger, C.; Harper, W.M.; Gregg, P.J. Unipolar or bipolar prosthesis for displaced intracapsular hip fracture in octogenarians: A randomised prospective study. *J. Bone Jt. Surg. Ser. B* **1996**, *78*, 391–394. [CrossRef]
38. Leon, D.A. Trends in European life expectancy: A salutary view. *Int. J. Epidemiol.* **2011**, *40*, 271–277. [CrossRef] [PubMed]

39. Oldmeadow, L.B.; Edwards, E.R.; Kimmel, L.A.; Kipen, E.; Robertson, V.J.; Bailey, M.J. No rest for the wounded: Early ambulation after hip surgery accelerates recovery. *ANZ J. Surg.* **2006**, *76*, 607–611. [CrossRef] [PubMed]
40. Kristensen, M.T.; Bandholm, T.; Bencke, J.; Ekdahl, C.; Kehlet, H. Knee-extension strength, postural control and function are related to fracture type and thigh edema in patients with hip fracture. *Clin. Biomech.* **2009**, *24*, 218–224. [CrossRef] [PubMed]
41. Sherrington, C.; Lord, S.R.; Herbert, R.D. A randomised trial of weight-bearing versus non-weight-bearing exercise for improving physical ability in inpatients after hip fracture. *Aust. J. Physiother.* **2003**, *49*, 15–22. [CrossRef] [PubMed]
42. Kronborg, L.; Bandholm, T.; Palm, H.; Kehlet, H.; Kristensen, M.T. Feasibility of progressive strength training implemented in the acute ward after hip fracture surgery. *PLoS ONE* **2014**, *9*, e0093332. [CrossRef] [PubMed]
43. Lamb, S.E.; Morse, R.E.; Evans, J.G. Mobility after proximal femoral fracture: The relevance of leg extensor power, postural sway and other factors. *Age Ageing* **1995**, *24*, 308–314. [CrossRef] [PubMed]
44. Jagos, H.; Pils, K.; Haller, M.; Wassermann, C.; Chhatwal, C.; Rafolt, D.; Rattay, F. Mobile gait analysis via eSHOEs instrumented shoe insoles: A pilot study for validation against the gold standard GAITRite®. *J. Med. Eng. Technol.* **2017**, *41*, 375–386. [CrossRef]
45. Marin, L.; Vandoni, M.; Zaza, G.; Febbi, M.; Pedrotti, L.; Chiodaroli, M.; Lovecchio, N.; Manzoni, F. The effects of insole-based visual feedback on weight-bearing in patients undergoing total hip replacement. *Int. J. Environ. Res. Public Health* **2021**, *18*, 3346. [CrossRef] [PubMed]

Journal of
Clinical Medicine

MDPI

Article

Bone Scintigraphy for Guidance of Targeted Treatment of Vertebral Compression Fractures

Elite Arnon-Sheleg [1,2], Daniel Weiner [2], Saeda Haj [3], Alon Rod [3] and Nimrod Rahamimov [2,3,*]

1 Department of Radiology and Nuclear Medicine, Galilee Medical Center, Nahariya 2210001, Israel
2 Azrieli Faculty of Medicine, Bar-Ilan University, Safed 5290002, Israel
3 Department of Orthopedics B and Spine Surgery, Galilee Medical Center, Nahariya 2210001, Israel; alonr@gmc.gov.il (A.R.)
* Correspondence: nimrodr@gmc.gov.il or nim205@gmail.com; Tel.: +972-505351635

Abstract: Background: Vertebral compression fractures (VCFs) are prevalent in the elderly population and might be the source of back pain if they are fresh and yet unhealed. In many cases, it is a diagnostic challenge to differentiate fresh VCFs from healed united fractures, which retain similar radiographic characteristics but no longer generate pain. This information is crucial for appropriate management. The aim of this study was to evaluate the role of bone scintigraphy (BS) in identifying fresh VCFs appropriate for targeted treatment when compared to the findings of Computerized Tomography (CT). **Methods**: We retrospectively reviewed 190 patients with back pain suspected to stem from a recent VCF that underwent both a CT and a BS and compared the imaging patterns per vertebra. **Results**: The studies were concordant in the majority of cases (95.5%), diagnosing 84.4% normal vertebrae, 6.4% acute VCFs, and 4.7% chronic VCFs. However, in 37 patients, 45 occult acute VCFs were only detected on BS and not on CT. Multivariate logistic regression analysis revealed that these patients were older and had lower bone density compared to the rest of the study population. Additionally, 40 patients had acute VCFs visible on CT, but with no increased or low intensity uptake on BS. These cases were associated with a shorter time period between trauma and BS, a higher prevalence of male patients, and a higher bone density. Acute VCFs with no increased uptake or low levels of uptake were found only within the first six days of the trauma. **Conclusions**: BS detects radiologically occult fractures and can differentiate if a radiographically evident VCF is indeed clinically active, guiding possible treatment options. To avoid missing acute VCFs, BS should be performed six days or more after the injury.

Keywords: bone scintigraphy; computed tomography; vertebral compression fracture; occult fracture; osteoporosis

1. Introduction

Vertebral compression fractures (VCFs) are one of the hallmark fractures of osteoporosis and are prevalent in the elderly population. The radiographic appearance of recent (fresh) VCFs and healed (old) VCFs can be similar, but since in acute and symptomatic VCFs, interventional procedures such as percutaneous vertebroplasty (VP), kyphoplasty (KP), or spine fusion surgery may be indicated [1], further imaging studies are needed to determine the fracture's age and guide appropriate patient management [2].

Magnetic resonance imaging (MRI) is the imaging method of choice for determining a VCF's age [3,4]. Acute fractures exhibit a low signal intensity on T1-weighted sequences and a high signal intensity on T2-weighted sequences. The abnormal signal gradually disappears within 2–4 months [5].

Bone scintigraphy (BS) using Tc99m-MDP can also be an effective method for determining the age of VCFs and is utilized mainly when MRI is unavailable or contraindicated.

In BS, an acute VCF presents as an intense horizontal linear tracer uptake in a vertebral body. This pattern usually appears within the first 48 h and decreases in intensity or fades over a period of 6 to 24 months [6]. Blood pool scintigraphy performed early, up to 5 min after injection of Tc-99m MDP, can demonstrate areas of hyperemia, also indicating an acute process [7].

In recent years, several small retrospective studies have compared the appearance of VCFs on MRI and BS with discordant results [8–10]. In one study, 30 patients who had undergone both BS and MRI evaluation were reviewed retrospectively with good consistency between the studies [11]. In a study of 30 patients with multilevel vertebral compression fractures, BS was found to better localize the fresh fracture causing clinical symptoms than MRI [12]. The small numbers in these studies and the varying outcome measures make it difficult to conclude whether BS can safely replace MRI as a method for determining a fracture's age and clinical relevance.

The aim of this study was to suggest a treatment algorithm utilizing BS rather than MRI as a guide in the decision-making process, by describing the patterns and temporal dynamics of VCFs on BS as related to the fracture type, age, and patient characteristics in a large patient population when MRI is unavailable in the initial evaluation and treatment phase.

2. Materials and Methods

This study was conducted retrospectively and was approved by our medical center's institutional review board (approval number 0038-20-NHR). The need for written informed consent was waived.

2.1. Study Population

Included were 200 consecutive patients admitted to our hospital between March 2017 and April 2022 with suspected acute VCFs in the thoracic and lumbar spine demonstrated on CT, corresponding with A1-type fractures according to the AOSpine Thoracolumbar Spine Injury Classification System and having undergone a BS were included [13]. Non-A1 fractures, systemic conditions affecting the skeleton (such as disseminated multiple myeloma, metastatic disease, or endocrine illnesses other than osteoporosis), as well as a technically inappropriate CT or BS were excluded, leaving 190 patients for further analysis.

2.2. Data Collection

The demographic and clinical information collected including age, gender, previously diagnosed osteoporosis, previously recorded trauma, and date of the trauma were retrieved from our hospital's electronic health records (EHRs).

CT of the spine was acquired using one of two CT scanners (Philips Ingenuity 128 and Brilliance 64, Cleveland, OH, USA). The CT parameters were as follows: tube voltage, 120 kV; tube current, 120–190 mA; slice thickness, 2 mm; detector collimation, 64 × 0.625 mm or 128 × 0.625 mm; gantry rotation time, 1; and pitch, 0.8. All CT data were reconstructed to a slice thickness of 2 mm, with a 512 × 512 matrix using a soft-tissue kernel. No oral or intravenous (IV) contrast media were administered. Sagittal and coronal reformatted images with a slice thickness of 2 mm were routinely created. In 161 patients, the CT included the thoracic and lumbar spine, and in 29 patients, only the lumbar spine. A total of 2966 vertebrae were scanned in 190 patients.

The CT images were reviewed by a radiologist and a spine surgeon for the presence of vertebral fractures at the time of admission. A spine surgeon retrospectively reviewed the CT images for the purpose of this study, defined the fractures as acute or chronic, and classified them using the AOSpine Thoracolumbar Spine Injury Classification System (AO type). Only A-type VCFs (compression injury) were included in the study. Signs of degenerative disc changes, including end plate sclerosis, irregularity, and osteophytes were noted separately.

A description of the CT pattern was documented for each vertebra according to the following (Figure 1): (A) normal vertebra (no fracture); (B) acute VCF displaying CT signs of loss of height or anterior wedge deformity with endplate irregularity, cortical incontinuity, step defects, increased density zone of impaction, and soft-tissue edema or hematoma surrounding the vertebral body; (C) non-union of a VCF displaying a non-healed fracture with an intravertebral cleft, also known as Kümmell's disease; (D) ankylotic VCF displaying a transverse fracture below an ankylotic spine segment; (E) chronic VCF displaying loss of height or anterior wedge deformity with smooth cortical borders; and (F) following percutaneous vertebroplasty (Post VP) displaying cement within the vertebral body.

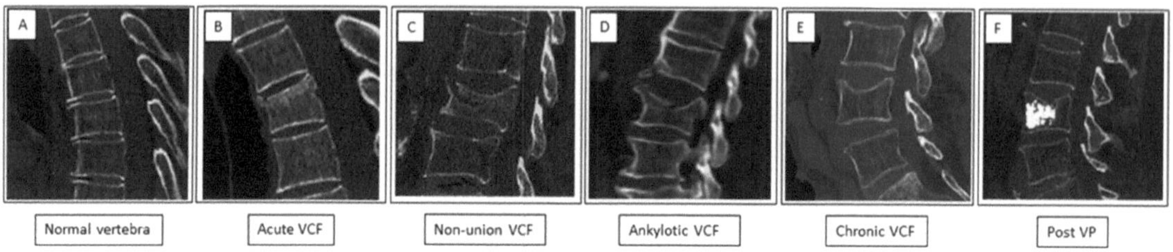

Figure 1. Patterns of vertebrae appearance on sagittal spine CT. (**A**) Normal vertebra—retained height and continuous cortex. (**B**) Acute VCF showing a "step defect" in the anterior border and a "zone of impaction" caused by impaction of the trabeculae. (**C**) Non-union fracture—a non-healed fracture with an intervertebral cleft (white arrow). (**D**) Ankylotic fracture—a transverse fracture below an ankylotic spine segment. (**E**) Chronic fracture showing loss of height and smooth cortical borders. (**F**) State after percutaneous vertebroplasty (Post VP)—chronic fracture with loss of height and hyperdense cement in the vertebral body.

The bone density was estimated for each patient using CT. Hounsfield units (HUs) were measured by placing a region of interest (ROI) in the intramedullary area of a lumbar vertebral body, preferably L3, unless fractured. Values measured below 118 HUs were consistent with osteopenia (T-score of −1.0 to −2.5). Values below 93 HUs were consistent with osteoporosis (T-score of −2.5 or less) [14].

BS was performed using one of two gamma cameras (Infinia Hawkeye and Optima 640, GE Medical Systems, Milwaukee, WI, USA) with a large field-of-view, dual-head, single-photon emission computed tomography (SPECT) system fitted with low-energy, high-resolution collimators. Whole-body planar acquisition was carried out using the continuous method in a 256 × 1024 matrix. SPECT images were obtained in a 128 × 128 matrix with a 20% window centered at 140 keV and were reconstructed with ordered subsets expectation maximization (OSEM), using 2 iterations. Early planar imaging of the spine and pelvis was performed 5–10 min after IV administration of 20–25 mCi (~740 MBq) of Tc99m-MDP (Jubilant DraxImage Inc, Canada) and late whole-body planar images and SPECT of the thoracic and lumbar spine were performed 2–4 h after injection. Early BS of the spine was performed in 185 patients (97%). All patients underwent late planar whole-body imaging and SPECT of the thoracic and lumbar spine with 2 fields of view (FOV). A total of 3230 vertebrae were scanned. All BS was reviewed by a board-certified nuclear medicine physician and findings on planar and SPECT images were documented for each vertebra. For early images, the presence or absence of increased blood pool was recorded. For late images, a 3-point visual score of the uptake pattern was documented according to the following: low intensity uptake, slightly above that of adjacent normal vertebra; intermediate intensity uptake, clearly above that of adjacent normal vertebra but below uptake in the sacroiliac joint (SIJ) or anterior superior iliac spine (ASIS); and high intensity uptake, similar or above uptake in the SIJ or ASIS.

Evaluation of the BS was performed unblinded to the findings on CT, which were used to accurately define the location of fractures and to distinguish between uptake caused by other etiologies such as osteophytes and degenerative changes. If the increased uptake was deemed to be the result of degenerative changes seen on the CT (rather than a fracture of the vertebral body), the uptake was excluded from the study.

2.3. Statistical Analysis

Data analysis was conducted using SPSS software, version 27.0 for Windows (IBM, New York, NY, USA). For normally distributed data, the results were presented as mean ± standard deviation and were analyzed using an unpaired Student's t-test. Categorical data were expressed as percentages to illustrate their distribution, and a p-value of less than 0.05 was considered to indicate statistical significance. To explore the relationship between bone density, sex, and age, Pearson's correlation test was employed. This test allowed for the assessment of the strength and direction of the linear relationship between these two continuous variables. Additionally, multivariate logistic regression analysis was performed to identify factors that could influence the likelihood of VCF detection. The variables included in this analysis were age, gender, the time elapsed between the trauma and scanning, and bone density. By incorporating these factors, the regression model aimed to determine the individual and combined effects on the odds of VCF detection provide a comprehensive understanding of the potential predictors in this clinical context.

3. Results

3.1. Patient Population

Two hundred consecutive patients were initially included. Ten patients were excluded from further analysis due to technically inappropriate or missing imaging studies or to etiology of fractures secondary to malignancy or multiple myeloma. A total of 2966 vertebrae were scanned in 190 patients.

The demographic data of the final study population of 190 patients are detailed in Table 1. Forty-three patients had documented osteoporosis on their electronic health records. In 108 patients (57%), a trauma event with a specific date was recorded; 19 patients (10%) had a known history of recent trauma within the previous two weeks but could not recall the exact date; and 63 patients (33%) had no history of a trauma event. In patients with a recorded trauma date, the mean time between the trauma and hospitalization was 6.1 days, and the mean time between the injury and BS was 8.3 days. All patients underwent CT within the first 48 h of admission. BS was acquired 48 h after the CT, except in four cases in which the study was performed on the same day or a day before the CT. The mean time interval between CT and BS was 3.1 days (see Table 1). An MRI study was not obtained in any of the patients.

Table 1. Patient characteristics.

		n	%	Mean	SD	Minimum	Maximum
Gender	male	60	31.6				
	female	130	68.4				
Age		190		75	11.2	36	98
Time between CT and BS		190		3.1	4.8	−1	33
Time between the trauma and hospitalization		108		6.1	10.7	0	61
Time between the trauma and BS		108		8.3	10.5	1	62

3.2. CT Findings

In CT, 84 patients (44.2%) had a single acute VCF, 48 patients (25.2%) had 2 VCFs, 26 patients (13.7%) had 3 acute VCFs, and 32 patients (16.8%) had more than 3 acute VCFs, with the highest number being 11 acute VCFs in a single patient. VCFs were observed in 439 vertebrae on CT, including 240 which had radiologic patterns of acute VCFs (54.7%), 162 chronic VCFs (36.9%), and 37 post VP VCFs (8.4%). Most of the VCFs were located between T11 and L4, with L1 being the most common location (Figure 2). Among the acute VCFs, 49 were non-union and 16 were fractures below an ankylotic segment.

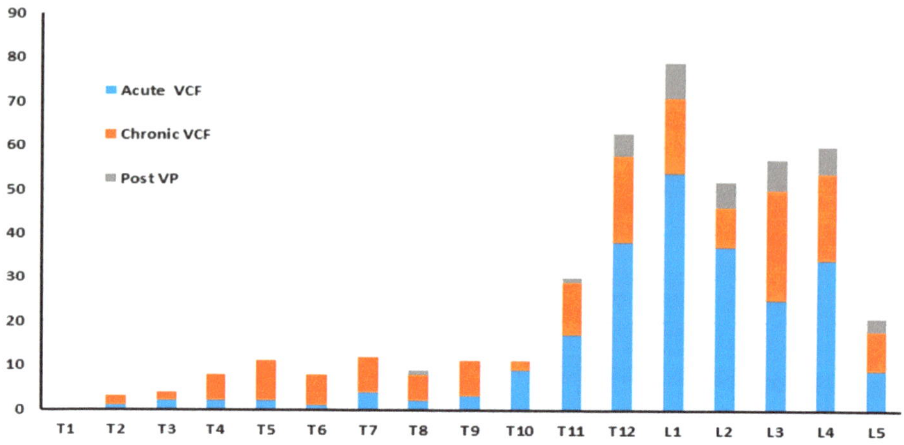

Figure 2. Distribution of VCFs according to type and location on CT.

3.3. Bone Density

The CT-measured mean bone density was 61.2 ± 32 HU, with a range of −21–164 HUs. Values above 118 HUs, considered normal, were found in 10 patients (5.2%). Values of 93 to 118 HUs, consistent with osteopenia, were found in 17 patients (8.9%), and values below 93 HUs, consistent with osteoporosis, were found in 163 patients (85.7%). The mean bone density in women was significantly lower compared to men (55.6 ± 31 HUs compared to 73.3 ± 31 HUs, $p < 0.001$) and lower values were found with increasing age of the patients in both men and women ($r = -0.368$, $p < 0.001$).

3.4. BS Findings

In BS, increased uptake, consistent with a vertebral fracture, was observed in 323 vertebrae. The uptake intensity was low in 81 (25%) vertebrae, intermediate in 107 (33%), and high in 135 (42%) vertebrae. Most of the vertebrae with an abnormal uptake were seen in the thoraco-lumbar region (Figure 3).

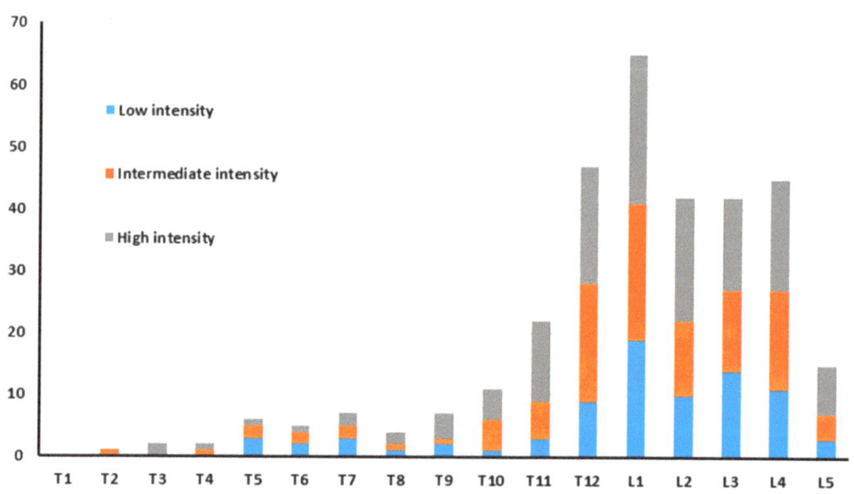

Figure 3. Distribution of VCFs according to uptake intensity and location on bone scintigraphy.

In early BS, increased blood pool was observed in 193 vertebrae (60%). In late BS, vertebrae showing hyperemia in early studies had higher uptake intensities; a total of 121 vertebrae (63%) had a high intensity uptake, 60 (31%) had intermediate, and 12 (6%) had low-level uptake. Increased late tracer uptake without hyperemia was found in 130 vertebrae (40%), with lower uptake intensities; a total of 14 vertebrae had high-intensity uptake (11%), 47 had intermediate (36%), and 69 had low-intensity uptake (53%). Hyperemia was more prevalent in the lower thoracic and lumbar spine (T11 to L5, 63%) compared to the high and mid-thoracic spine (T1 to T10, 42%).

In a subgroup of 108 patients with a known date of the traumatic event and 132 acute VCFs according to CT, BS uptake intensity was compared to the time period elapsed since the trauma. Acute VCFs with no increased uptake were found up to five days after trauma, and VCFs with low-intensity uptake were seen up to six days after trauma. Acute VCFs with intermediate- and high-intensity uptake were seen from the first day after trauma up to 38 and 62 days, respectively (Figure 4).

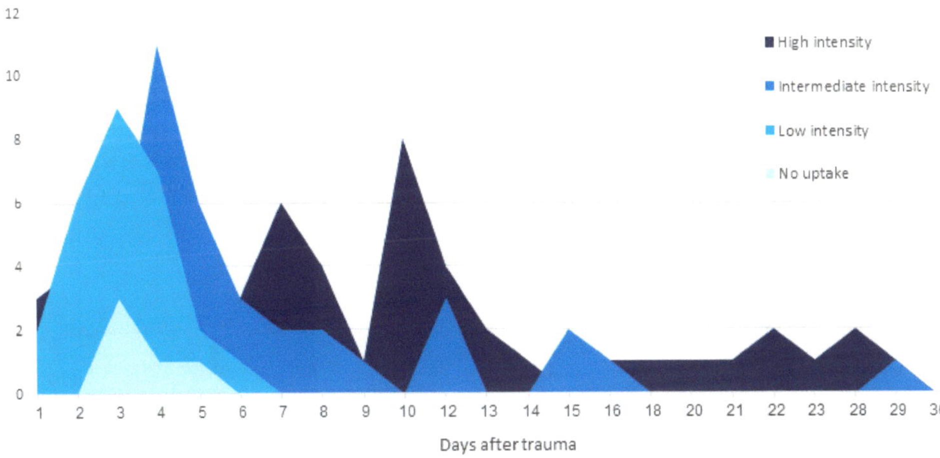

Figure 4. Radiotracer uptake intensity according to time after trauma.

Increased uptake in ribs, sacrum, and pelvis, consistent with acute fractures, were seen in the majority of the patients (160, 84%) in BS. Single-rib fractures were observed in 28 patients, multiple-rib fractures in 63 patients, sacral fractures in 55, and pelvic fractures in 14 patients.

3.5. Comparison of CT and BS Findings

The imaging patterns of CT and BS were compared in 2966 vertebrae. Table 2 and Figures 5–7 demonstrate the different combined patterns of CT and BS.

Table 2. Prevalence of combined CT and BS patterns (n = 2966).

CT Pattern	BS Uptake Intensity	Number	%
Normal	No increased uptake	2504	84.4
Normal	Low	3	0.1
Normal	Intermediate	6	0.2
Normal	High	14	0.5
Acute VCF	No increased uptake	7	0.2
Acute VCF	Low	43	1.4
Acute VCF	Intermediate	79	2.7
Acute VCF	High	111	3.7
Chronic VCF	No increased uptake	117	3.9
Chronic VCF	Low	23	0.8

Table 2. *Cont.*

CT Pattern	BS Uptake Intensity	Number	%
Chronic VCF	Intermediate	15	0.5
Chronic VCF	High	7	0.2
Post VP	No increased uptake	15	0.5
Post VP	Low	12	0.4
Post VP	Intermediate	7	0.2
Post VP	High	3	0.1

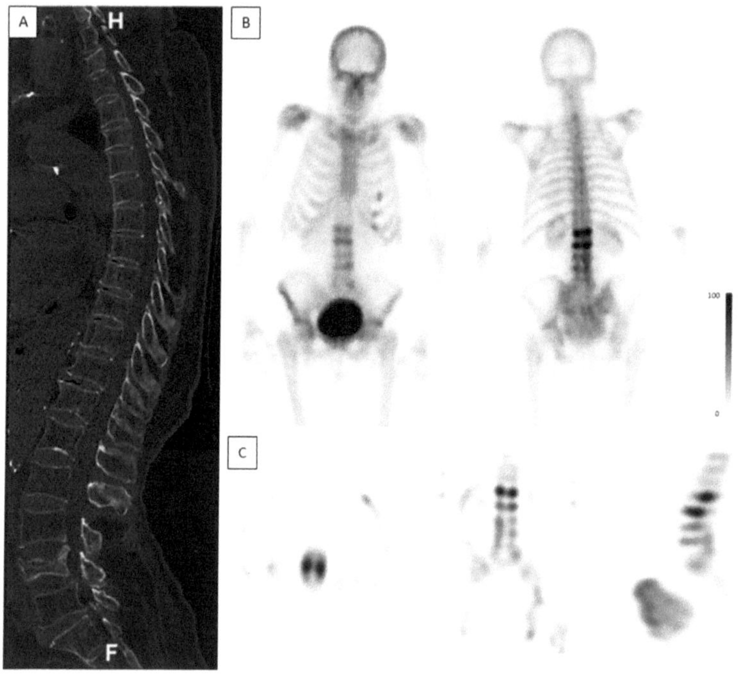

Figure 5. Occult fractures. A 78-year-old female complaining of back pain, without known trauma. CT was acquired on the day of admission and bone scintigraphy was performed 2 days after the CT. (**A**)—Sagittal spine CT shows a non-union fracture in L4. No other fractures are demonstrated. Bone density measured in L3 was 7 HUs, consistent with severe osteoporosis. (**B**)—Planar anterior and posterior bone scintigraphy shows high-intensity uptake in L2 and L3, suggestive of acute fractures. (**C**)—Axial, coronal, and sagittal SPECT show high-intensity uptake in L2 and L3.

Normal vertebrae—In the group of vertebrae with a normal appearance on CT, most had no increased uptake on BS (2504/2527, 99%). Increased uptake was seen in 23 (0.9%) vertebrae that appeared normal on CT, consistent with the diagnosis of an acute radiologically occult fracture (Figure 5). This pattern combination was observed in 17 patients. Multivariate logistic regression analysis of these patients indicated that an increase in age (OR = 0.913, 95% CI [0.840, 0.993], $p = 0.035$) and a decrease in bone density (OR = 0.969, 95% CI [0.939, 1.000], $p = 0.052$) were associated with a decrease in the odds of detection of a VCF on the CT. Notably, these associations remained statistically significant, even after controlling for gender and the time elapsed between the trauma and scanning. Gender and time elapsed from trauma had no significant impact on the likelihood of detection of an occult fracture.

Acute VCFs—Most vertebrae with acute fractures on CT had an increased uptake on BS (233/240, 97%), with 79 and 111 showing intermediate- and high-intensity uptake, respectively (Figure 6), and 43 showing low-intensity uptake (Figure 7). In seven acute VCFs, no increased uptake was seen on BS. The pattern combination of acute VCF with no increase or low-intensity uptake was observed in 40 patients. The clinical characteristics of these patients were compared to the group with intermediate- or high-intensity uptake. In univariate analyses, the time elapsed between the trauma and BS was significantly shorter in these patients (4.62 $\pm$ 6.18 vs. 9.68 $\pm$ 11.48 days, $p = 0.026$) and male gender was more prevalent (31.7% vs. 16.2%; $p = 0.015$). Bone density was higher, but not statistically significant (69.90 $\pm$ 34.92 vs. 58.87 $\pm$ 30.98, $p = 0.053$). Multivariate logistic regression analysis also found a significant difference in the time span elapsed from the traumatic event to BS, with a shorter time period in the low-uptake group (OR = 0.908, 95% CI [0.822, 1.003], $p = 0.057$). No association was found with patient's age.

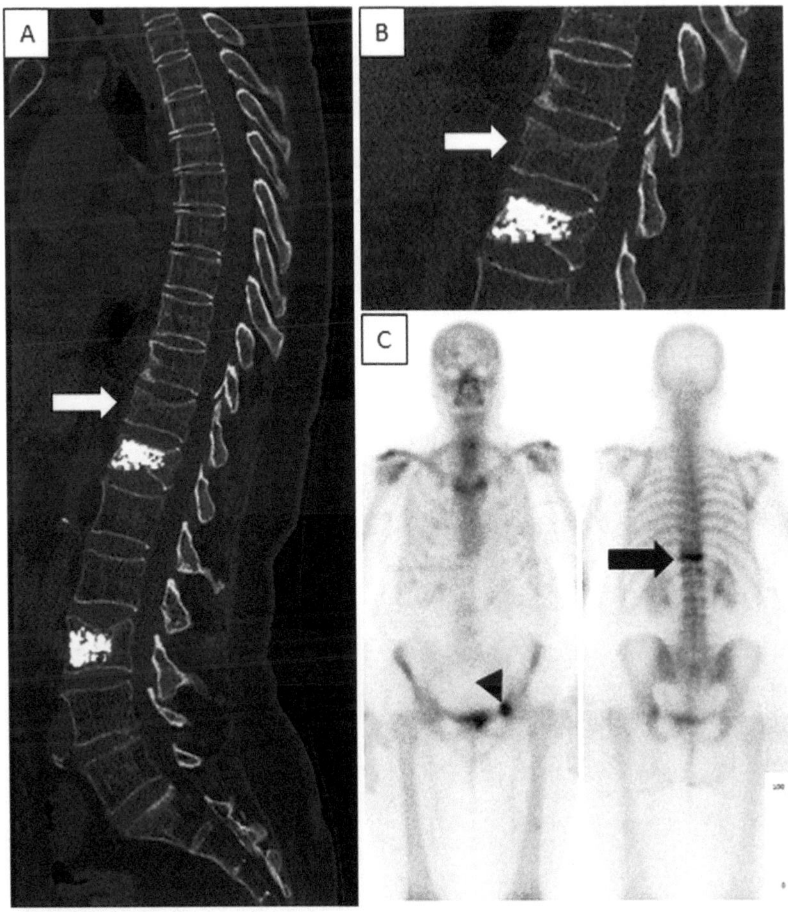

Figure 6. High-intensity uptake in an acute fracture, no uptake in chronic fractures post-vertebroplasty. A 77-year-old female after trauma. CT was acquired on the day of injury and bone scintigraphy was performed 3 days after the injury. (**A**,**B**)—Sagittal spine CT (enlarged in B) show an acute fracture in T11 (white arrow) and chronic fractures after vertebroplasty in T12 and L3. (**C**)—Planar anterior and posterior bone scintigraphy show high-intensity uptake in T11 (black arrow), indicating an acute fracture and no increased uptake in T12 and L3, consistent with chronic fractures. Note also, high-intensity uptake is seen in the anterior aspect of the left acetabulum (black arrow head), consistent with an acute fracture.

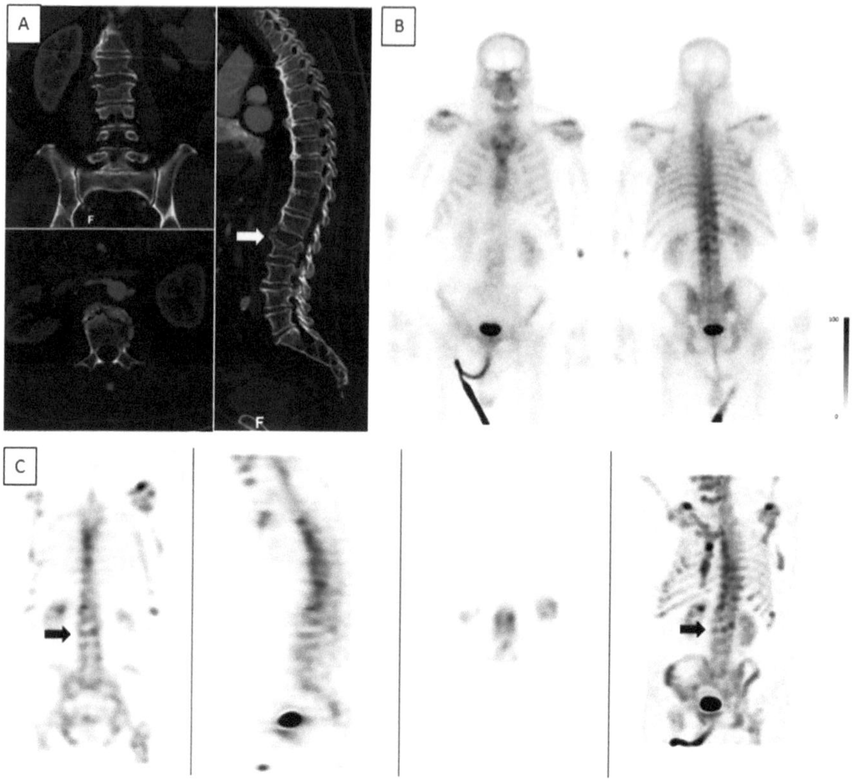

Figure 7. Low-intensity uptake in an acute ankylotic VCF. A 72-year-old male. CT was acquired on the day of injury and bone scintigraphy was performed 3 days after the injury. (**A**)—Coronal, axial, and sagittal spine CT show an acute ankylotic fracture in L2 and a fracture involving an osteophyte in L1 (white arrow). (**B**)—Planar anterior and posterior bone scintigraphy do not show any increased uptake in L2. (**C**)—Coronal, sagittal, axial, and MIP SPECT show only low-intensity uptake in L2 (black arrow).

Hyperemia was seen in the early BS images in 157 acute VCFs (65%). In 83 acute VCFs (35%), no hyperemia was observed.

In non-union VCFs, intermediate- and high-intensity uptakes were more prevalent (41 vertebrae, 84%), with few cases showing no increase in uptake or low-intensity uptake (8 vertebrae, 16%). In ankylotic VCFs, intermediate- and high-intensity uptakes were found in 12 vertebrae (63%) and low-intensity or no increase in uptake were observed in 7 vertebrae (37%). Univariate or multivariate logistic regression analysis were not possible due to the small number of cases.

Chronic VCFs—Among 162 vertebrae with chronic fractures according to CT, 117 did not display increased uptake (72%). Low-intensity uptake was observed in 23 vertebrae (14%), and high- and intermediate-intensity uptake was seen in 15 and 7 vertebrae (9% and 4%), respectively. The pattern combination of chronic VCFs with intermediate- or high-intensity uptake was observed in 20 patients, suggestive of an unstable or "active" fracture. Multivariate analysis of these patients' clinical characteristics showed a significantly lower bone density (43.55 vs. 63.26 HU, p = 0.009) and a trend towards female gender that was not statistically significant (p = 0.092).

Post VP—Most vertebrae in this group showed no increase (15, 40%) or a low-intensity uptake (12, 32%), and few demonstrated intermediate- and high-intensity uptake (7, 19% and 3, 8%, respectively).

4. Discussion

The present study identified and characterized 2966 vertebrae in 190 patients with 439 VCFs. The study population was mostly elderly and female. Only 5% of the patients had normal bone density, estimated using spine CT, and over 85% had osteoporosis according to these measurements. Most patients (55.8%) had more than one VCF, with 16.8% of them having three or more VCFs. In some cases, a combination of acute and chronic fractures was found. Most of the fractures were located in the thoraco-lumbar area.

In most patients, the CT results were retrospectively sufficient to determine whether a vertebra was normal or had either acute or chronic VCFs, but in 37 (19.5%) patients, BS added important information related to the fracture that could influence patient management, as radiologically occult fresh fractures were found in 23 normal-appearing vertebrae and in 22 vertebrae with the radiographic appearance of chronic fractures. These occult fractures were amenable to surgical intervention, which could potentially improve pain relief and facilitate patient mobilization [1].

The phenomenon of radiologically occult fractures, also known as "VCFs without radiologic collapse", has been described in several studies. Pham et al. described 16 osteoporotic subjects with acute, severe back pain, but no evidence of VCF on a lateral spine radiograph. MRI or BS showed findings consistent with acute fractures in an anatomic distribution, correlating with the clinical pain. The subjects were followed prospectively with radiographic changes, consistent with VCFs developing in 80% of subjects by the end of the study [15]. Additional studies and reviews have described this phenomenon on radiographs [16–20] but not on CT. Our study has demonstrated that occult fractures may also be present and missed on diagnostic, high-resolution CT or may be present in a vertebra with imaging characteristics of a chronic fracture. In multivariate logistic regression analysis, occult fractures in normal-appearing vertebrae on CT were associated with an increase in patient age and a decrease in bone density. This could be explained by the lower visibility of cortical disruption and the impaction of the trabeculae in osteoporotic vertebrae, which have thinner and less dense trabeculae and corteces. The patient's gender and the time elapsed between the traumatic event and scanning had no significant impact on the likelihood of detection of an occult fracture on BS.

In our study group, 40 patients had acute VCFs with no increase or low-intensity uptake on BS. These were observed up to 6 days after injury. According to the known literature, increased radiotracer uptake appears in vertebral fractures on BS during the osteoblastic activity phase, signifying the initiation of the healing process, usually during the first hours after injury. In many cases, fractures can be seen on BS much earlier than on radiographs or even CT, mainly in rib and sacral fractures [7]. In the seminal study by Matin et al. from 1979, the appearance of various fractures on BS over time was reported in 204 patients aged between 17 and 88 years, with a third of patients being over 65 years [21]. In their study, 80% of all fractures showed an abnormal uptake by 24 h, and 95% by 72 h after injury. Only in two patients, both over the age of 65 years, there was no increased uptake on BS in a known acute fracture by 72 h. While this study suggests that in the elderly population, scintigraphic abnormalities may appear later than in younger patients, it did not focus on vertebral fractures and had only a limited number of elderly patients. In our study, a higher percentage of patients had no uptake or low-grade uptake in acute VCFs for a longer period of time, suggesting that a longer lag period between the injury and BS is needed to prevent a false-negative diagnosis.

Another study by Spitz et al. from 1992 investigated the appearance of fractures on BS in 480 patients, including 123 fractures in the thoracic and lumbar spine and 357 fractures in other bones, including the radius, scaphoid, femoral neck, pelvis, and shaft of long bones [22]. In 18 patients, repeated scanning was conducted during the initial 24 h after injury. All acute fractures showed increasing accumulation of Tc-99m MDP at the fracture site in those 24 h and within 2 weeks after injury, but the magnitude of the increase was markedly different in different bones. Spine fractures showed the latest and slowest accumulation of Tc-99m MDP, with some fractures appearing only 10 to 12 days after the injury. The authors suggested that these findings are related to the amount of callus formation found in fractures adjacent to joints compared to vertebral fractures, and that a similar behavior can be seen in skull fractures that show minimal uptake on BS and almost no callus formation on radiographs. Multiple-regression analysis of their data did not find any correlation between the time of appearance of the fracture and the patient's age and gender, in contrast to Matin et al.'s study. The authors concluded that the rate of accumulation of Tc-99m MDP is only dependent on the fracture site, with slower accumulation in the spine and the shafts of long bones.

The appearance of vertebral fractures over time on BS has not been investigated in more recent years. Our results show that the time of appearance of increased tracer uptake is not dependent only on age, as suggested by Matin et al., or only on the timing of BS and the fracture location, as suggested by Spitz et al., but is influenced by multiple factors, including the injury to BS lag period, the patient's gender, and bone density. In the sub-group of ankylotic fractures with no uptake or low-grade uptake, we also observed a higher prevalence of males, but this was not statistically significant. Since diffuse idiopathic skeletal hyperostosis (DISH) occurs more in males [23,24], this may explain their higher prevalence in this group. A further study of this population is needed to elucidate the reasons for this phenomenon.

According to orthopedic guidelines, MRI is considered the gold-standard method for determining the acuity of a VCF, while the combination of CT and BS is reserved for claustrophobic patients or for MRI incompatibility [3,4,25]. Only one guideline refers to MRI and BS equally as "advanced imaging" that can reliably confirm the presence and location of acute VCFs that may be amenable to treatment [26]. Our study provides additional evidence demonstrating that in clinical scenarios when MRI is unavailable in the acute setting, a combination of spine CT and BS can be used for establishing the age of vertebral fractures and to detect additional occult fractures, supporting clinical decision-making. This is visualized in Figure 8, in which a diagnostic flow-chart algorithm is provided.

While BS is considered a sensitive method for detecting acute fractures and for determining a fracture's age [6,27], several studies report discordance between the results of MRI and BS concerning the establishment of the age of VCFs. A study by Masala et al. found that MRI and BS are concordant for fractures up to 4 months old [8]. Kim et al. found an overall concordance of only 55% between the methods. The concordance for single-level VCFs was very high (96%), with a significant drop in concordance in two-level (50%) and three-level fractures (only 36%) [9]. In a study by Dafydd et al. from 2014, the overall concordance was of 63%, with almost twice as many acute or subacute fractures found on BS [10]. These studies suggest that acute fractures appear on BS for a longer period of time than on MRI. In multilevel fractures, the different VCFs probably have different ages, with older fractures not apparent on MRI but still seen on BS. Therefore, it can be assumed that the information regarding the temporal dynamics is not equivalent in BS and MRI. Despite the discordance between the methods, BS was found to be a useful method for locating the painful vertebra before deciding on surgical treatment [28–31]. Most of these studies had a small number of up to 44 patients, none of them used an early blood pool phase, and SPECT/CT was used only in a single study. To the best of our knowledge, this is the first study comparing imaging patterns of VCFs in BS and CT at varying time points, using modern, state-of-the-art equipment.

In our study, an early blood pool phase scan was acquired in 97% of the patients, and all studies included SPECT of the thoracic and lumbar spine. The majority of acute VCFs, 65%, showed hyperemia. The fact that 83/240 (35%) of these fractures demonstrated no hyperemia may be explained by relatively older aged fractures. Early blood pool images are characterized by low-resolution and unfavorable target-to-background ratios and, in the thoracic spine, vertebral hyperemia is often obscured by uptake in the mediastinum. Therefore, it might be concluded that although hyperemia can be considered a definite sign of acute fracture, its sensitivity is low and its absence should not rule out an acute VCF.

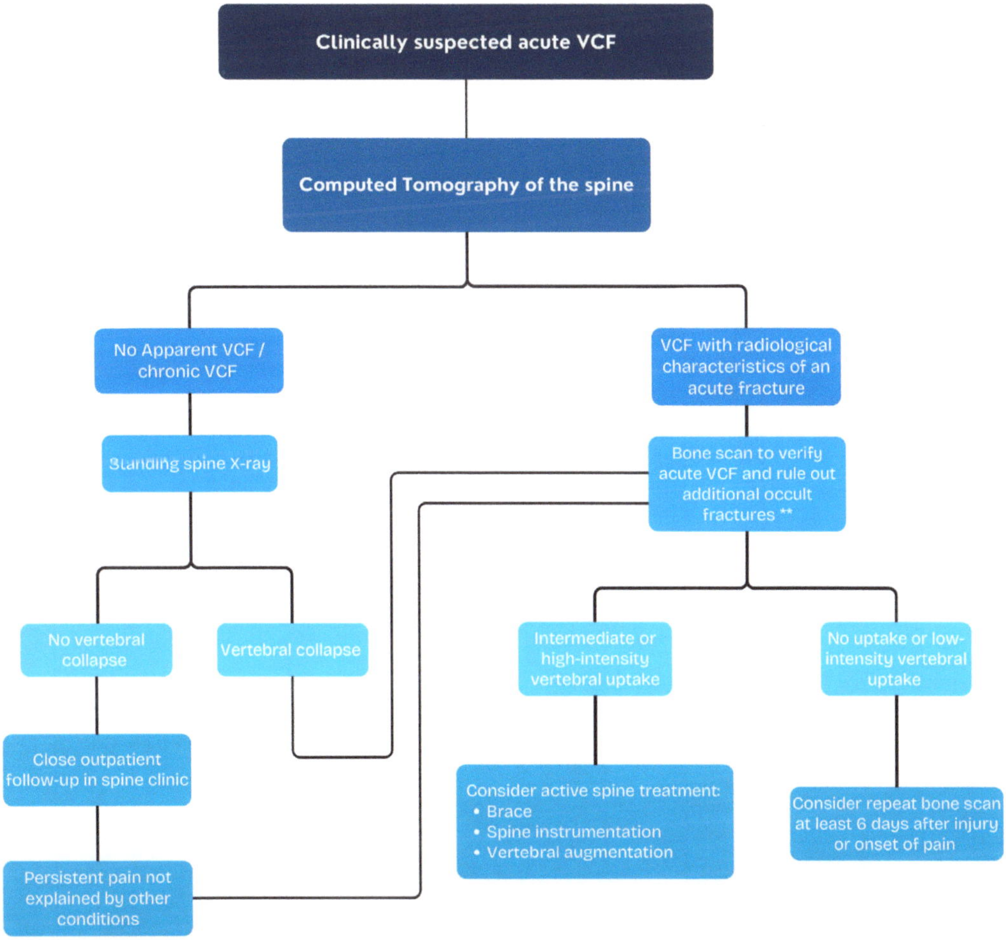

Figure 8. VCF diagnostic flow-chart. When MRI is unavailable or contraindicated. ** Bone scan should be obtained at least 48 h after injury or onset of pain.

SPECT studies are known to increase the sensitivity and specificity of BS [32]. In the current study, SPECT images were very helpful in detecting low-intensity uptakes that would have been missed using only planar images, as shown in Figure 7. They were also paramount for determining the exact location of the fractures and were easier to compare to the recently performed spine CT. The combined viewing of the SPECT and CT images was helpful in differentiating uptakes caused by degenerative changes vs. true fractures. If spine CT is not acquired prior to the bone scintigraphy in patients with suspected acute VCF, SPECT/CT should be performed when available.

The imaging patterns observed in the current study may be extrapolated in the future, after additional research, to other bone imaging scintigraphy methods such as F18-fluoride positron emission tomography (PET) or PET/MR.

Our study was limited by using retrospective data. More definite data may have been gained by repeating BS at decided time points during the first week after injury, but this was not clinically feasible. Estimation of osteopenia and osteoporosis in our patient population was performed using an opportunistic method applied to the previously acquired spine CT. Although this method was investigated and found to accurately represent mineral bone density [14], using dual x-ray absorptiometry would have been more precise.

Main Findings in This Study

In 19.5% of our patients, a BS added important information related to the fracture that could influence patient management.

A fresh VCF may be present in a vertebra with imaging characteristics of a chronic fracture.

A fresh VCF may be present with CT characteristics of a normal vertebra.

Although hyperemia can be considered a definite sign of an acute fracture, its sensitivity is low and its absence should not rule out an acute VCF

BS is equivalent to MRI as a corroborating modality in determining the age of VCFs found on radiographs or CT.

5. Conclusions

Bone scans, in the setting of vertebral compression fractures in the elderly population, add valuable information on the fracture's age, can detect occult fractures, and can subsequently affect patient management. The ideal timing of the scan should be considered as in some cases, no increased uptake or only low-intensity uptake was demonstrated in acute fractures up to six days after trauma.

Author Contributions: Conceptualization, N.R. and E.A.-S.; methodology, N.R. and E.A.-S.; formal analysis, A.R.; investigation, D.W. and S.H.; data curation, D.W., S.H. and A.R.; writing—original draft preparation, E.A.-S.; writing—review and editing, N.R.; All authors have read and agreed to the published version of the manuscript.

Funding: This research received no external funding.

Institutional Review Board Statement: Thid study was conducted in accordance with the Declaration of Helsinki and was approved by the Ethics Committee of The Galilee Medical Center, Nahariya, Israel (protocol code 0038-20-NHR, 21 April 2020).

Informed Consent Statement: Patient consent was waived due to this being a retrospective anonymous study evaluating regular treatment.

Data Availability Statement: Data used for this study may be obtained, on request, from the corresponding author.

Acknowledgments: We are grateful to Basem Hijazi for experimental design and statistical analysis, and Adi Shani for coordinating this study.

Conflicts of Interest: The authors declare no conflicts of interest.

References

1. Kondo, K.L. Osteoporotic vertebral compression fractures and vertebral augmentation. *Semin. Intervent. Radiol.* **2008**, *25*, 413–424. [CrossRef] [PubMed]
2. Rahamimov, N.; Arnon-Sheleg, E. Identifying Multi-Level Vertebral Compression Fractures Following a Convulsive Seizure. *Isr. Med. Assoc. J.* **2021**, *23*, 526–528. [PubMed]
3. McConnell, C.T.; Wippold, F.J.; Ray, C.E.; Weissman, B.N.; Angevine, P.D.; Fries, I.B.; Holly, L.T.; Kapoor, B.S.; Lorenz, J.M.; Luchs, J.S.; et al. ACR Appropriateness Criteria Management of Vertebral Compression Fractures. *J. Am. Coll. Radiol.* **2014**, *11*, 757–763. [CrossRef] [PubMed]
4. Hirsch, J.A.; Beall, D.P.; Chambers, M.R.; Andreshak, T.G.; Brook, A.L.; Bruel, B.M.; Deen, H.G.; Gerszten, P.C.; Kreiner, D.S.; Sansur, C.A.; et al. Management of vertebral fragility fractures: A clinical care pathway developed by a multispecialty panel using the RAND/UCLA Appropriateness Method. *Spine J.* **2018**, *18*, 2152–2161. [CrossRef] [PubMed]

5. Lin, H.-H.; Chou, P.-H.; Wang, S.-T.; Yu, J.-K.; Chang, M.-C.; Liu, C.-L. Determination of the painful level in osteoporotic vertebral fractures—Retrospective comparison between plain film, bone scan, and magnetic resonance imaging. *J. Chin. Med. Assoc.* **2015**, *78*, 714–718. [CrossRef] [PubMed]
6. Vali, R.; Bajno, L.; Kousha, M.; Martin, C. The Potential Role of Radionuclide Imaging in Osteoporotic Vertebral Fracture and Sacral Fracture. *Spine Res.* **2016**, *2*, 1. [CrossRef]
7. Ziessman, H.A.; O'Malley, J.P.; Thrall, J.H. *Nuclear Medicine: The Requisites in Radiology*; Mosby Elsevier: Maryland Heights, MO, USA, 2006; ISBN 0323029469.
8. Masala, S.; Schillaci, O.; Massari, F.; Danieli, R.; Ursone, A.; Fiori, R.; Simonetti, G. MRI and bone scan imaging in the preoperative evaluation of painful vertebral fractures treated with vertebroplasty and kyphoplasty. *In Vivo* **2005**, *19*, 1055–1060. [PubMed]
9. Kim, J.-H.; Kim, J.-I.; Jang, B.-H.; Seo, J.-G.; Kim, J.-H. The Comparison of Bone Scan and MRI in Osteoporotic Compression Fractures. *Asian Spine J.* **2010**, *4*, 89. [CrossRef] [PubMed]
10. Ap Dafydd, D.; Salem, S.; Zerizer, I.; Yan Mok, W.; Gishen, P.; Patel, M.C.; Patel, N.H.; Al-Nahhas, A.; Dunn, J.; Win, Z. The value of combined assessment of vertebral fractures with 99mTc MDP scintigraphy and MRI in selecting and planning percutaneous vertebroplasty. *Nucl. Med. Commun.* **2014**, *35*, 755–761. [CrossRef] [PubMed]
11. Zhao, Y.; Zhang, T.; Tang, P. Diagnostic value of SPECT/CT bone imaging in fresh osteoporotic vertebral compression fractures. *Hell. J. Nucl. Med.* **2022**, *25*, 138–142.
12. Okazaki, T.; Nakagawa, H.; Yagi, K.; Hayase, H.; Nagahiro, S.; Saito, K. Bone scintigraphy for the diagnosis of the responsible level of osteoporotic vertebral compression fractures in percutaneous balloon kyphoplasty. *Clin. Neurol. Neurosurg.* **2017**, *152*, 23–27. [CrossRef] [PubMed]
13. Vaccaro, A.R.; Oner, C.; Kepler, C.K.; Dvorak, M.; Schnake, K.; Bellabarba, C.; Reinhold, M.; Aarabi, B.; Kandziora, F.; Chapman, J.; et al. AOSpine thoracolumbar spine injury classification system: Fracture description, neurological status, and key modifiers. *Spine* **2013**, *38*, 2028–2037. [CrossRef] [PubMed]
14. Schreiber, J.J.; Anderson, P.A.; Rosas, H.G.; Buchholz, A.L.; Au, A.G. Hounsfield Units for Assessing Bone Mineral Density and Strength: A Tool for Osteoporosis Management. *J. Bone Jt. Surg.* **2011**, *93*, 1057–1063. [CrossRef] [PubMed]
15. Pham, T.; Azulay-Parrado, J.; Champsaur, P.; Chagnaud, C.; Legré, V.; Lafforgue, P. "Occult" Osteoporotic Vertebral Fractures. *Spine* **2005**, *30*, 2430–2435. [CrossRef] [PubMed]
16. Yang, X.; Mi, S.; Mahadevia, A.A.; Lin, X.; Shi, W.; Liu, A.; Li, L.; Wu, Z.; Murphy, K. Pain reduction in osteoporotic patients with vertebral pain without measurable compression. *Neuroradiology* **2008**, *50*, 153–159. [CrossRef] [PubMed]
17. McKiernan, F.E. The broadening spectrum of osteoporotic vertebral fracture. *Skeletal Radiol.* **2009**, *38*, 303–308. [CrossRef] [PubMed]
18. Kim, Y.J.; Chae, S.U.; Kim, G.D.; Park, K.H.; Lee, Y.S.; Lee, H.Y. Radiographic Detection of Osteoporotic Vertebral Fracture without Collapse. *J. Bone Metab.* **2013**, *20*, 89. [CrossRef] [PubMed]
19. Wáng, Y.X.J.; Che-Nordin, N. Some radiographically 'occult' osteoporotic vertebral fractures can be evidential if we look carefully. *Quant. Imaging Med. Surg.* **2019**, *9*, 1992–1995. [CrossRef] [PubMed]
20. Du, M.-M.; Che-Nordin, N.; Ye, P.-P.; Qiu, S.-W.; Yan, Z.-H.; Wang, Y.X.J. Underreporting characteristics of osteoporotic vertebral fracture in back pain clinic patients of a tertiary hospital in China. *J. Orthop. Transl.* **2020**, *23*, 152–158. [CrossRef]
21. Matin, P. The appearance of bone scans following fractures, including immediate and long-term studies. *J. Nucl. Med.* **1979**, *20*, 1227–1231. [PubMed]
22. Spitz, J.; Lauer, I.; Tittel, K.; Wiegand, H. Scintimetric evaluation of remodeling after bone fractures in man. *J. Nucl. Med.* **1993**, *34*, 1403–1409. [PubMed]
23. Fournier, D.E.; Leung, A.E.; Battié, M.C.; Séguin, C.A. Prevalence of diffuse idiopathic skeletal hyperostosis (DISH) and early-phase DISH across the lifespan of an American population. *Rheumatology* **2024**, *63*, 1153–1161. [CrossRef] [PubMed]
24. Ahmed, O.; Ramachandran, K.; Patel, Y.; Dhanapaul, S.; Meena, J.; Shetty, A.P.; Bhari Thippeswamy, P.; Kanna, R.M.; Rajasekaran, S. Diffuse Idiopathic Skeletal Hyperostosis Prevalence, Characteristics, and Associated Comorbidities: A Cross-Sectional Study of 1815 Whole Spine CT Scans. *Glob. Spine J.* **2022**, *14*, 219256822211368. [CrossRef] [PubMed]
25. Bravo, A.E.; Brasuell, J.E.; Favre, A.W.; Koenig, B.M.; Khan, A.A.; Beall, D.P. Treating Vertebral Compression Fractures: Establishing the Appropriate Diagnosis, Preoperative Considerations, Treatment Techniques, Postoperative Follow-Up and General Guidelines for the Treatment of Patients With Symptomatic Vertebral Compression Fractu. *Tech. Vasc. Interv. Radiol.* **2020**, *23*, 100701. [CrossRef] [PubMed]
26. Barr, J.D.; Jensen, M.E.; Hirsch, J.A.; McGraw, J.K.; Barr, R.M.; Brook, A.L.; Meyers, P.M.; Munk, P.L.; Murphy, K.J.; O'Toole, J.E.; et al. Position Statement on Percutaneous Vertebral Augmentation: A Consensus Statement Developed by the Society of Interventional Radiology (SIR), American Association of Neurological Surgeons (AANS) and the Congress of Neurological Surgeons (CNS), American Col. *J. Vasc. Interv. Radiol.* **2014**, *25*, 171–181. [CrossRef] [PubMed]
27. Martin, J.G.; Goldman, D.T.; Dabrowiecki, A.M.; Newsome, J.; Bercu, Z.L.; Gilliland, C. Additional Magnetic Resonance or Nuclear Scintigraphy Imaging Influences Approach to Vertebral Augmentation. *Spine* **2020**, *45*, E927–E932. [CrossRef] [PubMed]
28. Tang, Z.; Lei, Z.; Yang, H.; Chen, K. Value of Bone Scan Imaging in Determining Painful Vertebrae of Osteoporotic Vertebral Compression Fractures Patients With Contraindications to MRI. *Orthop. Surg.* **2012**, *4*, 172–176. [CrossRef] [PubMed]
29. Solá, M.; Pérez, R.; Cuadras, P.; Díaz, R.; Holgado, S.; Puyalto, P.; Iborra, M.; Fraile, M. Value of bone SPECT-CT to predict chronic pain relief after percutaneous vertebroplasty in vertebral fractures. *Spine J.* **2011**, *11*, 1102–1107. [CrossRef] [PubMed]

30. Jordan, E.; Choe, D.; Miller, T.; Chamarthy, M.; Brook, A.; Freeman, L.M. Utility of Bone Scintigraphy to Determine the Appropriate Vertebral Augmentation Levels. *Clin. Nucl. Med.* **2010**, *35*, 687–691. [CrossRef] [PubMed]
31. Maynard, A.S.; Jensen, M.E.; Schweickert, P.A.; Marx, W.F.; Short, J.G.; Kallmes, D.F. Value of bone scan imaging in predicting pain relief from percutaneous vertebroplasty in osteoporotic vertebral fractures. *AJNR. Am. J. Neuroradiol.* **2000**, *21*, 1807–1812. [PubMed]
32. Savelli, G.; Maffioli, L.; Maccauro, M.; De Deckere, E.; Bombardieri, E. Bone scintigraphy and the added value of SPECT (single photon emission tomography) in detecting skeletal lesions. *Q. J. Nucl. Med.* **2001**, *45*, 27–37.

Journal of
Clinical Medicine

MDPI

Review

An Umbrella Review and Updated Meta-Analysis of Imaging Modalities in Occult Scaphoid and Hip and Femoral Fractures

Patricia Jorisal [1,2,*], Callistus Bruce Henfry Sulay [3] and Gilbert Sterling Octavius [3]

1 Abdominal Radiology, Department of Radiology, Faculty of Universitas Pelita Harapan, Tangerang 12930, Indonesia
2 Department of Radiology, Siloam Hospital Kebon Jeruk, Jakarta 11530, Indonesia
3 Radiology Resident, Faculty of Universitas Pelita Harapan, Tangerang 12930, Indonesia
* Correspondence: patricia.raduph@gmail.com

Abstract: Background: Occult fractures may cause multiple morbidities. If occult fractures were detected earlier, complications may be preventable. This umbrella review and updated meta-analysis will aim to evaluate the use of imaging modalities in detecting occult scaphoid and hip fractures. **Methods:** The protocol for this study is available in the International Prospective Register of Systematic Reviews (PROSPERO) database (CRD42024525388). The literature search started and ended on 17 March 2024. We searched seven academic databases: MEDLINE, Cochrane Library, Pubmed, Science Direct, Google Scholar, WHO International Clinical Trials Registry Platform, and The Joanna Briggs Institute (JBI) database. The meta-analysis was conducted with the STATA program using the "midas" command. **Results:** There are four systematic reviews evaluating occult hip and femoral fractures with 6174 patients and two reviews evaluating occult scaphoid fractures with 1355 patients. The prevalence of occult scaphoid fracture and occult hip and femoral fractures is 23.87% (95% CI 18.25–29.49) and 44.8% (95% CI 39.38–51.4), respectively. Magnetic resonance imaging (MRI) had the best posterior probability of positive likelihood ratio (LR+) with 95% and 96% and negative likelihood ratio (LR-) with 0.15% and 1% for both occult scaphoid and hip fractures, respectively, assuming a 25% baseline. MRI could both confirm and exclude occult hip fractures while it can only confirm occult scaphoid fractures. Bone scans are inappropriate for either type of occult fractures The level of evidence for occult scaphoid fracture is weak while it is suggestive for occult hip fractures. **Conclusion:** The findings strengthen the use of MRI after an initially negative radiograph fracture for occult hip and femoral fractures, with a CT scan as a viable second option.

Keywords: occult fracture; magnetic resonance imaging; computed tomography; scaphoid; hip

1. Introduction

The definition of occult fractures, or negative radiograph fractures, is a fracture that is not initially seen in all available conventional radiography projections and a follow-up imaging (using conventional radiography or other modalities) reveals the cortical break in the bones [1]. Delayed diagnosis and treatment increase the likelihood of complications such as nonunion, avascular necrosis, and osteoarthritis in occult scaphoid fractures. Patients will also require further imaging while being splinted. This overtreatment results in a loss of productivity for the patients and a potential lawsuit for the clinical provider [2,3]. Although there is no increased mortality in occult hip fractures as compared to patients with apparent radiograph hip fractures [4], delaying the diagnosis of a proximal femur hip fracture can result in poorer patient outcomes. Earlier diagnosis of hip and femoral fractures will obviate the need for more extensive surgery [5].

The use of additional imaging for occult fractures is not new. However, the debate on what is the best next course of action after an initial negative radiograph persists. The American College of Radiology (ACR) recommends magnetic resonance imaging (MRI)

as the first line for detection of occult fractures. However, some authors argue against the routine use of MRI in the detection of occult fractures as it leads to overdiagnosis and overtreatment [6]. Another point of view is that the patient's preferences need to be incorporated into the decision-making, which hinges the diagnosis on multifactorial components and not just on the sensitivity and specificity of said imaging modalities [7].

There are also other modalities with strengths and limitations in diagnosing occult fractures, which may complement each other. For example, computed tomography (CT) may also replace MRI due to its more widespread availability in smaller centres compared to MRI despite its radiation penalty. There is also ultrasound, which is gaining increasing traction to be used as a radiation-free and widely available bedside tool to diagnose occult fracture, although the literature is very scarce. Lastly, nuclear studies or bone scans are very sensitive but the relative radiation level is sometimes unacceptable [8,9].

Therefore, this umbrella review and updated meta-analysis will aim to evaluate the use of imaging modalities in detecting occult scaphoid and hip fractures. To the best of our knowledge, this is the first attempt at an umbrella review and updated meta-analysis in this field, which will comprehensively summarize all the literature available on the pertaining topic.

2. Materials and Methods

2.1. Search Strategy and Study Selection

The literature search started and ended on 17 March 2024. We searched five academic databases: MEDLINE, Cochrane Library, Pubmed, Science Direct, and Google Scholar. The authors also searched the WHO International Clinical Trials Registry Platform and The Joanna Briggs Institute (JBI) database on the same day for ongoing clinical trials. The keywords used were related to the diagnostic tool ("X-ray, "cone beam computed tomography", "magnetic resonance imaging", "computed tomography", "bone scan", and "ultrasound") and the condition under study ("occult fracture", "suspected fracture", "non-displaced fracture", and "negative radiograph fracture"), as well as the word or filter "systematic review" and "meta-analysis". Supplementary Table S1 lists the Medical Subject Heading (MeSH) terms for each database. All records were entered into the Rayyan program, which manually screened them and automatically identified duplicates [10]. The initial search was conducted by authors GSO and CBHS, who imported all findings into Rayyan software. A separate evaluation of the initial searches was performed by author P.J. Each paper underwent individual assessment by GSO and CBHS, with conflicts resolved through group discussion and professional judgment from P.J. In instances where research from the same dataset had overlapping time points, we prioritized data that offered the most comprehensive information.

After the umbrella review was conducted, we found two anatomical sites of occult fractures included in our review, which were the hip or femur and scaphoid. A separate search strategy was conducted on the same day (25 March 2024) for these two anatomical sites using the same strategy as above and the MeSH terms were listed in Supplementary Tables S2 and S3. There are no other anatomical sites that could be included in this review which met the criteria. The search of the study was limited to one year before the latest systematic review until the present. For example, if the latest systematic review on scaphoid searched for 2020, we limited the search term from 2019 until 25 March 2024.

2.2. Eligibility Criteria

The authors followed the Preferred Reporting Items for Systematic reviews and Meta-Analyses (PRISMA) 2020 as well as the PRISMA Diagnostic Test Accuracy (PRISMA-DTA) guidelines [11,12]. The protocol for this study is available in the International Prospective Register of Systematic Reviews (PROSPERO) database (CRD42024525388).

This is an umbrella review and although the methodology had not been properly standardized [13,14], this review opted for an updated meta-analysis [15]. Therefore, the authors conducted a systematic search according to PRISMA 2020 guidelines for each topic found under the umbrella review. The studied population was all patients with occult fractures (defined as no cortical breaks or fracture lines seen on a plain radiograph series with a high clinical suspicion for fracture due to intense pain, swelling, inability to move the affected body parts, or other clinical suspicions) who underwent further imaging with reference standards. In this review, reference standards were considered adequate if they fulfilled one of the following criteria: (1) A follow-up plain radiograph series (with a minimum of two views) conducted at a minimum of six weeks apart after the initial injury; (2) clinical findings with an index test or repeated radiographs to formulate a reference standard; and (3) the use of advanced imaging that serves as a reference standard, which differs from the modality used as the index test (i.e., the use of a single computed tomography [CT] or MRI without any referenced index would not suffice). In a retrospective study, this review also considered studies that confirmed fractures with a clinical follow-up only, although this is not optimal.

2.3. Inclusion and Exclusion Criteria

The inclusion criteria were articles of any prospective or retrospective cohort studies that studied occult fractures in all ages with a reference index as delineated above. The search was also conducted for grey literature, including theses, dissertations, and conference abstracts. The exclusion criteria included case series, case reports, or animal research. Studies that did not perform the reference test according to our criteria were also excluded. To ensure that the literature was saturated, review study citations were looked up. We also manually searched and cited the literature to make sure that all pertinent studies were covered. There was no restriction on the language.

2.4. Data Extraction and Quality Assessment

Two authors (G.S.O. and C.B.H.S.) independently extracted the data, while all three authors verified its accuracy. We gathered pertinent data, including study identity (author and publication year), study characteristics (location, study design, and age of the participants), modalities used for the imaging, and the operational definition of fractures. The number of true positives (TP), false positives (FP), true negatives (TN), and false negatives (FN) were also extracted from each study.

As for the umbrella review, the A MeaSurement Tool to Assess Systematic Reviews 2 (AMSTAR 2) was used to evaluate each systematic review. A high-quality systematic review has no or one non-critical weakness, a moderate-quality systematic review means there is more than one non-critical weakness. One critical flaw with or without non-critical weakness placed the systematic review in low quality, while a critically low systematic review meant that there was more than one critical flaw with or without non-critical weakness [16].

To evaluate the risk of bias in the updated meta-analysis, we employed the Revised Tool for the Quality Assessment of Diagnostic Accuracy Studies (QUADAS-2). In QUADAS-2, there are no official cut-off scores, and bias risk is displayed graphically [17].

The scale was independently assessed by two reviewers, G.S.O. and C.B.H.S., with any discrepancies resolved internally and through the expertise of P.J. until consensus was achieved. In cases of missing or incomplete data, we reached out to the associated authors via email.

2.5. Stratification of Evidence

After the updated meta-analysis, a stratification of evidence was conducted according to this classification: Class I: Convincing—When there are over 1000 cases, the *p*-value is less than 10^{-6}, I2 is less than 50%, 95% prediction interval excludes the null hypothesis, there are no small-study effects, and no excess significance bias; Class II: Highly suggestive—When there are over 1000 cases, *p*-value is less than 10^{-6}, the largest study shows a statistically significant effect, but it does not meet all Class I criteria; Class III: Suggestive—When there are over 1000 cases, *p*-value is less than 10^{-3}, and it does not meet Class I or II criteria;

Class IV: Weak—When p-value is less than 0.05, but it does not meet Class I to III criteria; and Non-significant—When p-value is greater than 0.05 [14].

2.6. Data Synthesis

This review evaluated matrices of evidence and the calculation of the overall corrected covered area (CCA) according to Bracchiglione et al. [18] Each study in a given systematic review would be read one by one to ensure that they fulfil the inclusion criteria. This review calculated the point prevalence of occult fractures by dividing the number of occult fractures by the total number of patients being worked up for occult fractures. DerSimonian and Laird's random-effect model was chosen, and we calculated the 95% confidence interval (CI) using the Clopper–Pearson method [19]. We used prediction intervals to assess heterogeneity if more than 10 studies were included [20], and between-study heterogeneity was explored with a Galbraith plot [21]. Small-study effects were assessed with funnel plot analysis if there were more than ten studies included [22], Begg and Mazumdar's test for rank correlation [23], and Egger's test for a regression intercept [24]. Trim-and-fill analysis was done if there was an asymmetry in the funnel plot [25]. We also conducted a sensitivity analysis to assess one study's impact on the overall prevalence [26].

The sensitivity, specificity, LR+, LR−, PPV, and NPV of each study were calculated if no information was given in the article [27]. Model diagnostics were verified using a graphical representation of residual-based goodness of fit, bivariate normality, influence, and outlier detection analysis before moving forward with the meta-analysis. Sensitivity analyses would be used to confirm any outlier research. The level of interconnectedness would be represented by the bivariate box plot. We used the bivariate model of sensitivity and specificity to calculate the individual and pooled sensitivity and specificity [28]. Using the hierarchical summary receiver operating characteristic (HSROC), a summary receiver operating characteristic (SROC) was utilized to show and highlight the trade-off between sensitivity and specificity [29]. The area under the curve (AUC) was measured, and a value of 0.9–1 indicated excellent diagnostic accuracy, 0.8–0.9 indicated very good diagnostic accuracy, 0.7–0.8 indicated good diagnostic accuracy, 0.6–0.7 indicated sufficient diagnostic accuracy, and 0.5–0.6 meant poor diagnostic accuracy [30]. Heterogeneity was measured using the I2 index; a value of 0% indicated that there was no detectable heterogeneity, while a value of more than 50% was considered to be high heterogeneity [31]. To assess publication bias, a linear regression test of funnel plot asymmetry was performed; a slope coefficient of less than 0.1 signified a significant asymmetry. We used the Fagan plot, which is based on the likelihood ratio scattergram and the Bayes theorem, to determine the post-test probability. An arbitrary cut-off point was set at <-0.1 for LR− and $>+10$ for LR+, indicating significant changes in the probability ratio [32]. Furthermore, the probability modifying plots and predictive values were shown; curves that incline toward the (0,1) location were produced by test results with more informative positive results, and curves that incline toward the (1,0) line were produced by test results with more informative negative results [33]. The meta-analysis was carried out using the STATA program (Version 17.0, StataCorp, College Station, Texas, USA) using the "midas" commands. These commands could only synthesize data if there were at least four studies included [34].

3. Results

A total of 12,488 articles were initially identified, out of which 40 duplicates were promptly eliminated, leaving 12,448 unique articles for screening. Following the evaluation of titles and abstracts, 12,136 articles were excluded, and ultimately, six studies were included in the umbrella review (Supplementary Figure S1). Four reviews [35–38] evaluated occult hip and femur fractures with a combined total of 6174 patients and two reviews [39,40] evaluated occult scaphoid fractures with a combined total of 1355 patients. Amongst reviews evaluating hip and femur fractures, three of them achieve a high quality under AMSTAR-2 scoring, while one scores a critically low rating. Amongst scaphoid reviews, one scores a high quality and one scores a critically low rating (Table 1). There is a high overlap (12.94%) between the primary studies of occult hip and femur fractures, with 16 overlapping studies in two systematic reviews and three studies in three systematic reviews. The review conducted by Haj-Mirzaian (2020) [38] and Chatha (2011) [35] produced the largest overlap with 29.5% (Figure 1). Notable exclusions are presented in Supplementary Table S4.

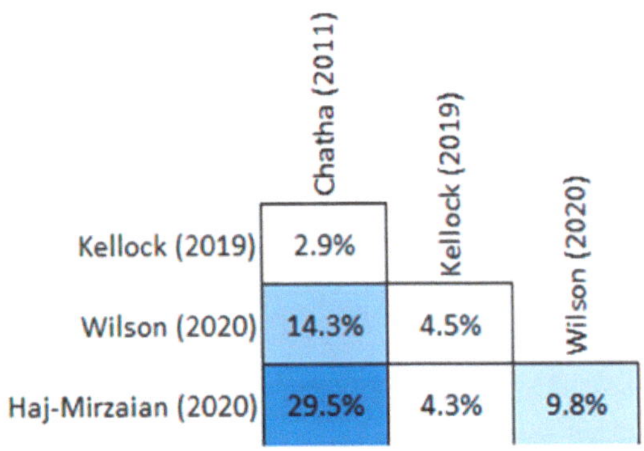

Figure 1. Graphical Representation of Overlap for OVErviews (GROOVE) of occult hip and femur fractures [35–38].

Table 1. Characteristics of systematic reviews and meta-analysis included in the umbrella review.

Author (Year)	Objectives	Anatomy	Setting and Context	Number of Databases Sourced and Searched	Date Range of Database Searching	Publication Date Range of Studies Included in the Review that Inform Each Outcome of Interest	Number of Studies	Types of Studies	Total Number of Patients	Country of Origin of Studies	Instruments Used to Appraise the Primary Studies	AMSTAR	Relevant Outcomes Reported	Methods of Synthesis	Publication Bias	Heterogeneity	Risk of Bias
Chatha (2011) [35]	To determine the role of CT and MRI in diagnosing occult fracture	Femur	N/A	5 (MEDLINE, EMBASE, CINAHL, Google Scholar, and the Cochrane Library)	31 October 2009	1989 to 2009	22	15 prospective and 7 retrospective	996	N/A	None	Critically low	MRI was an investigation of choice for occult proximal femoral fractures.	Qualitative	N/A	N/A	N/A
Kellock (2019) [36]	The diagnostic performance of CT for the detection of occult proximal femoral fracture	Femur	N/A	3 (Pubmed, Embase, and Web of Science)	1 December 2018	2005 to 2018	13	1 prospective, the rest are retrospective	1248	5 UK, 1 USA, 1 Israel, 3 Sweden, 1 Romania, 1 Denmark, 1 Canada	QUADAS-2	High Quality	The estimated summary sensitivity of CT for the detection of nondisplaced hip fracture was 94% (95% credible interval, 83–99%), and the specificity was 100% (95% credible interval, 99–100%) with an AUC of 0.981.	Meta-analysis	Present	Present	High risk of bias in the reference standard, with no single study achieving a good quality
Wilson (2019) [37]	Evaluate the diagnostic accuracy of limited MRI protocols for detecting radiographically occult proximal femoral fractures	Femur	All single-centre, academic hospitals	4 (MEDLINE, Embase, Cochrane Library and Scopus)	15 November 2019	1993–2019 (2012 to 2019 for meta-analysis; 1993 to 2016 for systematic review)	11 (only five for meta-analysis)	5 Prospective, 6 Retrospective (1 prospective and 4 retrospective for meta-analysis; 4 prospective and 2 retrospective for systematic review)	938	N/A	QUADAS-2	High Quality	The pooled and weighted summary sensitivity and specificity and the area under the summary ROC curve for limited MRI protocols in detecting radiographically occult hip fractures were 99% (95% CI, 91–100%), 99% (95% CI, 97–100%), and 100% (95% CI, 0.99–1), respectively.	Qualitative and Meta-Analysis	N/A	N/A	All studies included in the meta-analysis were low-risk
Haj-Mirzaian (2020) [38]	Determine the diagnostic performance of CT and bone scanning in the detection of occult fractures using MRI as the reference standard	Femoral head, femoral neck, intertrochanteric, or sub-trochanteric fractures	N/A	3 (Pubmed, EMBASE, and Cochrane Library)	27 September 2018	1993 to 2018	35	N/A	2992	N/A	ROB	High Quality	CT and bone scanning yielded comparable diagnostic performance in the detection of radiographically occult hip fracture ($p = 0.67$) with a sensitivity of 79% and 87%, respectively.	Meta-analysis	Present	Present	Low ROB = 27, Moderate ROB = 6, High ROB = 2

Table 1. *Cont.*

Author (Year)	Objectives	Anatomy	Setting and Context	Number of Databases Sourced and Searched	Date Range of Database Searching	Publication Date Range of Studies Included in the Review that Inform Each Outcome of Interest	Number of Studies	Types of Studies	Total Number of Patients	Country of Origin of Studies	Instruments Used to Appraise the Primary Studies	AMSTAR	Relevant Outcomes Reported	Methods of Synthesis	Publication Bias	Heterogeneity	Risk of Bias
Mallee (2015) [39]	identify the most suitable diagnostic imaging strategy for identifying clinically suspected fractures of the scaphoid bone in patients with normal radiographs	Scaphoid	People of all ages who presented at the hospital or clinics within one week of trauma with a clinically suspected scaphoid fracture and negative post-trauma radiographs	10 (Cochrane Register of Diagnostic Test Accuracy Studies, MEDLINE, EMBASE, the Database of Abstracts of Reviews of EHects, the Cochrane Central Register of Controlled Trials, the NHS Economic Evaluation Database, MEDION, ARIF, Current Controlled Trials, the World Health Organization (WHO) International Clinical Trials Registry Platform)	July 2012	1983–2011	11	9 Prospective, 3 Not Reported	1041	5 Netherlands, 2 Austria, 1 Turkey, 1 Denmark, 1 Ireland, 1 Norway	Not Specified	High Quality	Summary sensitivity and specificity of CT were 0.72 (95% confidence interval (CI) 0.36 to 0.92) and 0.99 (95% CI 0.71 to 1.00); for MRI, these were 0.88 (95% CI 0.64 to 0.97) and 1.00 (95% CI 0.38 to 1.00); for BS, these were 0.99 (95% CI 0.69 to 1.00) and 0.86 (95% CI 0.73 to 0.94). Indirect comparisons suggest that the diagnostic accuracy of BS was significantly higher than CT and MRI, and CT and MRI have comparable diagnostic accuracy.	Meta-analysis	Present	Could not be investigated formally	Five studies were considered "good quality", and six studies had "moderate quality".
Kwee (2018) [40]	To systematically review the literature on the performance of ultrasound in diagnosing radiographically occult scaphoid fracture.	Scaphoid	N/A	2 (MEDLINE and Embase databases)	No Limit–8 January 2018	2001–2013	7	Not Specified	314	1 Turkey, 2 Switzerland, 1 USA, 1 France, 1 Austria, 1 UK	QUADAS-2	Critically low	The sensitivity and specificity of ultrasound in diagnosing radiographically occult scaphoid fracture ranged from 77.8% to 100% and from 71.4% to 100% respectively, with pooled estimates of 85.6% (95% CI: 73.9%, 92.6%) and 83.3% (95% CI: 72.0%, 90.6%), respectively.	Meta-analysis	Not Assessed	Cannot be explored	Index Test: Low ROB: 6, High ROB: 1; Reference Standard: High ROB: 2, Unclear: 2; Low ROB: 3; Patient Selection and Flow and Timing: Low ROB 7.

An additional search for scaphoid occult fractures yielded four new articles [41–44] (Supplementary Figure S2). There were 23 studies with 1208 patients with suspected occult scaphoid fractures and 236 patients with eventual scaphoid fractures (Supplementary Table S7). Notable exclusions are presented in Supplementary Table S5. One study [45] was removed from a meta-analysis included in the umbrella review [40] as it did not fit the inclusion criteria. All studies were done prospectively with only thirteen studies explicitly mentioning that the studies employed consecutive sampling. Six studies [46–51] used ultrasound as the index test enrolling 270 patients, five studies [41,52–55] used a CT scan enrolling 297 patients, eight studies [42–44,54–58] used MRI enrolling 345 patients, seven studies [44,52,56,59–62] used bone scans enrolling 586 patients, and two studies [63,64] used cone-beam computed tomography (CBCT) enrolling 144 patients. Most patients are male, with females only ranging from 0% [53] to 64% [43]. The reference test was widely heterogeneous, ranging from retrospective clinical examination, a follow-up X-ray, bone scan, CT scan, MRI, or a combination of clinical and radiographic examinations. The machines and protocols used also varied widely (Supplementary Table S6). As a whole, the studies included for occult scaphoid fracture had relatively good qualities. However, only four studies [47,48,50,57] were free of bias, while the rest were at risk of some bias (Figure 2 and Table A1).

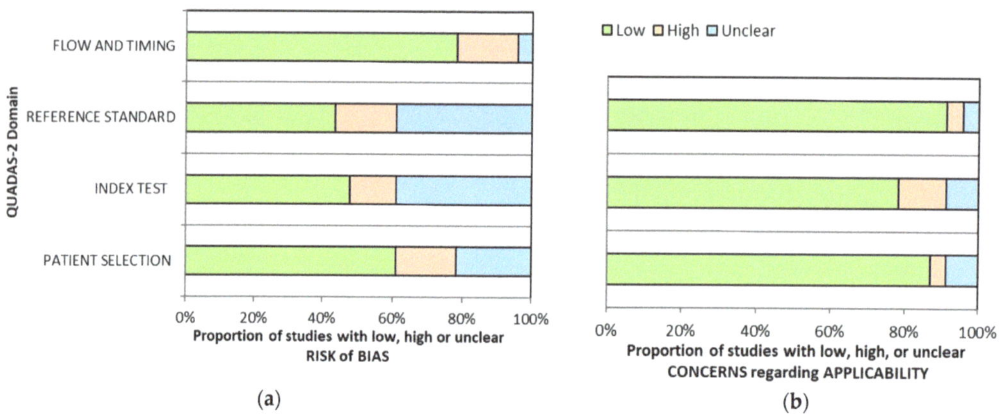

Figure 2. QUADAS-2 graphical representation of the risk-of-bias (**a**) and concerns regarding applicability (**b**) of occult scaphoid fractures.

The prevalence of occult scaphoid fracture is 23.87% (95% CI 18.25–29.49) (Supplementary Figure S3). The prediction interval, representing an absolute measure of heterogeneity, exhibits a prevalence rate of 17.8% to 30.2%. The Galbraith plot indicates some heterogeneity (Supplementary Figure S4). Begg and Mazumdar's test for rank correlation gives a p-value of <0.001, indicating possible evidence of publication bias. Egger's test for a regression intercept gives a p-value of 0.0005, indicating possible evidence of publication bias. The funnel plot indicates a small-studies effect as the results show asymmetry, not corrected by trim-and-fill (Supplementary Figure S5).

Bone scan had the highest sensitivity (98%; 95% confidence interval [CI] 90–100%) while CT scan (98%; 95% 86–100) had the highest specificity. Although MRI also has a 98% specificity, the 95% CI is much wider than CT scan. In this meta-analysis, MRI had the best posterior probability of LR+ and LR− amongst other imaging modalities, with 95% and 0.15%, respectively, assuming a baseline 25% prior probability. Heterogeneity exists amongst all imaging modalities, except for bone scan (I2 = 1 and p-value of 0.182). Publication bias does not exist for studies including ultrasound and bone scan. According to the likelihood ratio scattergram, ultrasound can be used as an exclusion and confirmation imaging modality, CT and MRI can only be used for confirmation of occult fracture, while bone scan can neither exclude nor confirm occult fracture. All of the imaging modalities have an excellent AUC, with bone scans having the best AUC value of 0.99 (95% CI 0.97–0.99). Although ultrasound has an AUC of 0.99, the 95% CI is very wide (0.2–1) (Supplementary Figure S6A–D). All of the imaging modalities only have weak evidence (Table 2).

Table 2. Pooled estimates of diagnostic performance of multimodality imaging for diagnosis of radiographically occult hip and femur and scaphoid fractures.

Parameter	Scaphoid				Hip and Femur	
	Ultrasound	CT Scan	MRI	Bone Scan	CT Scan	MRI
No. of studies	6	5	8	7	15	29
No. of patients	270	297	345	586	1329	1905
Sensitivity (%)	96 (66–100)	81 (64–91)	86 (68–94)	98 (90–100)	94 (80–99)	98 (97–99)
Specificity (%)	94 (66–99)	98 (86–100)	98 (28–100)	80 (44–95)	99 (96–100)	99 (98–99)
Positive likelihood ratio	16 (2.2–114.4)	41.7 (5.5–316.6)	48.7 (0.4–6437.6)	4.9 (1.3–17.9)	82.1 (22.6–298.5)	69 (41–116.1)
Posterior probability (%) assuming a 25% prior probability	84	93	95	62	96	96
Negative likelihood ratio	0.04 (0–0.47)	0.2 (0.1–0.39)	0.15 (0.06–0.35)	0.02 (0–0.16)	0.06 (0.01–0.22)	0.02 (0.01–0.03)
Posterior probability (%) assuming a 25% prior probability	1	6	0.15	1	2	1
Positive predictive value	0.95 (0.9–1)	0.82 (0.8–0.84)	0.86 (0.84–0.88)	0.97 (0.85–1)	82.1 (22.6–298.5)	69 (41–116.1)
Negative predictive value	0.93 (0.88–0.99)	0.97 (0.95–1)	0.98 (0.95–1)	0.81 (0.7–0.92)	0.06 (0.01–0.22)	0.02 (0.01–0.03)
Diagnostic odds ratio	387 (17–8879)	210 (31–1449)	334 (2–49,601)	213 (12–3743)	1425 (171–11851)	4185 (2009–8720)
Area under the curve	0.99 (0.2–1)	0.91 (0.17–1)	0.91 (0.89–0.94)	0.99 (0.97–0.99)	1 (0.99–1)	1 (0.99–1)
I^2 (%) and p-value	81 (59–100) and 0.003	85 (70–100) and 0.001	96 (93–99) and <0.0001	1 (0–100) and 0.182	92 (83–100) and <0.0001	100 (0–100) and 0.5
Publication bias	0.56	0.03	0.07	0.13	<0.001	<0.001
Likelihood ratio scattergram	LUQ; Exclusion and confirmation	RUQ; Confirmation only	RUQ; Confirmation only	RLQ; No exclusion or confirmation	LUQ; Exclusion and confirmation	LUQ; Exclusion and confirmation
Stratification of evidence	Weak	Weak	Weak	Weak	Suggestive	Suggestive

CT, computed tomography; MRI, magnetic resonance imaging; LUQ, left upper quadrant; RUQ, right upper quadrant; RLQ, right lower quadrant.

There are only two eligible studies that studied CBCT as their index test, hence the results will be qualitatively studied [63,64]. Both studies used MRI as their reference standard, with a total of 144 studies across both studies. Sensitivity is lower in Edlund's [64] study with 69% (95% CI 41–88%) as compared to Borel's [63] study with 100% (95% CI 75–100%). However, it should be noted that Edlund employed the MRI scan two weeks after the initial fracture, while Borel conducted the MRI scan one week after the initial fracture. Borel also found that CBCT had a specificity of 95% (95% CI: 75–100%), PPV of 96% (95% CI: 78–100%), and NPV of 100% (95% CI: 83–100%) [63]. Both studies conclude that CBCT is superior to radiography, but Edlund noted that CBCT cannot be used to exclude scaphoid fractures.

The model diagnostics are shown in Supplementary Figure S7A–D, where no studies appear to be outliers, as evidenced by the outlier detection, with a reasonable goodness-of-fit for MRI and bone scan studies. The goodness-of-fit is not linear in USG and CT studies. The bivariate normality assumption is not fulfilled, and some studies [41,44,46,47,49,52,53] seem to be more influential than others with a Cook's distance of >0.5. The bivariate box plot showed a skewness of the test performance measures toward a higher sensitivity with lower specificity for ultrasound, and vice versa for CT, MRI, and bone scan, providing indirect evidence of some threshold variability (Supplementary Figure S8A–D). Supplementary Figure S9A–D presents the paired forest plot description of empirical Bayes predicted versus observed study-specific sensitivity and specificity, indicating threshold variability as sensitivity increases and specificity decreases and vice versa.

The updated meta-analysis for occult hip and femur fracture yields an additional two articles [65,66], with three hand-searched articles [67–69]. Hence, there are five more new articles included in this updated meta-analysis (Supplementary Figure S10). Two [70,71] out of three [72] articles included in previous systematic reviews [36,38] had to be excluded as we believe the cohort is too similar. There were 45 studies with 3594 patients with suspected occult scaphoid fractures and 1523 patients with eventual scaphoid fractures (Supplementary Table S7). Notable exclusions are presented in Supplementary Table S8. Eleven studies were done prospectively with 29 studies being done retrospectively. The rest of the studies did not provide sufficient or direct information regarding the types of studies. Only fifteen studies explicitly mentioned that the studies were done consecutively, one being done non-consecutively, and the rest provided no information. Two studies [67,73] used ultrasound, three studies [74–76] employed bone scan as their index test, fifteen studies [65,66,68,69,77–87] used CT scans and the rest used MRI [72,74,75,77,78,88–111]. Most patients were female, ranging from 25% [95] to 95% [90] The reference test was heterogeneous, but most studies employed clinical and surgical follow-up. Only eight studies used MRI [65,67,68,73,76,82,87,88] as the reference test. The machines and protocols used also varied widely. As a whole, the studies included for occult hip and femoral fracture suffer from a moderate to high risk of bias and concerns of applicability. Only eight studies [72,73,82,87,106,108,110,111] were free of bias, while the rest were at risk of some bias (Figure 3 and Table A2).

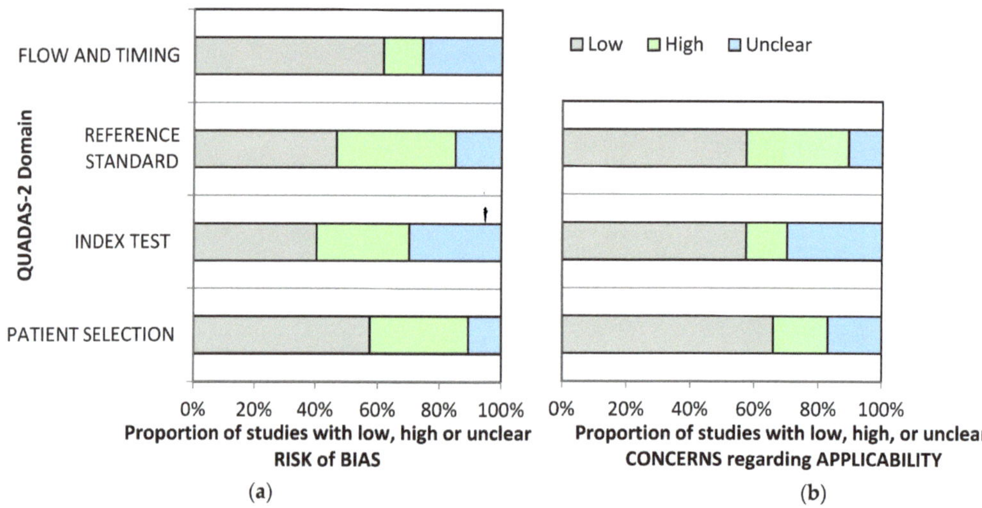

Figure 3. QUADAS-2 graphical representation of the risk-of-bias (**a**) and concerns regarding applicability (**b**) of occult hip and femoral fractures.

The prevalence of occult hip and femoral fractures is 44.8% (95% CI 39.38–51.4) (Supplementary Figure S11). The prediction interval, representing an absolute measure of heterogeneity, exhibits a prevalence rate of 38.2% to 51.4%. The Galbraith plot indicates some heterogeneity (Supplementary Figure S12). Begg and Mazumdar's test for rank correlation gives a *p*-value of 0.09, indicating little evidence of publication bias. Egger's test for a regression intercept gives a *p*-value of 0.0235, indicating possible evidence of publication bias. The funnel plot indicates a small-studies effect as the results show asymmetry, not corrected by trim-and-fill (Supplementary Figure S13).

Magnetic resonance imaging had the highest sensitivity (98%; 95% confidence interval [CI] 97–99%) while both CT scan and MRI had a high specificity (99%; 95% CI 96–100% and 99%; 95% CI 98–99%, respectively). In this meta-analysis, MRI had the best posterior probability of LR+ and LR− amongst other imaging modalities, with 96% and 100%, respectively, assuming a baseline 25% prior probability. Heterogeneity exists amongst all imaging modalities, although the heterogeneity is not statistically significant for MRI (I2 = 100 with a *p*-value of 0.5). Publication bias exists for both CT and MRI. According to the likelihood ratio scattergram, both CT scan and MRI can be used for exclusion and confirmation. Both imaging modalities have an excellent AUC with a very similar AUC value of 1 (0.99–1) (Supplementary Figure S14A,B). All of the imaging modalities have suggestive evidence (Table 2).

There are only two articles for ultrasonography and three for bone scan, hence they will be described qualitatively. In the ultrasound group, 124 patients were enrolled with 37 occult fractures [67,73]. Although both studies agree that ultrasonography is highly sensitive for occult hip and femoral fractures, with a sensitivity of 100% [73] and 96% (0.89–0.96) [67], the specificity differs wildly. Tsukamoto [67] found that ultrasound is highly specific with 0.98 (0.92–0.99), while Safran found a specificity of only 65% [73]. Nonetheless, both articles agree that ultrasonography can be used as an initial screening tool for patients with suspected occult hip and femoral fractures.

Three studies looked at the performance of bone scans in occult hip and femoral fractures. Out of all 139 patients enrolled across three studies, 50 had occult bone fractures. In these three studies, they agreed that MRI performs as well [76], if not better than bone scans [74,75]. These authors argue that MRI provides a faster scan (<15 min) and is well-tolerated by the patients, compared to delayed bone scans where not all centres provide imaging studies, and they are invasive and not cost effective [74–76].

The model diagnostics are shown in Supplementary Figure S15A,B, where no studies appear to be outliers, as evidenced by the outlier detection for MRI, with a reasonable goodness-of-fit for MRI. However, one study seems to be an outlier for the CT scan study [83]. Deletion of this study resulted in a more stable model diagnostics, with a reasonable goodness-of-fit assumption for CT scans. However, there is not much change in the diagnostic accuracy of CT scans after the deletion of that study, with the same specificity and a sensitivity of 95%. Hence, the study was kept. The bivariate box plot showed a moderately homogenous performance of high sensitivity and specificity, providing indirect evidence of little to no threshold variability (Supplementary Figure S16A,B). Supplementary Figure S17A,B present the paired forest plot description of empirical Bayes predicted versus observed study-specific sensitivity and specificity, indicating threshold variability as sensitivity increases and specificity decreases and vice versa.

4. Discussion

This updated meta-analysis finds that the prevalence of occult hip and femoral fracture is higher than occult scaphoid fracture, with 44.8% as compared to 23.87%, respectively. The rate of occult hip and femoral fracture is not that far off from a previous systematic review with 39% (95% CI 35–43) [38]. The rate of occult scaphoid fracture is also similar to currently published studies, with a rate of around 20–25% [112]. In the past, this figure was as low as 5–10% [2]. The more prevalent uses of advanced imaging and increased awareness about occult fractures may have contributed to the rise of earlier detections. The higher risk of occult fracture in the hip and femur compared to occult scaphoid fracture may partly have to do with the population. Patients who suffer from occult hip and femoral fractures are usually older people, cachectic, suffer from malnutrition, or have other comorbidities that predispose them to falls, such as osteoporosis, Parkinson's disease, dementia, or delirium [113,114]. Therefore, clinicians may find it difficult to ascertain with great confidence that an elderly individual, who may not fully cooperate, has a fracture when the initial radiographic result is negative. Meanwhile, those who suffer from occult fractures are usually younger, with a male predisposition, and with a clear history of trauma such as falling on outstretched hands, motor vehicle collision, or sports-related injuries [115].

Relying solely on sensitivity and specificity does not offer enough information to make informed decisions after receiving positive screening test results because of the occurrence of false positives [116]. There is also a trade-off between sensitivity and specificity, called the variability threshold, where if sensitivity rises, specificity falls, and vice versa [117]. Meanwhile, a limitation of utilizing the LR is its independence from prevalence, thereby impacting the accuracy of diagnostic tests. On the other hand, post-test probability, which is influenced by prevalence, emerges as a clinically more valuable parameter for assessing diagnostic test accuracy [118,119]. In this discussion, the focus will be heavily implied more on the posterior probability of LR+ and LR−.

In terms of post-test probability, MRI emerges as the best imaging modality to detect occult scaphoid and hip and femoral fractures. The next best imaging modality seems to be a CT scan for both fractures, but ultrasound has a better negative posterior probability than a CT scan. Our findings align with the ACR appropriateness criteria for both occult hip and scaphoid fractures, where MRI without IV contrast is typically employed as the first line and CT scan as an alternative [8,9]. In this analysis, the results show that the use of MRI, besides earlier detection of occult scaphoid fracture, can also exclude occult fractures. This finding is also supported by the ACR [8]. However, MRI cannot confidently exclude occult scaphoid fractures in this analysis, which is against the ACR document [8]. Some possibilities that may contribute to the discrepancies are the timing of imaging, the sampling methodologies, and the protocol, which will be discussed in-depth in the limitation section.

Despite numerous studies seemingly strengthening the argument for using earlier MRI to detect hip and scaphoid fractures, most centres are still reluctant to do so. One study finds that initial negative radiograph scaphoid fracture remains a persistent difficulty for the United Kingdom (UK) National Health Service (NHS), as numerous pathways demanding substantial resources rely on access to sophisticated imaging examinations. This difficulty is due to the constrained availability of advanced imaging in UK Emergency Departments for timely scanning of the scaphoid [120]. Numerous studies [5,121,122], including one randomized clinical trial for scaphoid fractures [123], have found that MRI is more cost-effective as compared to no further imaging or conventional follow-up radiographs for scaphoid fractures or CT scans for hip fractures.

Ultrasound in occult hip and femoral fractures is interesting as the previous systematic review excluded ultrasound as ultrasound was never used in clinical settings [39,124]. The primary radiographic signs often include scaphoid cortical disruption (a direct indication), radiocarpal fluid appearing hypoechoic due to hemarthrosis (with occasionally mixed echogenicity based on blood degradation stage), and effusion in the scaphoid–trapezium–trapezoid area (indirect indicators) [125]. The ACR appropriateness criteria also assign ultrasonography as "Usually Not Appropriate" for occult scaphoid fractures [8]. However, the assignment of this category is due to the lack of evidence, not due to evidence against its use [125]. Although it is inferior to MRI, its performance against CT scan as a second line is comparable, only falling short in the positive post-test probability department. Furthermore, ultrasound is more widely available, non-ionizing, and does not require special preparations (such as kidney function testing for contrast use in CT and MRI or sedation in paediatric patients undergoing MRI) [126]. Not all centres can afford CT scans or MRIs, and when they do, not all patients can afford them. Amongst all other imaging modalities for occult scaphoid fractures, ultrasound is the only diagnostic tool that can both exclude or confirm the fractures, with a low probability of publication bias. Although it is riddled with a high heterogeneity index, the use of ultrasound in occult scaphoid fracture merits further research.

The other imaging modalities mentioned in this analysis are CBCT and bone scan. While a bone scan is extremely sensitive, it is too costly and not appropriate for an emergency setting. Hence, it is not clinically viable and reflected in ACR appropriateness criteria for both occult hip and scaphoid fractures [8,9]. It is also worth mentioning that our analysis finds that bone scan has the lowest positive posterior probability and can neither confirm nor exclude occult scaphoid fractures. There is a low probability of heterogeneity and publication bias, which strengthens the arguments for reserving bone scans only in very special cases of occult scaphoid fractures. The use of CBCT is an emerging topic in the orthopaedics field. The main benefits compared to traditional CT lie in the fact that CBCT scanners enable quicker, more precise, quasi-three-dimensional imaging with significantly reduced radiation exposure, achieved through the utilization of smaller imaging devices [127]. It is also cheaper compared to CT scans [128]. One population-based, case-control study in France found that extremity CBCT in an emergency radiology department reduced the overall radiation dose, leading to an accelerated turnover, and it was feasible with a level of evidence of grade III [129]. The sentiment of the reduced dose is also expressed in another study, where they found that wrist CBCT involves a notably reduced scattered dose compared to wrist multi-sliced CT with similar diagnostic effectiveness. However, the use of CBCT entails a notably increased scattered radiation dosage to the neck, chest, and abdomen compared to scaphoid radiography from four views [130]. Similar to ultrasound, more studies are needed before the widespread clinical use of CBCT in occult fractures.

This umbrella review and updated meta-analysis suffers from several limitations. Firstly, there is a slight deviation in the protocol. Initially, the review aimed to include all occult fractures from all anatomical sites. However, the authors found that the scaphoid and hip are the two most extensive anatomical sites for occult fractures being studied, with no other systematic reviews on other anatomical sites. There is one systematic review on occult ankle fractures in the paediatric population, but further scrutiny found that not all included fractures were occult fractures [131]. Secondly, publications on some imaging modalities suffer from heterogeneity and publication bias. An attempt was made to meta-regress the findings to possibly elucidate the source of heterogeneity. However, several substantial missing data from the original publications made it difficult to uncover the sources of heterogeneity. Some sources of heterogeneity may include study methodology, the clinical context of the study (in-clinic vs. emergency department), study protocol (the reference test of choice and when the next follow-up is), the pre-test probability of each patient having occult fractures, the imaging protocols, and the number, experiences, and expertise of the interpreters. The fourth limitation is that most of the included studies suffer from some risk of bias, which may impede the clinical implementation of these imaging modalities in diagnosing occult fractures. The fifth limitation lies in the fact that the results of CBCT for occult scaphoid fractures and ultrasonography and bone scans for occult hip and femoral fractures cannot be synthesized into a meta-analysis, unlike the previous meta-analysis [38]. However, this limitation also underlines our strengths in reviewing every single manuscript for the inclusion and exclusion criteria. Despite being more time-consuming, our meta-analyses found that many primary articles that were previously included under very similar inclusion and exclusion criteria ended up not fulfilling the criteria. Lastly, despite a very thorough search, the stratification of evidence is still weak for occult scaphoid fractures and only suggestive for occult hip and femoral fractures.

5. Conclusions

The quest to find the best imaging modality for occult fractures has not ended here. Despite the limitations, our umbrella review and meta-analysis encompass the most recent literature around occult scaphoid and hip and femoral fractures. The findings strengthen the case for use of MRI after initially negative radiograph fracture for occult hip and femoral fractures, with a CT scan as a viable second option. However, the evidence is only suggestive at best. As for occult scaphoid fractures, MRI is still the first-line imaging choice with CT scan being the second option and ultrasonography being a potential candidate that needs further studies. Bone scans should be out of favour in detecting occult fractures and it may be worthwhile to conduct further studies on ultrasound in the detection of occult fractures. However, overall weak evidence for all imaging modalities of occult scaphoid fractures means that more evidence is needed.

The adoption of multimodality imaging into the guidelines does not ensure clinical translation. Although further large, prospective, multi-centre studies are welcomed, studies that explore the clinical inertia of using MRI as a first-line imaging modality to occult fractures or studies that explore the challenges faced by hospitals, clinicians, and their workload if all patients with occult fractures underwent MRI are also urgently needed. There is also a need for analysis that investigates the adverse impact of overdiagnosis when MRI is routinely implemented [132]. Lastly, although it seems intuitive that other modalities such as fludeoxyglucose (FDG)–positron emission tomography (PET) scan [133,134], PET/CT, PET/MRI scan [135], and single-photon emission computed tomography (SPECT) [136] may not be used for occult fractures, studies will still need to be done to determine definitively that these modalities are not needed in occult fractures or other indications and justifications for their use.

Supplementary Materials: The following supporting information can be downloaded at: https://www.mdpi.com/article/10.3390/jcm13133769/s1, File S1: PRISMA 2020 Checklist; Table S1: Medical subject heading (MeSH) terms used in each database for the umbrella study, Table S2: Medical subject heading (MeSH) terms used in each database for the hip or femoral fractures, Table S3: Medical subject heading (MeSH) terms used in each database for the scaphoid fractures, Table S4: Notable exclusions for the umbrella review, Table S5: Notable exclusions for the scaphoid fracture, Table S6: Machines and protocols used, Table S7: Descriptive characteristics of each study included in occult scaphoid fracture, Table S8: Notable exclusions for the hip fracture, Figure S1: PRISMA flowchart for selection of included studies in the umbrella review, Figure S2: PRISMA flowchart for selection of included studies in the systematic review of the occult fractures of the scaphoid, Figure S3: Meta-analysis of prevalence of occult scaphoid fracture, Figure S4: Galbraith plot of occult scaphoid fracture, Figure S5: Funnel plot of studies included in the prevalence of occult scaphoid fracture, Figure S6: The hierarchical summary receiver operating characteristic (HSROC) of ultrasound (A), CT (B), MRI (C), and bone scan (D) in detecting occult scaphoid fracture, Figure S7: Model diagnostics of each study for ultrasound (A), CT (B), MRI (C), and bone scan (D) in detecting occult scaphoid fracture, Figure S8: Bivariate boxplot of each study for ultrasound (A), CT (B), MRI (C), and bone scan (D) in detecting occult scaphoid fracture, Figure S9: Empirical Bayes prediction of sensitivity and specificity of each study for ultrasound (A), CT (B), MRI (C), and bone scan (D) in detecting occult scaphoid fracture, Figure S10: PRISMA flowchart for selection of included studies in the systematic review of the occult fractures of the hip, Figure S11: Meta-analysis of prevalence of occult hip and femoral fracture, Figure S12: Galbraith plot of occult scaphoid fracture, Figure S13: Funnel plot of studies included in the prevalence of occult hip and femoral fracture, Figure S14: The hierarchical summary receiver operating characteristic (HSROC) of CT (A) and MRI (B) in detecting occult hip and femoral fracture, Figure S15: Model diagnostics of each study for CT (A) and MRI (B) in detecting occult hip and femoral fracture, Figure S16: Model diagnostics of each study for CT (A) and MRI (B) in detecting occult hip and femoral fracture, Figure S17: Empirical Bayes prediction of sensitivity and specificity of each study for CT (A) and MRI (B) in detecting occult hip and femoral fracture.

Author Contributions: Conceptualization, P.J. and G.S.O.; methodology, G.S.O. and C.B.H.S.; software, G.S.O.; validation, P.J.; formal analysis, G.S.O.; investigation, G.S.O. and C.B.H.S.; data curation, P.J., C.B.H.S., and G.S.O.; writing—original draft preparation, P.J., C.B.H.S., and G.S.O.; writing—review and editing, P.J., C.B.H.S., and G.S.O.; visualization, G.S.O.; supervision, P.J.; project administration, P.J. All authors have read and agreed to the published version of the manuscript.

Funding: This research received no external funding.

Institutional Review Board Statement: Not applicable.

Informed Consent Statement: Not applicable.

Data Availability Statement: Available upon request.

Conflicts of Interest: The authors declare no conflicts of interest.

Appendix A

Table A1. QUADAS-2 graphical representation of the risk-of-bias and concerns regarding applicability of occult scaphoid fractures.

Study	Risk of Bias				Applicability Concerns			Conclusions
	Patient Selection	Index Test	Reference Standard	Flow and Timing	Patient Selection	Index Test	Reference Standard	
Yildirim (2013) [46]	☺	☺	?	☺	☺	☺	☺	At risk of bias
Platon (2011) [47]	☺	☺	☺	☺	☺	☺	☺	Low risk of bias
Fusetti (2005) [48]	☺	☺	☺	☺	☺	☺	☺	Low risk of bias
Senall (2004) [49]	☺	☺	☹	☺	☺	☺	☺	At risk of bias
Hauger (2002) [50]	☺	☺	☺	☺	☺	☺	☺	Low risk of bias
Herneth (2001) [51]	☺	?	?	☺	☺	☺	☺	At risk of bias
Xie (2020) [41]	☹	?	☺	☺	?	?	☺	At risk of bias
Kitsis (1989) [42]	☹	?	?	☺	☺	☺	☺	At risk of bias
Thorpe (1996) [43]	☺	?	?	☺	☺	☺	☺	At risk of bias
Fowler (1998) [44]	☺	?	☺	☺	☺	?	☺	At risk of bias
Borel (2017) [63]	☺	?	☺	☺	☺	☺	☺	At risk of bias
Edlund (2016) [64]	☺	☺	☺	☹	☺	☺	☺	At risk of bias
De Zwart (2012) [52]	?	☹	☹	☺	☺	☹	☺	At risk of bias
Beeres (2008) [56]	☺	☹	☹	☺	☺	☹	☺	At risk of bias
Ilica (2011) [53]	☹	☺	☺	☹	☺	☺	☺	At risk of bias
Mallee (2011) [54]	☺	?	☺	☺	☺	☺	☺	At risk of bias
Memasadeghi (2006) [55]	?	☺	?	☺	☺	☺	☺	At risk of bias
Breitenseher (1997) [57]	☺	☺	☺	☺	☺	☺	☺	Low risk of bias
Tiel-van Buul (1996) [58]	?	?	?	☺	☺	☺	☺	At risk of bias
Nielsen (1983) [62]	?	?	?	☺	☺	☺	☺	At risk of bias
O'Carroll (1982) [61]	☹	☹	☹	☹	☹	☹	☹	At risk of bias
Stordahl (1984) [60]	?	☺	?	?	?	☺	?	At risk of bias
Tiel-van Buul (1993) [59]	☺	☺	?	☺	☺	☺	☺	At risk of bias

☺ Low Risk; ☹ High Risk; ? Unclear Risk.

Table A2. QUADAS-2 graphical representation of the risk-of-bias and concerns regarding applicability of occult hip and femoral fractures.

Study	Risk of Bias				Applicability Concerns			Conclusions
	Patient Selection	Index Test	Reference Standard	Flow and Timing	Patient Selection	Index Test	Reference Standard	
Deutsch (1989) [89]	☹	☹	?	☺	?	?	?	At risk of bias
Rizzo (1993) [76]	☹	☹	?	☺	?	?	?	At risk of bias
Quinn and McCarthy (1993) [90]	☺	☹	☹	☺	☺	☹	☺	At risk of bias
Evans (1994) [75]	☺	☹	?	☺	?	?	?	At risk of bias
Haramati (1994) [91]	☹	☹	☹	☹	☹	☹	☹	At risk of bias
Bogost (1995) [92]	?	☹	☹	☺	?	☺	☺	At risk of bias
Stiris and Lilleas (1997) [93]	?	☹	☹	☺	?	☺	☺	At risk of bias
Rubin (1998) [74]	?	?	?	☺	☺	☺	☺	At risk of bias
Pandey (1998) [94]	☹	☹	☹	☹	☹	☹	☹	At risk of bias
Lim (2002) [95]	☺	☹	☹	☺	☺	☹	☹	At risk of bias
Oka and Monu (2004) [96]	☺	☹	☹	☺	☺	☹	☹	At risk of bias
Galloway (2004) [97]	☹	?	☺	?	☺	☺	☺	At risk of bias
Lee (2004) [98]	☹	?	☺	?	☺	☺	☺	At risk of bias
Alam (2005) [99]	☺	?	☺	☺	☺	☺	☺	At risk of bias
Frihagen (2005) [100]	☺	☹	☹	☺	☺	☹	☹	At risk of bias
Verbeeten (2005) [101]	☺	?	☺	☺	☺	☺	☺	At risk of bias

Table A2. *Cont.*

Study	Risk of Bias				Applicability Concerns			Conclusions
	Patient Selection	Index Test	Reference Standard	Flow and Timing	Patient Selection	Index Test	Reference Standard	
Lubovsky (2005) [88]	☹	?	☺	☹	☹	?	☺	At risk of bias
Dominguez (2005) [102]	☹	?	☺	☺	?	☺	☺	At risk of bias
Chana (2006) [103]	?	☹	☺	?	☺	☺	?	At risk of bias
Hossain (2007) [104]	?	?	☺	☺	☺	☺	☺	At risk of bias
Sankey (2009) [105]	☺	☹	☺	☺	☺	☺	☺	At risk of bias
Safran (2009) [73]	☺	☺	☺	☺	☺	☺	☺	Low risk of bias
Szewczyk (2012) [106]	☺	☺	☺	☺	☺	☺	☺	Low risk of bias
Iwata (2012) [107]	☺	?	☺	☺	☺	?	☺	At risk of bias
Dunker (2012) [80]	☺	☺	☹	☺	☺	☺	☹	At risk of bias
Ohishi (2012) [108]	☺	☺	☺	☺	☺	☺	☺	Low risk of bias
Geijer (2012) [79]	☺	☺	☹	?	☺	☺	☹	At risk of bias
Gill (2013) [77]	☹	☺	☹	?	☹	?	☹	At risk of bias
Heikal (2014) [81]	☺	☺	☹	☹	☺	☺	☹	At risk of bias
Haubro (2015) [82]	☺	☺	☺	☺	☺	☺	☺	Low risk of bias
Deleanu (2015) [83]	☺	?	☹	☹	☹	?	☹	At risk of bias
Collin (2016) [72]	☺	☺	☺	☺	☺	☺	☺	Low risk of bias
Rehman (2016) [78]	☺	?	☹	?	☺	?	☹	At risk of bias
Sadozai (2016) [84]	☺	☺	☹	?	☺	☺	☹	At risk of bias
Thomas (2016) [85]	☹	☺	☹	?	☺	☺	☹	At risk of bias
Lakshmanan (2017) [109]	☺	?	☺	☺	☺	?	☺	At risk of bias
Lord (2017) [110]	☺	☺	☺	☺	☺	☺	☺	Low risk of bias
Mandell (2018) [86]	☺	☺	☹	☺	☺	☺	☹	At risk of bias
Ross (2019) [111]	☺	☺	☺	☺	☺	☺	☺	Low risk of bias
Heynen (2019) [87]	☺	☺	☺	☺	☺	☺	☺	Low risk of bias
Haims (2020) [66]	☹	?	?	☺	☹	?	☺	At risk of bias
Lanotte (2019) [65]	☹	☺	?	☹	☹	☺	☺	At risk of bias
Kutaiba (2020) [68]	☹	☺	☺	?	?	?	☺	At risk of bias
Tsukamoto (2023) [67]	☹	☹	?	?	?	?	?	At risk of bias
Reddy (2015) [69]	☹	☺	☹	?	☹	?	☹	At risk of bias

☺ Low Risk; ☹ High Risk; ? Unclear Risk.

References

1. Ahn, J.M.; El-Khoury, G.Y. Occult Fractures of Extremities. *Radiol. Clin. North Am.* **2007**, *45*, 561–579. [CrossRef] [PubMed]
2. Yin, Z.G.; Zhang, J.B.; Kan, S.L.; Wang, X.G. Diagnostic accuracy of imaging modalities for suspected scaphoid fractures: Meta-analysis combined with latent class analysis. *J Bone Jt. Surg Br.* **2012**, *94*, 1077–1085. [CrossRef]
3. Busardò, F.P.; Frati, P.; Santurro, A.; Zaami, S.; Fineschi, V. Errors and malpractice lawsuits in radiology: What the radiologist needs to know. *Radiol. Med.* **2015**, *120*, 779–784. [CrossRef]
4. Beloosesky, Y.; Hershkovitz, A.; Guz, A.; Golan, H.; Salai, M.; Weiss, A. Clinical characteristics and long-term mortality of occult hip fracture elderly patients. *Injury* **2010**, *41*, 343–347. [CrossRef] [PubMed]
5. Yun, B.J.; Hunink, M.G.M.; Prabhakar, A.M.; Heng, M.; Liu, S.W.; Qudsi, R.; Raja, A.S. Diagnostic Imaging Strategies for Occult Hip Fractures: A Decision and Cost-Effectiveness Analysis. *Acad. Emerg. Med.* **2016**, *23*, 1161–1169. [CrossRef] [PubMed]
6. Bulstra, A.E.J.; van Boxel, M.F.; Crijns, T.J.; Kelly, J.; Obdeijn, M.C.; Kerkhoffs, G.M.M.J.; Doornberg, J.N.; Ring, D.; Jaarsma, R.L. Routine MRI Among Patients with a Suspected Scaphoid Fracture Risks Overdiagnosis. *Clin. Orthop. Relat. Res.* **2023**, *481*, 2309–2315. [CrossRef] [PubMed]
7. Bernstein, J. Letter to the Editor: Routine MRI Among Patients with a Suspected Scaphoid Fracture Risks Overdiagnosis. *Clin. Orthop. Relat. Res.* **2024**. [CrossRef] [PubMed]
8. Torabi, M.; Lenchik, L.; Beaman, F.D.; Wessell, D.E.; Bussell, J.K.; Cassidy, R.C.; Czuczman, G.J.; Demertzis, J.L.; Khurana, B.; Klitzke, A.; et al. ACR Appropriateness Criteria® Acute Hand and Wrist Trauma. *J. Am. Coll. Radiol.* **2019**, *16*, S7–S17. [CrossRef] [PubMed]
9. Ross, A.B.; Lee, K.S.; Chang, E.Y.; Amini, B.; Bussell, J.K.; Gorbachova, T.; Ha, A.S.; Khurana, B.; Klitzke, A.; Mooar, P.A.; et al. ACR Appropriateness Criteria® Acute Hip Pain-Suspected Fracture. *J. Am. Coll. Radiol.* **2019**, *16*, S18–S25. [CrossRef] [PubMed]
10. Ouzzani, M.; Hammady, H.; Fedorowicz, Z.; Elmagarmid, A. Rayyan—A web and mobile app for systematic reviews. *Syst. Rev.* **2016**, *5*, 210. [CrossRef] [PubMed]

11. Page, M.J.; McKenzie, J.E.; Bossuyt, P.M.; Boutron, I.; Hoffmann, T.C.; Mulrow, C.D.; Shamseer, L.; Tetzlaff, J.M.; Akl, E.A.; Brennan, S.E.; et al. The PRISMA 2020 statement: An updated guideline for reporting systematic reviews. *Syst. Rev.* **2021**, *10*, 89. [CrossRef] [PubMed]
12. Salameh, J.P.; Bossuyt, P.M.; McGrath, T.A.; Thombs, B.D.; Hyde, C.J.; Macaskill, P.; Takwoingi, Y. Preferred reporting items for systematic review and meta-analysis of diagnostic test accuracy studies (PRISMA-DTA): Explanation, elaboration, and checklist. *BMJ* **2020**, *370*, m2632. [CrossRef] [PubMed]
13. Aromataris, E.; Fernandez, R.; Godfrey, C.M.; Holly, C.; Khalil, H.; Tungpunkom, P. Summarizing systematic reviews: Methodological development, conduct and reporting of an umbrella review approach. *Int. J. Evid. Based Healthc.* **2015**, *13*, 132–140. [CrossRef] [PubMed]
14. Fusar-Poli, P.; Radua, J. Ten simple rules for conducting umbrella reviews. *Evid. Based Ment. Health* **2018**, *21*, 95–100. [CrossRef] [PubMed]
15. Choi, G.J.; Kang, H. Introduction to Umbrella Reviews as a Useful Evidence-Based Practice. *J. Lipid Atheroscler.* **2023**, *12*, 3–11. [CrossRef] [PubMed]
16. Shea, B.J.; Reeves, B.C.; Wells, G.; Thuku, M.; Hamel, C.; Moran, J.; Moher, D.; Tugwell, P.; Welch, V.; Kristjansson, E.; et al. AMSTAR 2: A critical appraisal tool for systematic reviews that include randomised or non-randomised studies of healthcare interventions, or both. *BMJ* **2017**, *358*, j4008. [CrossRef] [PubMed]
17. Whiting, P.F.; Rutjes, A.W.S.; Westwood, M.E.; Mallett, S.; Deeks, J.J.; Reitsma, J.B.; Leeflang, M.M.G.; Sterne, J.A.C.; Bossuyt, P.M.M.; QUADAS-2 Group. QUADAS-2: A revised tool for the quality assessment of diagnostic accuracy studies. *Ann. Intern. Med.* **2011**, *155*, 529–536. [CrossRef] [PubMed]
18. Bracchiglione, J.; Meza, N.; Bangdiwala, S.I.; de Guzmán, E.N.; Urrútia, G.; Bonfill, X.; Madrid, E. Graphical Representation of Overlap for OVErviews: GROOVE tool. *Res. Synth. Methods* **2022**, *13*, 381–388. [CrossRef] [PubMed]
19. Nyaga, V.N.; Arbyn, M.; Aerts, M. Metaprop: A Stata command to perform meta-analysis of binomial data. *Arch. Public Health* **2014**, *72*, 39. [CrossRef] [PubMed]
20. Borenstein, M. Research Note: In a meta-analysis, the I(2) index does not tell us how much the effect size varies across studies. *J. Physiother.* **2020**, *66*, 135–139. [CrossRef] [PubMed]
21. Gao, J.; Yang, L.; Zhao, J.; Wang, L.; Zou, J.; Wang, C.; Fan, X. Comparison of problem-based learning and traditional teaching methods in medical psychology education in China: A systematic review and meta-analysis. *PLoS ONE* **2020**, *15*, e0243897. [CrossRef] [PubMed]
22. Page, M.; Higgins, J.; Sterne, J. Chapter 13: Assessing risk of bias due to missing results in a synthesis. In *Cochrane Handbook for Systematic Reviews of Interventions*, 2nd ed.; Higgins, J.P.T., Thomas, J., Chandler, J., Cumpston, M., Li, T., Page, M.J., Welch, V.A., Eds.; John Wiley & Sons: Chichester, UK, 2019; pp. 349–374.
23. Begg, C.B.; Mazumdar, M. Operating characteristics of a rank correlation test for publication bias. *Biometrics* **1994**, *50*, 1088–1101. [CrossRef] [PubMed]
24. Egger, M.; Smith, G.D.; Schneider, M.; Minder, C. Bias in meta-analysis detected by a simple, graphical test. *BMJ* **1997**, *315*, 629. [CrossRef] [PubMed]
25. Duval, S.; Tweedie, R. Trim and fill: A simple funnel-plot-based method of testing and adjusting for publication bias in meta-analysis. *Biometrics* **2000**, *56*, 455–463. [CrossRef] [PubMed]
26. Deeks, J.J.; Higgins, J.P.T.; Altman, D.G. Chapter 10: Analysing data and undertaking meta-analyses. In *Cochrane handbook for Systematic Reviews of Interventions*, 2nd ed.; Higgins, J.P.T., Thomas, J., Chandler, J., Cumpston, M., Li, T., Page, M.J., Welch, V.A., Eds.; John Wiley & Sons: Chichester, UK, 2019; pp. 241–284.
27. MedCalc Software Ltd. Diagnostic Test Evaluation Calculator (Version 22.016). 2023. Available online: https://www.medcalc.org/calc/diagnostic_test.php (accessed on 29 December 2023).
28. Reitsma, J.B.; Glas, A.S.; Rutjes, A.W.; Scholten, R.J.; Bossuyt, P.M.; Zwinderman, A.H. Bivariate analysis of sensitivity and specificity produces informative summary measures in diagnostic reviews. *J. Clin. Epidemiol.* **2005**, *58*, 982–990. [CrossRef] [PubMed]
29. Rutter, C.M.; Gatsonis, C.A. A hierarchical regression approach to meta-analysis of diagnostic test accuracy evaluations. *Stat. Med.* **2001**, *20*, 2865–2884. [CrossRef] [PubMed]
30. Lee, Y.H. Overview of the Process of Conducting Meta-analyses of the Diagnostic Test Accuracy. *J. Rheum. Dis.* **2018**, *25*, 3–10. [CrossRef]
31. Higgins, J.P.; Thompson, S.G. Quantifying heterogeneity in a meta-analysis. *Stat. Med.* **2002**, *21*, 1539–1558. [CrossRef] [PubMed]
32. Stengel, D.; Bauwens, K.; Sehouli, J.; Ekkernkamp, A.; Porzsolt, F. A likelihood ratio approach to meta-analysis of diagnostic studies. *J. Med. Screen.* **2003**, *10*, 47–51. [CrossRef]
33. Li, J.; Fine, J.P.; Safdar, N. Prevalence-dependent diagnostic accuracy measures. *Stat. Med.* **2007**, *26*, 3258–3273. [CrossRef] [PubMed]
34. Dwamena, B.; Sylvester, R.; Carlos, R.C. MIDAS: Stata module for meta-analytical integration of diagnostic test accuracy studies. *Stata J.* **2007**, *12*, 605–622.
35. Chatha, H.; Ullah, S.; Cheema, Z. Review article: Magnetic resonance imaging and computed tomography in the diagnosis of occult proximal femur fractures. *J. Orthop. Surg.* **2011**, *19*, 99–103. [CrossRef] [PubMed]

36. Kellock, T.T.; Khurana, B.; Mandell, J.C. Diagnostic Performance of CT for Occult Proximal Femoral Fractures: A Systemati Review and Meta-Analysis. *AJR Am. J. Roentgenol.* **2019**, *213*, 1324–1330. [CrossRef] [PubMed]
37. Wilson, M.P.; Nobbee, D.; Murad, M.H.; Dhillon, S.; McInnes, M.D.F.; Katlariwala, P.; Low, G. Diagnostic Accuracy of Limited MR Protocols for Detecting Radiographically Occult Hip Fractures: A Systematic Review and Meta-Analysis. *AJR Am. J. Roentgeno* **2020**, *215*, 559–567. [CrossRef] [PubMed]
38. Haj-Mirzaian, A.; Eng, J.; Khorasani, R.; Raja, A.S.; Levin, A.S.; Smith, S.E.; Johnson, P.T.; Demehri, S. Use of Advanced Imaging for Radiographically Occult Hip Fracture in Elderly Patients: A Systematic Review and Meta-Analysis. *Radiology* **2020**, *296* 521–531. [CrossRef] [PubMed]
39. Mallee, W.H.; Wang, J.; Poolman, R.W.; Kloen, P.; Maas, M.; de Vet, H.C.; Doornberg, J.N. Computed tomography versus magnetic resonance imaging versus bone scintigraphy for clinically suspected scaphoid fractures in patients with negative plain radiographs. *Cochrane Database Syst. Rev.* **2015**. [CrossRef] [PubMed]
40. Kwee, R.M.; Kwee, T.C. Ultrasound for diagnosing radiographically occult scaphoid fracture. *Skelet. Radiol.* **2018**, *47*, 1205–1212 [CrossRef]
41. Xie, C.; Ather, S.; Mansour, R.; Gleeson, F.; Chowdhury, R. Dual-energy CT in the diagnosis of occult acute scaphoid injury: A direct comparison with MRI. *Eur. Radiol.* **2021**, *31*, 3610–3615. [CrossRef] [PubMed]
42. Kitsis, C.; Taylor, M.; Chandey, J.; Smith, R.; Latham, J.; Turner, S.; Wade, P. Imaging the problem scaphoid. *Injury* **1998**, *29* 515–520. [CrossRef] [PubMed]
43. Thorpe, A.P.; Murray, A.D.; Smith, F.W.; Ferguson, J. Clinically suspected scaphoid fracture: A comparison of magnetic resonance imaging and bone scintigraphy. *Br. J. Radiol.* **1996**, *69*, 109–113. [CrossRef] [PubMed]
44. Fowler, C.; Sullivan, B.; Williams, L.A.; McCarthy, G.; Savage, R.; Palmer, A. A comparison of bone scintigraphy and MRI in the early diagnosis of the occult scaphoid waist fracture. *Skelet. Radiol.* **1998**, *27*, 683–687. [CrossRef] [PubMed]
45. Hodgkinson, D.W.; Nicholson, D.A.; Stewart, G.; Sheridan, M.; Hughes, P. Scaphoid fracture: A new method of assessment. *Clin Radiol.* **1993**, *48*, 398–401. [CrossRef] [PubMed]
46. Yıldırım, A.; Unlüer, E.E.; Vandenberk, N.; Karagöz, A. The role of bedside ultrasonography for occult scaphoid fractures in the emergency department. *Ulus. Travma Acil. Cerrahi. Derg.* **2013**, *19*, 241–245. [CrossRef] [PubMed]
47. Platon, A.; Poletti, P.-A.; Van Aaken, J.; Fusetti, C.; Della Santa, D.; Beaulieu, J.-Y.; Becker, C.D. Occult fractures of the scaphoid The role of ultrasonography in the emergency department. *Skelet. Radiol.* **2011**, *40*, 869–875. [CrossRef] [PubMed]
48. Fusetti, C.; A Poletti, P.; Pradel, P.H.; Garavaglia, G.; Platon, A.; Della Santa, D.R.; Bianchi, S. Diagnosis of occult scaphoid fracture with high-spatial-resolution sonography: A prospective blind study. *J. Trauma* **2005**, *59*, 677–681. [PubMed]
49. Senall, J.A.; Failla, J.M.; Bouffard, J.A.; van Holsbeeck, M. Ultrasound for the early diagnosis of clinically suspected scaphoid fracture. *J. Hand Surg. Am.* **2004**, *29*, 400–405. [CrossRef] [PubMed]
50. Hauger, O.; Bonnefoy, O.; Moinard, M.; Bersani, D.; Diard, F. Occult fractures of the waist of the scaphoid: Early diagnosis by high-spatial-resolution sonography. *AJR Am. J. Roentgenol.* **2002**, *178*, 1239–1245. [CrossRef] [PubMed]
51. Herneth, A.M.; Siegmeth, A.; Bader, T.R.; Ba-Ssalamah, A.; Lechner, G.; Metz, V.M.; Grabenwoeger, F. Scaphoid fractures: Evaluation with high-spatial-resolution US initial results. *Radiology* **2001**, *220*, 231–235. [CrossRef] [PubMed]
52. de Zwart, A.; Rhemrev, S.J.; Kingma, L.M.; Meylaerts, S.A.; Arndt, J.-W.; Schipper, I.B.; Beeres, F.J. Early CT compared with bone scintigraphy in suspected schapoid fractures. *Clin. Nucl. Med.* **2012**, *37*, 981. [CrossRef]
53. Ilica, A.T.; Ozyurek, S.; Kose, O.; Durusu, M. Diagnostic accuracy of multidetector computed tomography for patients with suspected scaphoid fractures and negative radiographic examinations. *Jpn. J. Radiol.* **2011**, *29*, 98–103. [CrossRef] [PubMed]
54. Mallee, W.; Doornberg, J.N.; Ring, D.; van Dijk, C.N.; Maas, M.; Goslings, J.C. Comparison of CT and MRI for diagnosis of suspected scaphoid fractures. *J. Bone Jt. Surg. Am.* **2011**, *93*, 20–28. [CrossRef] [PubMed]
55. Memarsadeghi, M.; Breitenseher, M.J.; Schaefer-Prokop, C.; Weber, M.; Aldrian, S.; Gäbler, C.; Prokop, M. Occult scaphoid fractures: Comparison of multidetector CT and MR imaging--initial experience. *Radiology* **2006**, *240*, 169–176. [CrossRef] [PubMed]
56. Beeres, F.J.; Rhemrev, S.J.; den Hollander, P.; Kingma, L.M.; Meylaerts, S.A.; le Cessie, S.; Bartlema, K.A.; Hamming, J.F.; Hogervorst, M. Early magnetic resonance imaging compared with bone scintigraphy in suspected scaphoid fractures. *J. Bone Jt. Surg. Br.* **2008**, *90*, 1205–1209. [CrossRef] [PubMed]
57. Breitenseher, M.J.; Metz, V.M.; A Gilula, L.; Gaebler, C.; Kukla, C.; Fleischmann, D.; Imhof, H.; Trattnig, S. Radiographically occult scaphoid fractures: Value of MR imaging in detection. *Radiology* **1997**, *203*, 245–250. [CrossRef] [PubMed]
58. Tiel-van Buul, M.M.; Roolker, W.; Verbeeten, B.W.; Broekhuizen, A.H. Magnetic resonance imaging versus bone scintigraphy in suspected scaphoid fracture. *Eur. J. Nucl. Med.* **1996**, *23*, 971–975. [CrossRef] [PubMed]
59. Tiel-van Buul, M.M.; van Beek, E.J.; Broekhuizen, A.H.; Bakker, A.J.; Bos, K.E.; van Royen, E.A. Radiography and scintigraphy of suspected scaphoid fracture. A long-term study in 160 patients. *J. Bone Jt. Surg. Br.* **1993**, *75*, 61–65. [CrossRef] [PubMed]
60. Stordahl, A.; Schjøth, A.; Woxholt, G.; Fjermeros, H. Bone scanning of fractures of the scaphoid. *J. Hand Surg. Br.* **1984**, *9*, 189–190. [CrossRef] [PubMed]
61. O'Carroll, P.F.; Doyle, J.; Duffy, G. Radiography and scintigraphy in the diagnosis of carpal scaphoid fractures. *Ir. J. Med. Sci.* **1982**, *151*, 211–213. [CrossRef] [PubMed]
62. Nielsen, P.T.; Hedeboe, J.; Thommesen, P. Bone scintigraphy in the evaluation of fracture of the carpal scaphoid bone. *Acta Orthop. Scand.* **1983**, *54*, 303–306. [CrossRef]

63. Borel, C.; Larbi, A.; Delclaux, S.; Lapegue, F.; Chiavassa-Gandois, H.; Sans, N.; Faruch-Bilfeld, M. Diagnostic value of cone beam computed tomography (CBCT) in occult scaphoid and wrist fractures. *Eur. J. Radiol.* **2017**, *97*, 59–64. [CrossRef] [PubMed]
64. Edlund, R.; Skorpil, M.; Lapidus, G.; Bäcklund, J. Cone-Beam CT in diagnosis of scaphoid fractures. *Skelet. Radiol.* **2016**, *45*, 197–204. [CrossRef] [PubMed]
65. Lanotte, S.J.; Larbi, A.; Michoux, N.; Baron, M.-P.; Hamard, A.; Mourad, C.; Malghem, J.; Cyteval, C.; Berg, B.C.V. Value of CT to detect radiographically occult injuries of the proximal femur in elderly patients after low-energy trauma: Determination of non-inferiority margins of CT in comparison with MRI. *Eur. Radiol.* **2020**, *30*, 1113–1126. [CrossRef] [PubMed]
66. Haims, A.H.; Wang, A.; Yoo, B.J.; Porrino, J. Negative predictive value of CT for occult fractures of the hip and pelvis with imaging follow-up. *Emerg Radiol.* **2021**, *28*, 259–264. [CrossRef] [PubMed]
67. Tsukamoto, H.; Kijima, H.; Saito, K.; Saito, H.; Miyakoshi, N. Diagnostic accuracy of ultrasonography for occult femoral neck fracture. *J. Clin. Orthop. Trauma* **2023**, *36*, 102087. [CrossRef] [PubMed]
68. Kutaiba, N.; Lamanna, A.; Malara, F.; Yap, L.P. Use of computed tomography and magnetic resonance imaging for occult neck of femur fractures: A single-centre study. *Emerg. Med. Australas.* **2020**, *32*, 980–985. [CrossRef] [PubMed]
69. Reddy, T.; McLaughlin, P.D.; Mallinson, P.I.; Reagan, A.C.; Munk, P.L.; Nicolaou, S.; Ouellette, H.A. Detection of occult, undisplaced hip fractures with a dual-energy CT algorithm targeted to detection of bone marrow edema. *Emerg. Radiol.* **2015**, *22*, 25–29. [CrossRef] [PubMed]
70. Collin, D.; Geijer, M.; Göthlin, J.H. Computed tomography compared to magnetic resonance imaging in occult or suspect hip fractures. A retrospective study in 44 patients. *Eur. Radiol.* **2016**, *26*, 3932–3938. [CrossRef]
71. Collin, D.; Göthlin, J.H.; Nilsson, M.; Hellström, M.; Geijer, M. Added value of interpreter experience in occult and suspect hip fractures: A retrospective analysis of 254 patients. *Emerg. Radiol.* **2016**, *23*, 229–234. [CrossRef] [PubMed]
72. Collin, D.; Geijer, M.; Göthlin, J.H. Prevalence of exclusively and concomitant pelvic fractures at magnetic resonance imaging of suspect and occult hip fractures. *Emerg. Radiol.* **2016**, *23*, 17–21. [CrossRef] [PubMed]
73. Safran, O.; Goldman, V.; Applbaum, Y.; Milgrom, C.; Bloom, R.; Peyser, A.; Kisselgoff, D. Posttraumatic painful hip: Sonography as a screening test for occult hip fractures. *J. Ultrasound Med.* **2009**, *28*, 1447–1452. [CrossRef] [PubMed]
74. Rubin, S.J.; Marquardt, J.D.; Gottlieb, R.H.; Meyers, S.P.; Totterman, S.M.; O'Mara, R.E. Magnetic resonance imaging: A cost-effective alternative to bone scintigraphy in the evaluation of patients with suspected hip fractures. *Skelet. Radiol.* **1998**, *27*, 199–204. [CrossRef]
75. Evans, P.D.; Wilson, C.; Lyons, K. Comparison of MRI with bone scanning for suspected hip fracture in elderly patients. *J. Bone Jt. Surg Br.* **1994**, *76*, 158–159. [CrossRef]
76. Rizzo, P.F.; Gould, E.S.; Lyden, J.P.; Asnis, S.E. Diagnosis of occult fractures about the hip. Magnetic resonance imaging compared with bone-scanning. *JBJS* **1993**, *75*, 395–401. [CrossRef]
77. Gill, S.K.; Smith, J.; Fox, R.; Chesser, T.J. Investigation of occult hip fractures: The use of CT and MRI. *Sci. World J.* **2013**, *2013*, 830319. [CrossRef]
78. Rehman, H.; Clement, R.G.; Perks, F.; White, T.O. Imaging of occult hip fractures: CT or MRI? *Injury* **2016**, *47*, 1297–1301. [CrossRef]
79. Geijer, M.; Dunker, D.; Collin, D.; Göthlin, J.H. Bone bruise, lipohemarthrosis, and joint effusion in CT of non-displaced hip fracture. *Acta Radiol.* **2012**, *53*, 197–202. [CrossRef]
80. Dunker, D.; Collin, D.; Göthlin, J.H.; Geijer, M. High clinical utility of computed tomography compared to radiography in elderly patients with occult hip fracture after low-energy trauma. *Emerg. Radiol.* **2012**, *19*, 135–139. [CrossRef] [PubMed]
81. Heikal, S.; Riou, P.; Jones, L. The use of computed tomography in identifying radiologically occult hip fractures in the elderly. *Ann. R Coll. Surg. Engl.* **2014**, *96*, 234–237. [CrossRef] [PubMed]
82. Haubro, M.; Stougaard, C.; Torfing, T.; Overgaard, S. Sensitivity and specificity of CT- and MRI-scanning in evaluation of occult fracture of the proximal femur. *Injury* **2015**, *46*, 1557–1561. [CrossRef]
83. Deleanu, B.; Prejbeanu, R.; Tsiridis, E.; Vermesan, D.; Crisan, D.; Haragus, H.; Predescu, V.; Birsasteanu, F. Occult fractures of the proximal femur: Imaging diagnosis and management of 82 cases in a regional trauma center. *World J. Emerg. Surg.* **2015**, *10*, 55. [CrossRef] [PubMed]
84. Sadozai, Z.; Davies, R.; Warner, J. The sensitivity of ct scans in diagnosing occult femoral neck fractures. *Injury* **2016**, *47*, 2769–2771. [CrossRef] [PubMed]
85. Thomas, R.W.; Williams, H.L.; Carpenter, E.C.; Lyons, K. The validity of investigating occult hip fractures using multidetector CT. *Br. J. Radiol.* **2016**, *89*, 20150250. [CrossRef] [PubMed]
86. Mandell, J.C.; Weaver, M.J.; Khurana, B. Computed tomography for occult fractures of the proximal femur, pelvis, and sacrum in clinical practice: Single institution, dual-site experience. *Emerg. Radiol.* **2018**, *25*, 265–273. [CrossRef] [PubMed]
87. Heynen, B.; Tamigneaux, C.; Pasoglou, V.; Malghem, J.; Vande Berg, B.; Kirchgesner, T. MRI detection of radiographically occult fractures of the hip and pelvis in the elderly: Comparison of T2-weighted Dixon sequence with T1-weighted and STIR sequences. *Diagn. Interv. Imaging* **2019**, *100*, 169–175. [CrossRef] [PubMed]
88. Lubovsky, O.; Liebergall, M.; Mattan, Y.; Weil, Y.; Mosheiff, R. Early diagnosis of occult hip fractures MRI versus CT scan. *Injury* **2005**, *36*, 788–792. [CrossRef] [PubMed]
89. Deutsch, A.L.; Mink, J.H.; Waxman, A.D. Occult fractures of the proximal femur: MR imaging. *Radiology* **1989**, *170*, 113–116. [CrossRef] [PubMed]

90. Quinn, S.F.; McCarthy, J.L. Prospective evaluation of patients with suspected hip fracture and indeterminate radiographs: Use of T1-weighted MR images. *Radiology* **1993**, *187*, 469–471. [CrossRef] [PubMed]
91. Haramati, N.; Staron, R.B.; Barax, C.; Feldman, F. Magnetic resonance imaging of occult fractures of the proximal femur. *Skelet Radiol.* **1994**, *23*, 19–22. [CrossRef] [PubMed]
92. Bogost, G.A.; Lizerbram, E.K.; Crues, J.V., III. MR imaging in evaluation of suspected hip fracture: Frequency of unsuspected bone and soft-tissue injury. *Radiology* **1995**, *197*, 263–267. [CrossRef] [PubMed]
93. Stiris, M.G.; Lilleås, F.G. MR findings in cases of suspected impacted fracture of the femoral neck. *Acta. Radiol.* **1997**, *38*, 863–866. [CrossRef] [PubMed]
94. Pandey, R.; McNally, E.; Ali, A.; Bulstrode, C. The role of MRI in the diagnosis of occult hip fractures. *Injury* **1998**, *29*, 61–63. [CrossRef] [PubMed]
95. Lim, K.B.; Eng, A.K.; Chng, S.M.; Tan, A.G.; Thoo, F.L.; Low, C.O. Limited magnetic resonance imaging (MRI) and the occult hip fracture. *Ann. Acad. Med. Singap.* **2002**, *31*, 607–610. [PubMed]
96. Oka, M.; Monu, J.U. Prevalence and patterns of occult hip fractures and mimics revealed by MRI. *AJR Am. J. Roentgenol.* **2004**, *182*, 283–288. [CrossRef] [PubMed]
97. Galloway, H.R.; Meikle, G.R.; Despois, M. Patterns of injury in patients with radiographic occult fracture of neck of femur as determined by magnetic resonance imaging. *Australas. Radiol.* **2004**, *48*, 21–24. [CrossRef] [PubMed]
98. Lee, Y.P.; Griffith, J.F.; Antonio, G.E.; Tang, N.; Leung, K.S. Early magnetic resonance imaging of radiographically occult osteoporotic fractures of the femoral neck. *Hong Kong Med. J.* **2004**, *10*, 271–275.
99. Alam, A.; Willett, K.; Ostlere, S. The MRI diagnosis and management of incomplete intertrochanteric fractures of the femur. *J Bone Jt. Surg. Br.* **2005**, *87*, 1253–1255. [CrossRef] [PubMed]
100. Frihagen, F.; Nordsletten, L.; Tariq, R.; Madsen, J.E. MRI diagnosis of occult hip fractures. *Acta Orthop.* **2005**, *76*, 524–530. [CrossRef] [PubMed]
101. Verbeeten, K.M.; Hermann, K.L.; Hasselqvist, M.; Lausten, G.S.; Joergensen, P.; Jensen, C.M.; Thomsen, H.S. The advantages of MRI in the detection of occult hip fractures. *Eur. Radiol.* **2005**, *15*, 165–169. [CrossRef] [PubMed]
102. Dominguez, S.; Liu, P.; Roberts, C.; Mandell, M.; Richman, P.B. Prevalence of traumatic hip and pelvic fractures in patients with suspected hip fracture and negative initial standard radiographs--a study of emergency department patients. *Acad. Emerg. Med.* **2005**, *12*, 366–369. [CrossRef] [PubMed]
103. Chana, R.; Noorani, A.; Ashwood, N.; Chatterji, U.; Healy, J.; Baird, P. The role of MRI in the diagnosis of proximal femoral fractures in the elderly. *Injury* **2006**, *37*, 185–189. [CrossRef] [PubMed]
104. Hossain, M.; Barwick, C.; Sinha, A.K.; Andrew, J.G. Is magnetic resonance imaging (MRI) necessary to exclude occult hip fracture? *Injury* **2007**, *38*, 1204–1208. [CrossRef] [PubMed]
105. Sankey, R.A.; Turner, J.; Lee, J.; Healy, J.; Gibbons, C.E. The use of MRI to detect occult fractures of the proximal femur: A study of 102 consecutive cases over a ten-year period. *J. Bone Jt. Surg. Br.* **2009**, *91*, 1064–1068. [CrossRef] [PubMed]
106. Szewczyk-Bieda, M.; Thomas, N.; Oliver, T.B. Radiographically occult femoral and pelvic fractures are not mutually exclusive: A review of fractures detected by MRI following low-energy trauma. *Skelet. Radiol.* **2012**, *41*, 1127–1132. [CrossRef] [PubMed]
107. Iwata, T.; Nozawa, S.; Dohjima, T.; Yamamoto, T.; Ishimaru, D.; Tsugita, M.; Maeda, M.; Shimizu, K. The value of T1-weighted coronal MRI scans in diagnosing occult fracture of the hip. *J. Bone Jt. Surg. Br.* **2012**, *94*, 969–973. [CrossRef] [PubMed]
108. Ohishi, T.; Ito, T.; Suzuki, D.; Banno, T.; Honda, Y. Occult hip and pelvic fractures and accompanying muscle injuries around the hip. *Arch. Orthop. Trauma Surg.* **2012**, *132*, 105–112. [CrossRef]
109. Lakshmanan, P.; Sharma, A.; Lyons, K.; Peehal, J.P. Are occult fractures of the hip and pelvic ring mutually exclusive? *J. Bone Jt. Surg. Br.* **2007**, *89*, 1344–1346. [CrossRef] [PubMed]
110. Lord, C.; Leach, S.; Skiadas, V.T. (Eds.) MRI for suspected hip fracture: How many sequences are enough? *ESSR* **2017**, *2017*. [CrossRef]
111. Ross, A.B.; Chan, B.Y.; Yi, P.H.; Repplinger, M.D.; Vanness, D.J.; Lee, K.S. Diagnostic accuracy of an abbreviated MRI protocol for detecting radiographically occult hip and pelvis fractures in the elderly. *Skelet. Radiol.* **2019**, *48*, 103–108. [CrossRef] [PubMed]
112. Turan, A.; Kose, O.; Aktan, C.; Unal, M.; Acar, B.; Sindel, M. Radiographic analysis of anatomic risk factors for scaphoid fractures; A case-control study. *Clin. Imaging* **2018**, *51*, 341–346. [CrossRef]
113. Wiklund, R.; Toots, A.; Conradsson, M.; Olofsson, B.; Holmberg, H.; Rosendahl, E.; Gustafson, Y.; Littbrand, H. Risk factors for hip fracture in very old people: A population-based study. *Osteoporos. Int.* **2016**, *27*, 923–931. [CrossRef]
114. Oztürk, A.; Ozkan, Y.; Akgöz, S.; Yalçýn, N.; Ozdemir, R.M.; Aykut, S. The risk factors for mortality in elderly patients with hip fractures: Postoperative one-year results. *Singap. Med. J.* **2010**, *51*, 137–143.
115. Wells, M.E.; Nicholson, T.C.; Macias, R.A.; Nesti, L.J.; Dunn, J.C. Incidence of Scaphoid Fractures and Associated Injuries at US Trauma Centers. *J. Wrist Surg.* **2021**, *10*, 123–128. [CrossRef] [PubMed]
116. Trevethan, R. Sensitivity, Specificity, and Predictive Values: Foundations, Pliabilities, and Pitfalls in Research and Practice. *Front. Public Health* **2017**, *5*, 308890. [CrossRef] [PubMed]
117. Trikalinos, T.A.; Balion, C.M.; Coleman, C.I.; Griffith, L.; Santaguida, P.L.; Vandermeer, B.; Fu, R. Chapter 8: Meta-analysis of test performance when there is a "gold standard". *J. Gen. Intern. Med.* **2012**, *27* (Suppl. 1), S56–S66. [CrossRef] [PubMed]
118. Leeflang, M.M.; Bossuyt, P.M.; Irwig, L. Diagnostic test accuracy may vary with prevalence: Implications for evidence-based diagnosis. *J. Clin. Epidemiol.* **2009**, *62*, 5–12. [CrossRef] [PubMed]

119. Moons, K.G.; Biesheuvel, C.J.; Grobbee, D.E. Test research versus diagnostic research. *Clin. Chem.* **2004**, *50*, 473–476. [CrossRef]
120. Snaith, B.; Walker, A.; Robertshaw, S.; Spencer, N.J.B.; Smith, A.; Harris, M.A. Has NICE guidance changed the management of the suspected scaphoid fracture: A survey of UK practice. *Radiography* **2021**, *27*, 377–380. [CrossRef] [PubMed]
121. Dorsay, T.A.; Major, N.M.; Helms, C.A. Cost-effectiveness of immediate MR imaging versus traditional follow-up for revealing radiographically occult scaphoid fractures. *AJR Am. J. Roentgenol.* **2001**, *177*, 1257–1263. [CrossRef] [PubMed]
122. Rua, T.; Malhotra, B.; Vijayanathan, S.; Hunter, L.; Peacock, J.; Shearer, J.; Goh, V.; McCrone, P.; Gidwani, S. Clinical and cost implications of using immediate MRI in the management of patients with a suspected scaphoid fracture and negative radiographs results from the SMaRT trial. *Bone Jt. J.* **2019**, *101*, 984–994. [CrossRef]
123. Rua, T.; Gidwani, S.; Malhotra, B.; Vijayanathan, S.; Hunter, L.; Peacock, J.; Turville, J.; Razavi, R.; Goh, V.; McCrone, P.; et al. Cost-Effectiveness of Immediate Magnetic Resonance Imaging In the Management of Patients With Suspected Scaphoid Fracture: Results From a Randomized Clinical Trial. *Value Health.* **2020**, *23*, 1444–1452. [CrossRef] [PubMed]
124. Groves, A.M.; Kayani, I.; Syed, R.; Hutton, B.F.; Bearcroft, P.P.; Dixon, A.K.; Ell, P.J. An international survey of hospital practice in the imaging of acute scaphoid trauma. *AJR Am. J. Roentgenol.* **2006**, *187*, 1453–1456. [CrossRef] [PubMed]
125. Ortiz, A.F.H.; Guevara, S.Z.; Ramírez, S.M.; Rojas, J.C.; Malo, R.G.; Beaujon, L.F.; Ochoa, M.M.; Zarate, J.F.; Niño, M.F.; Aguilar, M.O. What is the role of ultrasonography in the early diagnosis of scaphoid fractures? *Eur. J. Radiol. Open.* **2021**, *8*, 100358. [CrossRef] [PubMed]
126. Muljadi, R.; Koesbandono Octavius, G.S. A systematic review and meta-analysis of diagnostic test accuracy of chest ultrasound in diagnosing pediatric pulmonary tuberculosis. *Pediatr. Pulmonol.* **2024**. [CrossRef]
127. Bailey, J.; Solan, M.; Moore, E. Cone-beam computed tomography in orthopaedics. *Orthop. Trauma* **2022**, *36*, 194–201. [CrossRef]
128. Compton, N.; Murphy, L.; Lyons, F.; Jones, J.; MacMahon, P.; Cashman, J. Tomosynthesis: A new radiologic technique for rapid diagnosis of scaphoid fractures. *Surgeon* **2018**, *16*, 131–136. [CrossRef] [PubMed]
129. Jacques, T.; Morel, V.; Dartus, J.; Badr, S.; Demondion, X.; Cotten, A. Impact of introducing extremity cone-beam CT in an emergency radiology department: A population-based study. *Orthop. Traumatol. Surg. Res.* **2021**, *107*, 102834. [CrossRef]
130. Hughes, J.; Harris, M.; Snaith, B.; Benn, H. Comparison of scattered entrance skin dose burden in MSCT, CBCT, and X-ray for suspected scaphoid injury: Regional dose measurements in a phantom model. *Radiography* **2022**, *28*, 811–816. [CrossRef] [PubMed]
131. Najaf-Zadeh, A.; Nectoux, E.; Dubos, F.; Happiette, L.; Demondion, X.; Gnansounou, M.; Herbaux, B.; Martinot, A. Prevalence and clinical significance of occult fractures in children with radiograph-negative acute ankle injury. A meta-analysis. *Acta Orthop.* **2014**, *85*, 518–524. [CrossRef] [PubMed]
132. Leopold, S.S. Editor's Spotlight/Take 5: Routine MRI Among Patients With a Suspected Scaphoid Fracture Risks Overdiagnosis. *Clin. Orthop. Relat. Res.* **2023**, *481*, 2303–2308. [CrossRef]
133. Jarraya, M.; Hayashi, D.; Roemer, F.W.; Crema, M.D.; Diaz, L.; Conlin, J.; Marra, M.D.; Jomaah, N.; Guermazi, A. Radiographically occult and subtle fractures: A pictorial review. *Radiol. Res. Pract.* **2013**, *2013*, 370169. [CrossRef] [PubMed]
134. Ravenel, J.G.; Gordon, L.L.; Pope, T.L.; Reed, C.E. FDG-PET uptake in occult acute pelvic fracture. *Skelet. Radiol.* **2004**, *33*, 99–101. [CrossRef] [PubMed]
135. Gholamrezanezhad, A.; Basques, K.; Batouli, A.; Matcuk, G.; Alavi, A.; Jadvar, H. Clinical Nononcologic Applications of PET/CT and PET/MRI in Musculoskeletal, Orthopedic, and Rheumatologic Imaging. *AJR Am. J. Roentgenol.* **2018**, *210*, W245–W263. [CrossRef] [PubMed]
136. Allainmat, L.; Aubault, M.; Noël, V.; Baulieu, F.; Laulan, J.; Eder, V. Use of hybrid SPECT/CT for diagnosis of radiographic occult fractures of the wrist. *Clin. Nucl. Med.* **2013**, *38*, e246–e251. [CrossRef] [PubMed]

Journal of
Clinical Medicine

MDPI

Systematic Review

Is There Any Purpose in Routine Syndesmotic Screw Removal? Systematic Literature Review

Błażej G. Wójtowicz [1,*], Katarzyna Chawrylak [2], Jędrzej Lesman [1] and Marcin Domżalski [1]

[1] Department of Orthopedics and Traumatology of the Musculoskeletal System, WAM University Clinical Hospital, Central Veterans Hospital, Żeromskiego 113 St., 90-549 Lodz, Poland; jedreklesman@yahoo.pl (J.L.); marcin.domzalski@umed.lodz.pl (M.D.)

[2] Department of Surgical Oncology, Medical University of Lublin, Radziwiłłowska 13 St., 20-080 Lublin, Poland; 56646@student.umlub.pl

* Correspondence: wojtblaz@gmail.com

Abstract: Introduction: The aim of this systematic review is to examine the recent evidence comparing the removal and non-removal of syndesmotic screws in tibiofibular syndesmosis injuries in terms of functional, clinical, and radiographic outcomes. **Methods**: A comprehensive literature review was conducted to identify clinical studies on syndesmotic screw removal and its outcomes, searching the Cochrane Library and PubMed Medline for publications from 1 January 2004 to 12 February 2024. Studies were included if they involved tibiofibular syndesmotic screw fixation, assessed screw removal or retention, described clinical outcomes, and were original research with at least fifteen patients per group. **Results**: Most reviewed articles (18 out of 27; 67%) found no significant differences between the routine removal and retention of syndesmotic screws post-fixation. Four retrospective studies (15%) suggested that retaining screws might result in worse outcomes compared to removal. Two studies (7%) indicated that removing screws could introduce additional risks. One study (4%) observed that post-removal, there is some fibula–tibia separation without affecting the medial clear space. Another study (4%) noted that intraosseous screw breakage might increase the need for implant removal due to pain. Additionally, no significant differences in ankle function were found among groups with varying intervals of screw removal. **Conclusions**: The current literature does not definitively support routine removal of syndesmotic screws. Given the potential complications and financial costs, routine removal should not be performed unless specifically indicated.

Keywords: syndesmosis; syndesmotic screw; malleoli fracture; tibiofibular syndesmosis

1. Introduction

Malleoli fractures are one of the most common orthopedic injuries. Associated injuries to the tibiofibular syndesmosis may account for approximately 20% of cases [1]. It is believed that the tibiofibular syndesmosis heals after two to three months, and the screw that fixes the syndesmosis is not needed after this period [2]. From a biomechanical point of view, screw fixation is associated with issues in restoring fibular rotation, leading to increased distal tibiofibular space, which can limit ankle mobility [3]. Additionally, anatomical factors such as limited preinjury range of motion in dorsiflexion can impact the degree of mobility limitation when using syndesmotic screws [4]. The timeframe for these limitations can vary, but studies indicate that they may persist at least until the follow-up periods, which are typically around two years postoperation [3,4]. There are differing opinions on the optimal number of screws or the use of suture-buttons, and how many cortical layers the screws should traverse to effectively stabilize the syndesmosis [3]. Recent studies suggest that suture-button fixation provides superior early postoperative outcomes compared to traditional screw fixation, although no long-term superiority has been definitively established. The choice between these methods often depends on individual case assessments and surgeon preference. Screw fixation traditionally involves the screw passing through three or four cortices, but the precise protocol can vary. The suture-button technique, on the other hand, generally does not require crossing as many cortical layers and tends to involve fewer complications related to implant removal [3]. There is also no clear opinion on whether the syndesmotic screw should be removed routinely and, if so, when is the best time for removal. Therefore, the decision to remove the syndesmotic screw is often based on the surgeon's own beliefs [5–9]. In the past, several studies have evaluated the routine removal of syndesmotic screws (Table 1) [10,11]. Most of them showed no significant difference in results between the screws retained or removed. The aim of this systematic review is to examine the recent evidence comparing the removal and non-removal of syndesmotic screws in tibiofibular syndesmosis injuries in terms of functional, clinical, and radiographic outcomes.

Table 1. Characteristics of studies evaluating the routine removal of syndesmotic screws.

Author, Year of the Study	Type of Study	Strength of Evidence	Number of Patients	Key Findings
Jacobsen 1994 [10]	Retrospective	4	66	About 75% of patients reported improvement after removal.
Kaye 1989 [11]	Retrospective	4	30	• No screw broke prior to removal. • Calcification of the interosseous membrane observed in 6 patients. • Distal tibiofibular synostosis developed in 4 patients. • Transfixation screws provided satisfactory stability of the syndesmosis. • Permitted stable healing of the interosseous membrane and distal ligaments after ankle fracture.

2. Materials and Methods

2.1. Search Strategy

A comprehensive literature review was conducted to identify clinical studies investigating syndesmotic screw removal and assessing patients' clinical, radiographic, or functional outcomes. The search was carried out in the Cochrane Library and PubMed Medline electronic databases, covering studies published from 1 January 2004 to 12 February 2024. The search terms used included "syndesmosis" OR "syndesmotic" OR "transsyndesmotic" OR "distal tibiofibular" AND "screw" AND "remove". The publication date range was chosen to ensure the retrieval of the most recent findings on syndesmotic screw removal in ankle fracture patients. Articles that reported on postoperative outcomes following syndesmotic screw fixation, irrespective of screw number, size, or position, were considered eligible for inclusion.

2.2. Selection

The first criterion was that studies must have been published within the past 20 years. This criterion was set to avoid outdated data that might not reflect current medical practices and understandings. Studies published more than 20 years ago were excluded.

The next step involved verifying that the study involved tibiofibular syndesmotic screw fixation. This ensured that the procedure in question was relevant to the research focus. Studies that did not involve tibiofibular syndesmotic screw fixation were excluded.

The researchers then assessed whether the study included patients where the syndesmotic screw was either removed or retained. This was crucial to focus on the specific intervention being studied. Studies where neither removal nor retention of the syndesmotic screw was assessed were excluded.

The study was required to describe the outcomes of the intervention, including clinically important results such as physical examinations, measurements, and complications.

This ensured that the study provided useful and detailed outcomes for the analysis. Studies that did not describe the outcomes of the screw removal or retention were excluded.

It was necessary for the study to be an original study with a prospective or retrospective comparative design, excluding case series and meta-analyses. This criterion ensured high methodological quality. Case series were excluded due to their lower level of scientific evidence and higher risk of bias, often involving only a few individuals. The review focused on studies with at least 15 patients in each group, with most studies considering over 50 patients in total, making case series less significant.

Meta-analyses were excluded because they often included the same original studies already in this review, leading to the duplication of results and potential distortion of data interpretation. Ensuring a minimum of fifteen patients in each group provided a sufficient sample size for reliable results. Additionally, studies performed on the same group of patients at different times were excluded to avoid duplicative data that might skew the analysis.

Inclusion Criteria:

- Studies published within the past 20 years.
- Studies involving tibiofibular syndesmotic screw fixation.
- Studies assessing the intervention of the removal or retention of the syndesmotic screw.
- Studies describing outcomes of the intervention, including clinically important results.
- Original studies with a prospective or retrospective comparative design.
- Studies with a minimum of fifteen patients in each group.

Exclusion Criteria:

- Studies older than 20 years.
- Case series, reviews, or meta-analyses.
- Studies with fewer than fifteen patients in each group.
- Studies involving the same group of patients at different times.

2.3. Assessment of Quality

One reviewer (B.W.) assessed the methodological quality of each included study in terms of study design, type of intervention, follow-up time, and similarity of surgical procedures. A study was considered to be prospective if it started before the first patient was enrolled. In contrast, a study was considered to be retrospective if it started after the first patient was enrolled.

2.4. Data Extraction

Specific data extracted from the research were recorded in sheets. The specific data extracted included the country in which the study was primarily conducted, study duration, number of eligible patients, type of surgical intervention, number of patients who underwent syndesmotic screw removal, patient-oriented outcomes, and scales. These worksheets were subsequently compared, and any discrepancies were resolved through a review of the original study and discussions to achieve consensus.

3. Results

A total of 198 articles were retrieved through the search process. After screening the titles and abstracts, 163 articles were excluded. Among the remaining 35 articles, an additional 8 were eliminated after reading the full text. These exclusions were based on the articles being either case reports [12], systematic reviews [5–7,9], meta-analyses [8], or studies in which syndesmotic screws were not removed. Of the twenty-seven articles that remained, five were identified as randomized controlled trials (RCTs), while the remaining twenty-two studies were retrospective or cohort studies (see Figure 1).

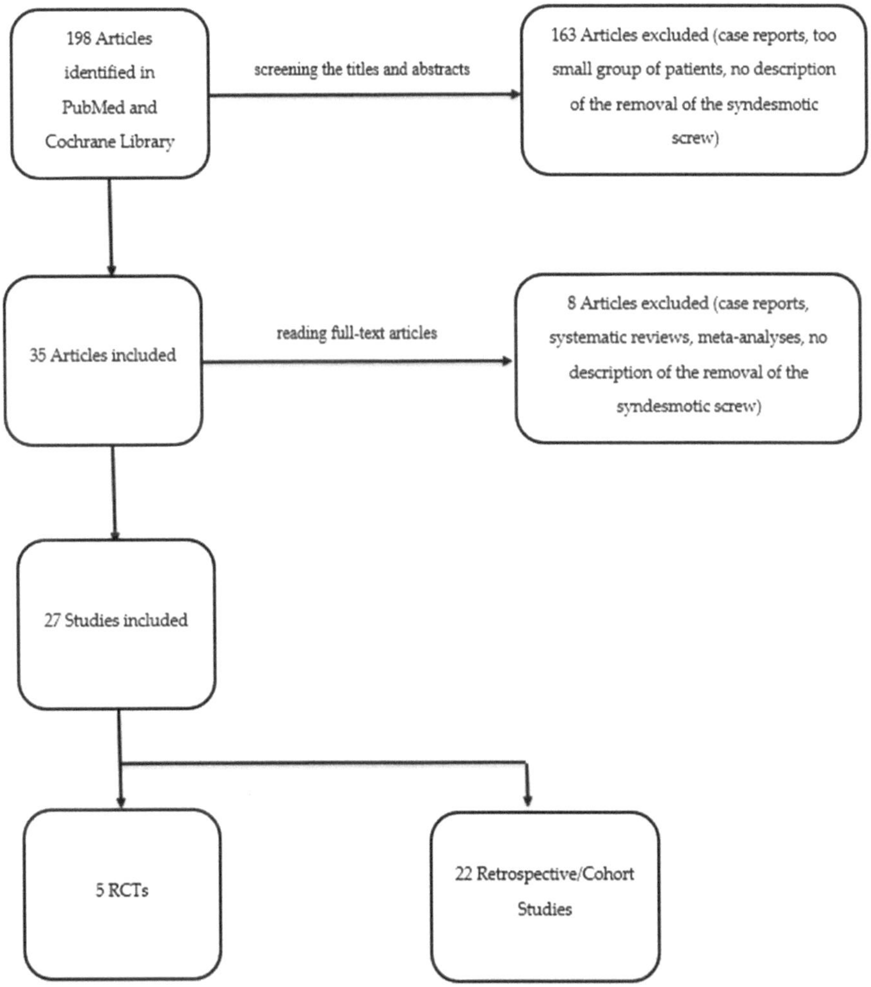

Figure 1. Search strategy flow chart according to PRISMA checklist. RCT—randomized controlled trial.

The findings from both the RCTs and non-randomized investigations are outlined in Table 2.

The majority of these articles indicated no significant variance between the routine removal and retention of syndesmotic screws following tibiofibular syndesmosis fixation (18 out of 27; 67%) [13–30]. Only four retrospective studies suggested that retaining syndesmotic screws might yield inferior outcomes compared to their removal (4 out of 27; 15%) [31–34]. Additionally, some studies suggested that removing syndesmotic screws could pose additional risks for patients (2 out of 27; 7%) [35,36]. After the removal of syndesmotic screws, there is some separation between the fibula and tibia, but the medial clear space remains unaffected (1/27 cases; 4%) [37]. It appears that syndesmotic screw breakage might pose greater challenges than previously understood. In particular, intraosseous breakage could lead to increased rates of implant removal due to pain (1/27 cases; 4%) [38]. Additionally, there are no notable discrepancies in ankle function among the groups with different intervals of syndesmotic screw removal (1/27 cases; 4%) (Figure 2) [39]. A meta-analysis was considered impossible due to the heterogeneity of the data.

Table 2. Characteristics of studies included in this review. AAOS—American Academy of Orthopedic Surgeons Scale; AOFAS—American Orthopaedic Foot and Ankle Society Scale; AP—Anteroposterior; CRPS—Complex Regional Pain Syndrome; CS—Clear Space; CT—Computed Tomography; EQ-5D—EuroQol-5 Dimension; FAOS—Foot and Ankle Outcome Score; i.v.—In Venous; IQR—Interquartile Range; MCS—Medial Clear Space; MO—Ankle Mortise Radiograph; ODR—On-Demand Removal; OL—Tibia–Fibula Overlap; OMAS—Olerud–Molander Scale; RODEO—Routine versus On-Demand Removal of the Syndesmotic Screw; RR—Routine Removal; SD—Standard Deviation; SF12-MCS—Short-Form-12 Mental Component Summary; SF12-PCS—Short-Form-12 Physical Component Summary; SMFA—Short Musculoskeletal Function Assessment; SSI—Surgical Site Infection; VAS—Visual Analog Scale.

Author, Year of the Study	Type of Study	Strength of Evidence	Number of Patients	Number of Participants Undergoing Screw Removal	Main Outcomes	Complications	Specific Findings
Andersen 2015 [35]	Retrospective Cohort	4	161	161	• Incidence of complications following routine syndesmotic screw removal: 6%.	• Wound infection in 8 (5%) patients. • Serious infections requiring hospitalization and intravenous antibiotics: 3 patients. • Surgical revisions needed: 2 patients. • Treated by oral antibiotics: 5 patients. • *Staphylococcus aureus* identified in 6/8 cases with positive culture. • Postoperative infection associated with more pain (5.3 vs. 2.3; $p = 0.02$). • Postoperative infection associated with lower satisfaction (4.7 vs. 7.6; $p = 0.014$).	• Data do not support routine removal. • Recommend routine antibiotic prophylaxis if removal chosen—single dose Cefalotin at 2 g i.v.
Bell 2006 [13]	Retrospective Cohort	4	30	23	• No statistically significant variance in ankle scores between groups. • Occurrence of screw breakage consistent in retained group after six months. • Osteolysis occurrence consistent in retained group after six months.	• Complications in five patients postoperatively. • Syndesmotic screw removed: malposition of medial malleolar screw in one patient, requiring repositioning after 2 days. • Syndesmotic screw removed: superficial wound infection in one patient, resolving on oral antibiotics after 1 week. • Syndesmotic screws left in situ: superficial wound infection in one patient, resolving on oral antibiotics after 2 weeks.	• Functional outcomes similar: ankle scores of 88 ± 5.50 (screws removed) vs. 86 ± 7.46 (screws retained). • No significant difference in ankle scores ($p = 0.79$). • Pain-free walking: 11/23 (48%) with screws removed, 2/7 (29%) with screws retained ($p > 0.05$). • Return to work without restrictions: 13/23 (57%) with screws removed, 4/7 (57%) with screws retained ($p > 0.05$). • No significant difference in range of motion deficit between groups in flexion/extension and inversion/eversion ($p > 0.05$).

Table 2. *Cont.*

Author, Year of the Study	Type of Study	Strength of Evidence	Number of Patients	Number of Participants Undergoing Screw Removal	Main Outcomes	Complications	Specific Findings
Boyle 2014 [14]	Randomized Controlled Trial	1	51	26	No statistically significant difference in ankle scores. Persistent screw breakage in the retained group after six months. Ongoing osteolysis in the retained group after six months.	No intra-operative complications. Recurrent diastasis and broken syndesmotic screw in one patient (screw retention group) four months postoperatively, managed with revision surgery. Wound infection in two patients (screw removal group) after screw removal.	Mean removal time: 116 days (range: 81 to 177). No significant effect of removal time on • OMAS ($p = 0.507$). • AOFAS ankle–hindfoot score ($p = 0.860$). • AAOS foot and ankle score ($p = 0.818$). • Pain VAS ($p = 0.596$). • Ankle dorsiflexion ($p = 0.818$). • Ankle plantarflexion ($p = 0.911$). • Calf girth ($p = 0.221$). • Tibiofibular clear space ($p = 0.279$).
Egol 2010 [15]	Retrospective Cohort	4	79	11	No statistical differences in outcomes between • Removed screws and intact screws. • Broken screws and intact screws.	Asymptomatic nonunion of medial malleolus. Symptomatic fibular nonunion, treated with secondary plating and bone graft. Delayed fibular union. Three draining wounds, treated with antibiotics. One arthrodesis after early deep infection. No differences in complication rates between syndesmotic fixation and non-fixation groups.	Comparison of screws: failed/removed (n = 26) vs. intact (n = 53). No statistical difference in • Pain ($p = 0.87$). • Function ($p = 0.82$). • Range of ankle motion ($p = 0.20$). Comparison of failed/removed screws (n = 26) vs. no syndesmotic injury (n = 268): • More no pain reports in the no-syndesmotic-injury group ($p = 0.049$). • Trend towards greater function in no-syndesmotic-injury group ($p = 0.068$).

Table 2. *Cont.*

Author, Year of the Study	Type of Study	Strength of Evidence	Number of Patients	Number of Participants Undergoing Screw Removal	Main Outcomes	Complications	Specific Findings
Gennis 2015 [16]	Retrospective Cohort	4	166	58	No statistically significant difference in radiographic displacement outcomes: • Syndesmosis. • Mortise Comparison: screw removal vs. intact or broken screws.	• No data.	Removal of syndesmotic screws at 3 months: • Slightly lower OL (< 1 mm) on mortise radiographs. • Greater CS (0.5 mm) on mortise radiographs. No talar subluxation observed. Differences were not statistically significant. Mortise remained intact regardless of screw status: • Removed. • Loosened or broken. • Retained solid.
Hamid 2009 [17]	Retrospective Cohort	4	52	15	No statistical difference in clinical outcomes: • Syndesmosis screw removal vs. no removal. Broken screws appeared to have the most favorable outcomes.	• Two patients (5%) with retained screws had local tenderness.	Mean VAS: 2.02 (SD: 2.70) in screw-retained group vs. 0.074 (SD: 0.97) in screw-removed group (p = 0.268). Mean AOFAS score: 85.59 (SD: 13.83) in screw-retained group vs. 85.80 (SD: 11.33) in screw-removed group ($p = 0.714$).
Huevel 2023 [18]	Randomized Controlled Trial	1	109	77 (24 on demand)	No functional difference between on-demand and routine removal for syndesmotic injuries during four-year follow-up. Findings corroborate the primary RODEO trial. On-demand removal should be considered standard practice following syndesmotic screw fixation.	Pain: 7 patients. Stiffness: 2 patients. Broken or loosened screw: 3 patients. Desire for removal without further explanation: 3 patients. Combination of complications: 9 patients.	Median OMAS score: • RR group: 85.0. • ODR group: 90.0 ($p = 0.384$). Secondary outcome measures: AOFAS: • RR group: 88.0. • ODR group: 90.0 ($p = 0.722$). FAOS: • RR group: 87.5. • ODR group: 92.9 ($p = 0.399$). EQ-5D: • RR group: 0.87. • ODR group: 0.96 ($p = 0.092$).

Table 2. *Cont.*

Author, Year of the Study	Type of Study	Strength of Evidence	Number of Patients	Number of Participants Undergoing Screw Removal	Main Outcomes	Complications	Specific Findings
Hoines 2004 [19]	Randomized Controlled Trial	1	64	32 (2 on demand)	No difference in functional outcomes between single-quadcortical-screw-removal group and two-tricortical-screw-retention group.	Three tricortical syndesmosis screws removed in 2 patients due to spontaneous loosening and telescoping after 3 months. High incidence of deep surgical site infections (6.3%) with biodegradable screws considered coincidental and unrelated to fixation method.	OMAS at 3 months: • Tricortical group: 77 points. • Quadricortical group: 66 points ($p = 0.025$). OMAS after 1 year: • Tricortical group: 92.6 points. • Quadricortical group: 85.7 points ($p = 0.192$). Pain significantly lower in tricortical group after 3 months ($p = 0.017$). No significant difference in pain after 1 year.
Hsu 2011 [39]	Retrospective Cohort	4	52	52	• No notable differences in ankle function across groups with varying intervals of syndesmotic screw removal.	Syndesmotic screw breakage: • Within three months: 3 patients (15.0%) in group 2. • Beyond three months: 2 patients (15.4%) in group 3 (at 6 and 12 months). • Group 1: No screw breakage. Statistically significant overall rate of screw breakage among the three groups ($p = 0.034$). No significant difference in breakage between • Group 1 and group 2 ($p = 0.125$). • Group 1 and group 3 ($p = 0.157$). • Group 2 and group 3 ($p = 0.375$).	No statistical difference in ankle function among the four groups ($p = 0.051$). No significant difference in ankle function between syndesmotic diastasis with or without associated ankle fractures ($p = 0.410$). No significant difference in ankle function among the three groups with different intervals of syndesmotic screw removal ($p = 0.191$). No significant difference in ankle function between patients with or without syndesmotic screw breakage ($p = 0.343$). No significant difference in ankle function between patients with or without syndesmotic diastasis recurrence ($p = 0.218$).

Table 2. *Cont.*

Author, Year of the Study	Type of Study	Strength of Evidence	Number of Patients	Number of Participants Undergoing Screw Removal	Main Outcomes	Complications	Specific Findings
Huang 2022 [20]	Retrospective Cohort	4	63	63	Diastasis observed at end of follow-up after syndesmotic screw removal. Diastasis developed prior to screw removal, not as a result of it.	All included patients followed similar rehabilitation protocols. No major complications or dropouts.	OL decreased by an average of 2.0 mm ± 2.8 mm (range: −10.1 to 5.0 mm; $p < 0.001$). CS increased by an average of 0.8 mm ± 1.3 mm (range: −1.8 to 5.8 mm; $p < 0.001$). MCS increased by an average of 0.1 mm ± 1.3 mm (range: −2.8 to 3.6 mm; $p = 0.495$). Significant changes in OL and CS; no significant change in MCS.
Ibrahim 2022 [38]	Retrospective Cohort	4	43	21	Syndesmotic screw breakage is more challenging than previously acknowledged. Intraosseous breakage may be linked to increased implant removals due to pain. Placing screws at least 20 mm above the tibiotalar joint might reduce intraosseous breakage risk. Increased screw placement height could minimize the need for implant removal postoperatively.	• No data.	Screws placed further from the tibiotalar joint had a lower risk of intraosseous breakage (OR: 0.818, $p = 0.002$). Screws placed at a height of 20 mm or greater were more likely to break in the clear space (OR: 12.1, $p = 0.002$). No significant association between breakage location and screw diameter, length, or angulation.
Juarez-Jimenez 2018 [36]	Retrospective Cohort	4	207	207	• Frequency of complications associated with syndesmotic screw removal was lower in this study compared to existing literature.	Five patients with complications observed (2.41%). Wound dehiscence: 2 cases. Superficial infection: 2 cases (1.92%). Subsequent diastasis of the syndesmosis with pain due to instability: 1 case (0.48%).	Prevalence of complications related to syndesmotic screw removal in our hospital was lower than reported in the surgical literature. Syndesmotic screw removal is considered a safe procedure with low risk for infection and post-traumatic ankle instability.

Table 2. *Cont.*

Author, Year of the Study	Type of Study	Strength of Evidence	Number of Patients	Number of Participants Undergoing Screw Removal	Main Outcomes	Complications	Specific Findings
Jordan 2011 [37]	Retrospective Cohort	4	86	86	Diastasis of the fibula from the tibia observed after transsyndesmotic screw removal. Medial clear space remained unchanged.	• No data.	CS: Pre-screw removal (12.5 weeks): • AP view: 4.63 mm (SD ± 1.62). • MO view: 4.73 mm (SD ± 1.58). Post-screw removal: • AP view: 5.41 mm (SD ± 1.67). • MO view: 5.53 mm (SD ± 1.47). • Statistically significant increase in both views ($p \leq 0.000$). MCS: Pre-screw removal (12.5 weeks): • AP view: 2.84 mm (SD ± 0.64). • MO view: 2.99 mm (SD ± 0.61). Post-screw removal: • AP view: 2.97 mm (SD ± 0.67). • MO view: 3.05 mm (SD ± 0.66). • Significant increase in AP view ($p = 0.034$); no significant change in MO view. Overlap of the lateral (OL): Pre-screw removal (12.5 weeks): • AP view: 5.83 mm (SD ± 2.54). • MO view: 2.29 mm (SD ± 2.17). Post-screw removal: • AP view: 5.02 mm (SD ± 2.53). • MO view: 1.32 mm (SD ± 2.58). • Statistically significant decrease in both views ($p \leq 0.000$).

Table 2. *Cont.*

Author, Year of the Study	Type of Study	Strength of Evidence	Number of Patients	Number of Participants Undergoing Screw Removal	Main Outcomes	Complications	Specific Findings
Kaftadziev 2015 [21]	Retrospective Cohort	4	82	23	Patients with retained screws had significantly better outcomes compared to those with routinely removed screws. Improved outcomes were primarily attributed to the subset of patients with broken screws.	• Patients with complications were excluded.	Three cortices: 66 patients (80%). Quadricortical fixation: 16 patients (20%). No correlation with clinical outcomes or screw fractures. Syndesmotic screw usage: single screw—71 patients (86%). Mean AOFAS scores: • Intact screw (I): 83. • Broken screw (B): 92.5. • Removed screw (R): 85.5. • Significant difference overall (p = 0.0496), mainly between groups I and B. No significant differences between groups I and R or B and R. VAS results: No significant differences in patient satisfaction (p = 0.34).
Kolodziej 2010 [22]	Retrospective Cohort	4	33	13	• Removal of the syndesmotic screw did not significantly improve functional outcome.	Delayed wound healing: 2 patients. Skin changes around upper ankle and lower leg: 1 patient, indicative of post-thrombotic syndrome.	AOFAS score (mean): • Screw removal group: 89 points (range: 80 to 100). • Screw breakage group: 85 points (range: 80 to 98). • Intact screw group: 87 points (range: 77 to 100). No significant differences between groups ($p > 0.05$).

Table 2. *Cont.*

Author, Year of the Study	Type of Study	Strength of Evidence	Number of Patients	Number of Participants Undergoing Screw Removal	Main Outcomes	Complications	Specific Findings
Manjoo 2010 [31]	Retrospective Cohort	4	106	25	• Intact screws: slightly worse functional outcomes compared to broken, loosened, or removed screws.	Indications for screw removal: • Tenderness over screw prominence. • Less than 10° of ankle dorsiflexion.	Tibiofibular clear space: • Fractured, loose, or removed screws: 4.1 ± 0.2 mm. • Intact screws: 3.1 ± 0.2 mm. • $p = 0.005$. Medial clear space: • Intact screws: 3.1 ± 0.2 mm. • Broken, loose, or removed screws: 3.1 ± 0.1 mm. • $p = 0.9$. Tibiofibular overlap: • Intact screws: 7.0 ± 0.3 mm. • Broken, loose, or removed screws: 6.9 ± 0.3 mm. • $p = 0.69$.
Moon 2020 [23]	Retrospective Cohort	4	56	28	No difference in clinical outcomes between • Screw removal group and screw retention group within three months. • Screw breakage/loosening group and no issues group.	Group sizes: 9 (recurrence of diastasis) vs. 47 (no recurrence). AOFAS scores: 70.33 ± 6.22 (recurrence) vs. 76.50 ± 10.26 (no recurrence), p = 0.808. SF12-PCS scores: 49.85 ± 3.83 (recurrence) vs. 47.40 ± 8.01 (no recurrence), $p = 0.948$. SF12-MCS scores: 44.47 ± 4.47 (recurrence) vs. 46.97 ± 5.80 (no recurrence), $p = 0.407$. No significant differences based on screw size, number, or position.	Group sizes: 28 patients each (group A: screws removed in 3 months; group B: screws retained until 4 months). AOFAS scores: 75.10 ± 10.40 (group A) vs. 77.07 ± 10.60 (group B)—Not statistically significant. SF12-PCS scores: 45.78 ± 5.68 (group A) vs. 47.33 ± 5.83 (group B)—Not statistically significant. SF12-MCS scores: 48.45 ± 4.30 (group A) vs. 48.50 ± 10.04 (group B)—Not statistically significant.

Table 2. *Cont.*

Author, Year of the Study	Type of Study	Strength of Evidence	Number of Patients	Number of Participants Undergoing Screw Removal	Main Outcomes	Complications	Specific Findings
Moore 2006 [24]	Randomized Controlled Trial	1	120	7	• No difference in outcomes between retained and removed screws.	Two patients: late postoperative infections. Required hardware removal. Treated with intravenous antibiotics.	Group 1: • Five patients (8%) had screw breakage. • One required screw removal due to pain. • Three had loss of reduction (noncompliance with weight-bearing restrictions before 6 weeks). • Two had loss of fixation at the screw. Group 2: • Four patients (7%) had broken screws. • No loss of reduction with four cortices of fixation. • Four patients (7%) had painful, prominent hardware, requiring screw removal.
Omrani 2019 [25]	Retrospective Cohort	4	60	18	Removing syndesmotic screws and allowing weight-bearing: potential benefit for anatomical alignment. Timely removal of screws: no improvement in foot functional outcomes.	• No data.	18 patients (30%) with syndesmosis malreduction on initial postoperative CT. After screw removal (12 weeks), weight-bearing, and rehabilitation (4 weeks): 13 of 18 patients (72.2%) showed appropriate reduction on final CT scans.
Pogliacomi 2018 [26]	Retrospective Cohort	4	90	65	• Syndesmotic screw removal: possibly unnecessary.	• Patients with complications were excluded.	Group 1: 65 patients (72%), group 2: 25 patients (28%). Group 1: Screw removal after a mean of 7 weeks (range: 6–8 weeks). Group 2: 8 patients had broken screws; results similar to others. No significant differences in OMAS and AOFAS scores ($p < 0.05$). Tibiofibular clear space: similar in both groups, measured immediately and 1 year later ($p < 0.05$). All fractures healed after a mean of 3.5 months.

Table 2. *Cont.*

Author, Year of the Study	Type of Study	Strength of Evidence	Number of Patients	Number of Participants Undergoing Screw Removal	Main Outcomes	Complications	Specific Findings
Sanda 2023 [32]	Retrospective Cohort	4	144	93	Patients who chose screw removal reported better satisfaction with mobility and daily activities. Removal group experienced reduced pain. Complications in the removal group: infection, loss of reduction. Potential negative impact on quality of life and mobility due to complications.	• No data.	Postoperative screw removal improved mobility and daily activity performance. Reduced postoperative pain and anxiety in the screw removal group. No significant difference in overall quality of life between screw removal and conservative treatment groups.
Sanders 2021 [27]	Randomized Controlled Trial	1	152	85 (18 on demand)	On-demand screw removal had similar functional outcomes to routine removal. Routine removal group had significantly more complications (12 of 73) compared to on-demand removal group.	Significantly more complications in RR group (12/73) vs. ODR group (1/79) ($p = 0.007$). RR group complications: 5, wound dehiscence; 2, superficial SSI 2, deep SSI; 1, diastasis after removal; 1, synovitis; 1, increase in stiffness. Four RR patients had syndesmotic fixation complications: 2 deep infections (1 causing flare-up post-removal, 1 leading to diastasis), 1 superficial SSI (wound dehiscence post-removal), 1 synovitis case (persisting post-removal).	Median OMAS at 12 months: 85 (IQR: 60–95) for RR; 80 (IQR: 65−100) for ODR. Noninferiority test: effect size within equivalent bounds of −10 to 10 scale points ($p < 0.001$). ODR not inferior to RR based on intention-to-treat and per-protocol analyses.

Table 2. *Cont.*

Author, Year of the Study	Type of Study	Strength of Evidence	Number of Patients	Number of Participants Undergoing Screw Removal	Main Outcomes	Complications	Specific Findings
Schepers 2014 [28]	Retrospective Cohort	4	93	81	• No difference in outcome scores among early, late, and no removal of the syndesmotic screw.	• Six patients developed wound complications post-surgery. • One 54-year-old male with a tri-malleolar Weber B fracture developed CRPS, AOFAS score: 19, OMAS score: 10, VAS score: 7, and single screw length: 36.6 mm.	AOFAS, OMAS, and VAS outcomes were not influenced by the number of engaged cortices or screw diameter. Two screws more frequently used in uni-malleolar fractures (27%) vs. bi- and tri-malleolar fractures (7%) ($p = 0.033$). Higher frequency of two screws in Weber C-type (24%) vs. B-type fractures (5%) ($p = 0.007$). Increased stiffness reported in OMAS subdomain for patients where screws were not removed or removed after 8 weeks (60%) compared to those removed within 8 weeks (29%) ($p = 0.017$). No significant effect on overall outcome between early and delayed removal groups.
Song 2014 [33]	Prospective, Prognostic Case Series	4	25	25	Initial malreduction rate: 36% following syndesmosis screw placement. 89% of malreduced syndesmoses corrected spontaneously after screw removal. Syndesmotic screw removal may assist in achieving final anatomical reduction in the distal tibiofibular joint.	Patient with continued malreduction despite screw removal: 21-year-old male. Fracture type: Weber B with medial malleolus fracture. Stabilization: Two 3.5 mm tricortical syndesmotic screws.	Initial postoperative CT: 9 patients (36%) with tibiofibular syndesmosis malreduction. Post-screw removal CT: 8 of 9 (89%) with initial malreduction showed adequate reduction. Statistical significance: Significant reduction in malreduction ($t = 3.333$, $p < 0.001$). Malreduction rates: Initial rate of 36% (9/25), post-screw removal rate of 4% (1/25).
Tucker 2013 [29]	Retrospective Cohort	4	63	43	Retention of screw: No significant reduction in functional capacity. Cost-effectiveness: Provides added cost-effectiveness.	• No data.	Mean OMAS scores—Retained group: 81.5 ± 19.3; removed group: 75 ± 12.9 ($p = 0.107$). Functional scores: Higher in retained group across OMAS domains. Pain levels: Lower in retained group. Adjusted for gender: Significant results ($p = 0.046$).

Table 2. *Cont.*

Author, Year of the Study	Type of Study	Strength of Evidence	Number of Patients	Number of Participants Undergoing Screw Removal	Main Outcomes	Complications	Specific Findings
Weening 2005 [30]	Retrospective Cohort	4	51	30	• OMAS and SMFA scores: no significant difference between removed and retained screws.	Malreduction causes: • Fibular fracture malreduction in 2 patients. • Tibiofibular misalignment in 6 patients.	Multivariable model: no significance for age, number of cortices, medial malleolar fracture, ankle dislocation, appropriateness of screw fixation, or screw removal. Medial malleolar fracture: no significant difference in SMFA-functional index (12.7 ± 13.6 vs. 9.9 ± 14.9, $p = 0.64$) and OMAS (73.5 ± 25.9 vs. 70.0 ± 20.5, $p = 0.82$). Ankle dislocation: trend toward decreased function (12.9 ± 8.9 vs. 8.1 ± 7.2, $p = 0.09$). Screw insertion appropriateness: no significant difference in SMFA-functional index (9.1 ± 14.3 vs. 15.1 ± 14.1, $p = 0.68$).
Yang 2021 [34]	Retrospective Cohort	4	113	113	Longer screw retention: might be necessary to prevent syndesmotic diastasis recurrence in tri-malleolar fractures without posterior malleolar fixation. Posterior malleolar fragment: even small fragments should be considered a risk factor for recurrent syndesmotic instability.	• Superficial infection: two patients, one in Group I and one in Group II.	Functional outcomes: no significant difference among groups. Recurrence rates: • Group I: 10.6%. • Group II: 20.9%. • Group III: 8.7%. Recurrence rate significance: not statistically significant ($p = 0.264$). Tibiofibular clear space changes: greater interval change in group II ($p = 0.028$).

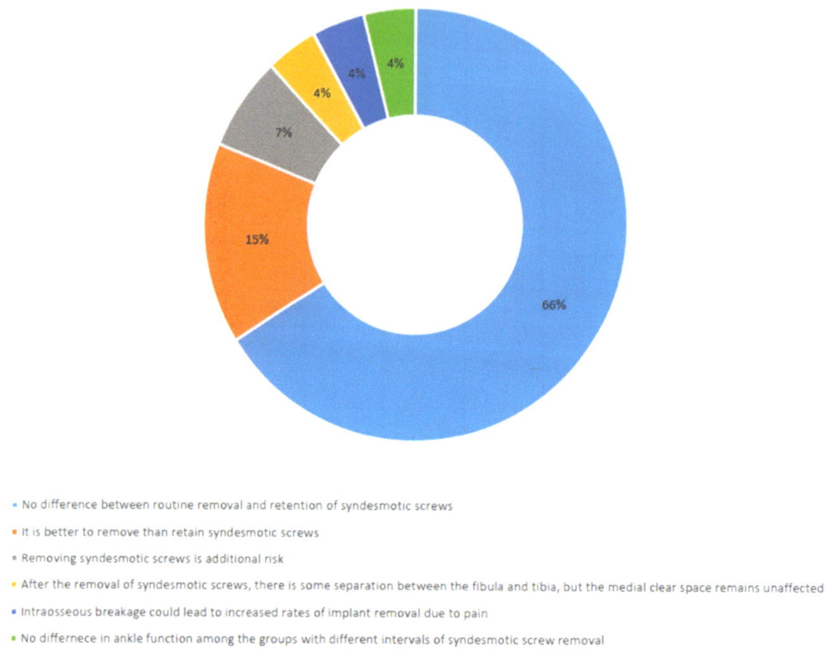

Figure 2. Summary conclusions from reviewed studies.

4. Discussion

A comprehensive review of the existing literature did not reveal notable differences in functional outcomes when syndesmotic screws are removed following tibiofibular syndesmosis stabilization. This indicates that the removal of these screws does not significantly impact the overall functional recovery of patients, as supported by current research.

Several studies have examined the relationship between syndesmotic screw removal and functional outcomes post-stabilization. Despite variations in methodology and sample sizes, a consistent trend shows no substantial change in functional recovery after screw removal.

This suggests insufficient justification for routinely removing syndesmotic screws. Findings from five RCTs also indicated no significant functional differences between removing the screws and leaving them in place.

4.1. Retain and Remove Outcomes

Thirteen retrospective studies involving a total of 855 patients did not show any significant statistical differences in ankle joint function between patients who had syndesmotic screws removed and those who retained their screws after tibiofibular syndesmosis fixation. Moon et al. conducted a study to determine whether the removal of syndesmotic screws before weight-bearing ambulation impacts clinical outcomes in patients with distal tibiofibular syndesmosis injuries. The study included 56 patients divided into groups based on whether their screws were removed (n = 28) or retained (n = 28) and whether they experienced recurrence of diastasis (n = 9) or not (n = 47). Results showed no significant differences in the American Orthopaedic Foot and Ankle Society scale (AOFAS) and Short-Form Health Survey-12 (SF-12) between screw-removed and -retained groups. However, the recurrence of diastasis was significantly higher in the screw-removed group (p = 0.025). The study concluded that removing syndesmotic screws before weight-bearing is unnecessary, as it does not influence clinical outcomes [23]. Jordan et al. aimed to evaluate the radiographic changes in tibiofibular position and the ankle mortise after the removal of trans-syndesmotic screws in patients with displaced ankle fractures. The retrospective study included 86 patients who underwent open reduction with syndesmosis screw stabilization. The key findings indicated a significant increase in tibiofibular clear space (from 4.63 mm to 5.41 mm) and a decrease in tibiofibular overlap (from 5.83 mm to 5.02 mm) post-screw removal, suggesting a high correlation of loss of syndesmotic integrity. Despite these radiographic changes, the medial clear space remained relatively stable, indicating that while there is a common occurrence of tibiofibular diastasis upon screw removal, the ankle mortise maintains its stability [37].

Kaftandziev et al. stated that the aim of their study was to compare clinical outcomes between patients who retained the syndesmosis screw and those who had it removed following the open reduction and internal fixation of malleolar fractures associated with syndesmosis disruption. The study included patients treated from January 2011 to December 2012, excluding those with incomplete data or specific postoperative complications. The findings showed no statistically significant difference in clinical outcomes between patients with the screw retained and those with the screw removed. However, patients with a syndesmotic screw fracture had better clinical outcomes. Routine removal of the syndesmosis screw is not recommended based on these results [21]. Hamid et al. demonstrated in their study the comparison of clinical and radiological outcomes in patients with Weber B or C ankle fractures and associated syndesmosis injuries, focusing on the condition of the syndesmosis screw (intact, broken, or removed). The study included 52 patients out of a possible 142 who met the inclusion criteria and returned for assessment at least one year post-surgery. Of these, 27 had intact screws, 10 had broken screws, and 15 had undergone elective screw removal. The findings revealed that the mean AOFAS scores were 83.07 in the intact screw group, 92.40 in the broken screw group, and 85.80 in the removed screw group. Interestingly, patients with broken screws exhibited the best clinical outcomes. The study concluded that there was no significant difference in outcomes between patients with intact and removed screws and suggested against the routine removal of syndesmosis screws, whether intact or broken [17]. Hsu et al. aimed to investigate the outcomes of syndesmotic screw fixation in the treatment of syndesmotic diastasis. They conducted a retrospective study on 52 adult patients treated for syndesmotic diastasis with a trans-syndesmotic cancellous screw, following strict inclusion criteria and excluding patients with pilon fractures or insufficient follow-up. Patients were grouped based on the timing of syndesmotic screw removal: six weeks, three months, and an average of nine months. The study compared recurrence rates of syndesmotic diastasis, incidence of screw breakage, and ankle function among these groups. The findings revealed that syndesmotic diastasis recurrence rates were 15.8% in the six-week removal group, 15.0% in the three-month group, and 0% in the nine-month group, though this difference was not statistically significant. Screw breakage occurred in 15.0% of patients within three months and 15.4% beyond three months, with no breakages in the six-week group. Overall, 82.7% of patients had satisfactory outcomes, and ankle function did not significantly differ among the groups, regardless of screw breakage or syndesmotic diastasis recurrence. The study concluded that while early removal of the syndesmotic screw might prevent its breakage, it could increase the risk of syndesmotic diastasis recurrence [39]. One possible explanation for the finding that timing did not affect functional outcomes could be the inherent stability provided by the syndesmotic fixation itself. Syndesmotic screws are primarily used to maintain proper alignment and stability of the tibiofibular syndesmosis during the initial phases of healing following injury. Once the ligaments have sufficiently healed and the syndesmosis has regained stability, the necessity of the screws for maintaining alignment diminishes.

Furthermore, the absence of a significant impact of timing on functional outcomes may also be attributed to the body's natural healing processes. Over time, the surrounding soft tissues, ligaments, and muscles adapt and strengthen, contributing to the overall stability of the ankle joint. This inherent healing capacity may compensate for any minor disruptions caused by the timing of syndesmotic screw removal.

Additionally, it is important to consider the rehabilitation protocol employed post-surgery. Regardless of the timing of screw removal, patients typically undergo structured rehabilitation programs aimed at restoring strength, flexibility, and function. These rehabilitation efforts likely play a crucial role in facilitating functional recovery, potentially mitigating any differences attributable to the timing of screw removal.

Two retrospective studies examining 250 patients show slightly worse results in patients who had syndesmotic screws left in place.

Sanda et al. aimed to evaluate whether the removal of syndesmotic screws post distal tibiofibular diastasis repair improves patient outcomes in terms of quality of life, mobility, and daily living activities, and whether it is a cost-effective solution. The study included patients with uni-malleolar or bi-malleolar ankle fractures, who were evaluated using standardized questionnaires approximately two months post-surgery. Out of the participants, 93 had their screws removed, while 51 retained them. The results showed that patients with screw removal reported better mobility (7.8 vs. 6.7) and ability to perform daily activities (8.1 vs. 6.5) and experienced less pain (5.3 vs. 6.8). Additionally, these patients had higher scores on the SF 6 physical domain (55.9 vs. 53.3) and lower anxiety levels (5.8 vs. 7.3). However, overall quality of life and willingness to recommend the treatment did not significantly differ between the groups. Thus, screw removal post-surgery enhances specific aspects of recovery, but the overall quality of life remains comparable [32]. Yang et al. intended to assess the outcomes of fixation for bi-malleolar and tri-malleolar ankle fractures with syndesmotic injury, particularly assessing the effects of early versus delayed removal of syndesmotic screws. The study focused on whether removing these screws at 6 to 8 weeks or at 3 months postoperatively offers more benefits. Patients who underwent open reduction and internal fixation for these fractures between January 2013 and December 2017 were analyzed, with a minimum follow-up of 24 months. Patients were categorized into three groups based on the timing of syndesmotic screw removal: group I (bi-malleolar fractures with removal at 6 to 8 weeks), group II (tri-malleolar fractures with removal at 6 to 8 weeks), and group III (tri-malleolar fractures with removal at 3 months). The study included 113 patients. Results indicated no significant difference in ankle functional outcomes among the groups. However, recurrence of syndesmotic instability was observed to be higher in group II (20.9%) compared to group I (10.6%) and group III (8.7%). Despite the lack of statistical significance in recurrence rates, group II showed a significant interval change in tibiofibular clear space compared to the other groups, suggesting potential benefits of delayed screw removal [34].

Ibrahim et al. studied the incidence and predictors of intraosseous screw breakage in syndesmotic stabilization and its association with implant removal due to pain. They retrospectively reviewed patients at a level 1 trauma center from 2011 to 2018, identifying 43 patients with 58 broken screws. The study aimed to determine the incidence of intraosseous screw breakage, identify clinical and radiographic predictors, and assess if IO breakage was associated with higher rates of painful implant removal. Findings showed that 74.4% of screw breakages occurred intraosseously, significantly linked with subsequent removal due to pain ($p = 0.034$). Only screw height from the tibial plafond significantly predicted breakage location, with screws placed 20 mm or more from the tibiotalar joint being less likely to break intraosseously (OR: 0.818, $p = 0.002$). The study highlighted the clinical importance of screw placement in preventing painful complication [38].

4.2. Complications

Two retrospective studies involving 368 patients demonstrate that reoperation, such as routine removal of syndesmotic screws, is associated with an increased risk for the patient. Infectious complications are primarily reported, with the incidence of complications ranging from 1.4% to 6%.

4.3. Limitation

The present study also has several limitations. Primarily, this review included a limited number of RCTs, resulting in weaker evidence. Furthermore, conducting a meta-analysis would be challenging due to the diversity of data analyzed across the studies mentioned.

To establish a unified consensus based on a reliable meta-analysis, additional replicable RCTs would be required. Although an RCT protocol was designed by Dingmans et al. in 2018, there remains an insufficient number of such studies available [40].

5. Conclusions

The current literature does not provide definitive evidence supporting the superiority of routinely removing syndesmotic screws over retaining them. Considering the heightened risk of complications and the additional financial burden associated with routine removal, it is advisable not to perform this procedure unless specifically indicated. Further RCTs are required to determine whether there are any differences in functional and clinical outcomes between patients who undergo syndesmotic screw removal and those who retain them following tibiofibular syndesmosis fixation. The routine versus on-demand removal of the syndesmotic screw (RODEO) trial, an international protocol for RCTs, serves as an example of such a study aimed at assessing the efficacy of routine syndesmotic screw removal [40].

Author Contributions: Conceptualization, B.G.W., J.L. and M.D.; methodology, B.G.W., K.C., J.L. and M.D.; software, J.L. and M.D.; validation, B.G.W., K.C. and J.L.; formal analysis, J.L. and M.D.; investigation, B.G.W., J.L. and K.C.; resources, B.G.W., J.L. and M.D.; data curation, B.G.W. and J.L.; writing—original draft preparation, B.G.W. and K.C.; writing—review and editing, J.L. and M.D.; visualization, B.G.W., K.C., J.L. and M.D.; supervision, J.L. and M.D.; project administration, B.G.W. and K.C.; funding acquisition, B.G.W., K.C., J.L. and M.D. All authors have read and agreed to the published version of the manuscript.

Funding: This research received no external funding.

Institutional Review Board Statement: Not applicable.

Informed Consent Statement: Not applicable.

Data Availability Statement: The data presented in this study are available on request from the corresponding author (B.G.W.).

Conflicts of Interest: The authors declare no conflicts of interest.

References

1. Dattani, R.; Patnaik, S.; Kantak, A.; Srikanth, B.; Selvan, T.P. Injuries to the tibiofibular syndesmosis. *J. Bone Joint Surg. Br.* **2008**, *90*, 405–410. [CrossRef]
2. Yang, Z.; Chen, J.; Liu, X.; Wang, B.; Zhao, X.; Guan, P. Clinical study of a steel cable fixation for distal tibiofibular syndesmosis injury. *Medicine* **2023**, *102*, e35691. [CrossRef] [PubMed]
3. Zhang, P.; Liang, Y.; He, J.; Fang, Y.; Chen, P.; Wang, J. A systematic review of suture-button versus syndesmotic screw in the treatment of distal tibiofibular syndesmosis injury. *BMC Musculoskelet. Disord.* **2017**, *18*, 286. [CrossRef] [PubMed]
4. Needleman, R.L.; Skrade, D.A.; Stiehl, J.B. Effect of the syndesmotic screw on ankle motion. *Foot Ankle* **1989**, *10*, 17–24. [CrossRef]
5. Desouky, O.; Elseby, A.; Ghalab, A.H. Removal of Syndesmotic Screw After Fixation in Ankle Fractures: A Systematic Review. *Cureus* **2021**, *13*, e15435. [CrossRef] [PubMed]
6. Dingemans, S.A.; Rammelt, S.; White, T.O.; Goslings, J.C.; Schepers, T. Should syndesmotic screws be removed after surgical fixation of unstable ankle fractures? A systematic review. *Bone Joint J.* **2016**, *98*, 1497–1504. [CrossRef]
7. Walley, K.C.; Hofmann, K.J.; Velasco, B.T.; Kwon, J.Y. Removal of Hardware After Syndesmotic Screw Fixation: A Systematic Literature Review. *Foot Ankle Spec.* **2017**, *10*, 252–257. [CrossRef] [PubMed]
8. Khurana, A.; Kumar, A.; Katekar, S.; Kapoor, D.; Vishwakarma, G.; Shah, A.; Singh, M.S. Is routine removal of syndesmotic screw justified? A meta-analysis. *Foot* **2021**, *49*, 101776. [CrossRef] [PubMed]
9. Schepers, T. To retain or remove the syndesmotic screw: A review of literature. *Arch. Orthop. Trauma Surg.* **2011**, *131*, 879–883. [CrossRef]
10. Jacobsen, S.; Honnens de Lichtenberg, M.; Jensen, C.M.; Tørholm, C. Removal of internal fixation—The effect on patients' complaints: A study of 66 cases of removal of internal fixation after malleolar fractures. *Foot Ankle Int.* **1994**, *15*, 170–171. [CrossRef]
11. Kaye, R.A. Stabilization of ankle syndesmosis injuries with a syndesmosis screw. *Foot Ankle* **1989**, *9*, 290–293. [CrossRef]
12. Bafna, K.R.; Jordan, R.; Yatsonsky, D., II; Dick, S.; Liu, J.; Ebraheim, N.A. Revision of Syndesmosis Screw Fixation. *Foot Ankle Spec.* **2020**, *13*, 138–143. [CrossRef] [PubMed]
13. Bell, D.P.; Wong, M.K. Syndesmotic screw fixation in Weber C ankle injuries—Should the screw be removed before weight bearing? *Injury* **2006**, *37*, 891–898. [CrossRef]

14. Boyle, M.J.; Gao, R.; Frampton, C.M.; Coleman, B. Removal of the syndesmotic screw after the surgical treatment of a fracture of the ankle in adult patients does not affect one-year outcomes: A randomised controlled trial. *Bone Joint J.* **2014**, *96*, 1699–1705. [CrossRef] [PubMed]
15. Egol, K.A.; Pahk, B.; Walsh, M.; Tejwani, N.C.; Davidovitch, R.I.; Koval, K.J. Outcome after unstable ankle fracture: Effect of syndesmotic stabilization. *J. Orthop. Trauma* **2010**, *24*, 7–11. [CrossRef] [PubMed]
16. Gennis, E.; Koenig, S.; Rodericks, D.; Otlans, P.; Tornetta, P., III. The Fate of the Fixed Syndesmosis Over Time. *Foot Ankle Int.* **2015**, *36*, 1202–1208. [CrossRef]
17. Hamid, N.; Loeffler, B.J.; Braddy, W.; Kellam, J.F.; Cohen, B.E.; Bosse, M.J. Outcome after fixation of ankle fractures with an injury to the syndesmosis: The effect of the syndesmosis screw. *J. Bone Joint Surg. Br.* **2009**, *91*, 1069–1073. [CrossRef] [PubMed]
18. van den Heuvel, S.; Penning, D.; Sanders, F.; van Veen, R.; Sosef, N.; van Dijkman, B.; Schepers, T.; RODEO Collaborator group. Functional outcome of routine versus on-demand removal of the syndesmotic screw. *Bone Jt. Open* **2023**, *4*, 957–963. [CrossRef] [PubMed]
19. Høiness, P.; Strømsøe, K. Tricortical versus quadricortical syndesmosis fixation in ankle fractures: A prospective randomized study comparing two methods of syndesmosis fixation. *J. Orthop. Trauma* **2004**, *18*, 331–337. [CrossRef]
20. Huang, C.T.; Huang, P.J.; Lu, C.C.; Shih, C.L.; Cheng, Y.M.; Chen, S.J. Syndesmosis Changes before and after Syndesmotic Screw Removal: A Retrospective Radiographic Study. *Medicina* **2022**, *58*, 445. [CrossRef]
21. Kaftandziev, I.; Spasov, M.; Trpeski, S.; Zafirova-Ivanovska, B.; Bakota, B. Fate of the syndesmotic screw—Search for a prudent solution. *Injury* **2015**, *46* (Suppl. 6), S125–S129. [CrossRef] [PubMed]
22. Kołodziej, Ł.; Kaczmarczyk, M.; Bohatyrewicz, A.; Budzyński, T. Czy usuniecie śruby wzrostowej poprawia kliniczny wynik leczenia operacyjnego złamań kostek goleni ze współistniejacym uszkodzeniem wiezozrostu piszczelowo-strzałkowego? [Does removal of the syndesmotic screw improve clinical results of operative treatment of ankle fractures with concomitant syndesmosis injury?]. *Chir. Narzadow Ruchu Ortop. Pol.* **2010**, *75*, 143–146. (In Spanish)
23. Moon, Y.J.; Kim, D.H.; Lee, K.B. Is it necessary to remove syndesmotic screw before weight-bearing ambulation? *Medicine* **2020**, *99*, e19436. [CrossRef] [PubMed]
24. Moore, J.A., Jr.; Shank, J.R.; Morgan, S.J.; Smith, W.R. Syndesmosis fixation: A comparison of three and four cortices of screw fixation without hardware removal. *Foot Ankle Int.* **2006**, *27*, 567–572. [CrossRef] [PubMed]
25. Amouzadeh Omrani, F.; Kazemian, G.; Salimi, S. Evaluation of Syndesmosis Reduction after Removal Syndesmosis Screw in Ankle Fracture with Syndesmosis Injury. *Adv. Biomed. Res.* **2019**, *8*, 50. [CrossRef] [PubMed] [PubMed Central]
26. Pogliacomi, F.; Artoni, C.; Riccoboni, S.; Calderazzi, F.; Vaienti, E.; Ceccarelli, F. The management of syndesmotic screw in ankle fractures. *Acta Biomed.* **2018**, *90*, 146–149. [CrossRef] [PubMed] [PubMed Central]
27. Sanders, F.R.K.; Birnie, M.F.; Dingemans, S.A.; van den Bekerom, M.P.J.; Parkkinen, M.; van Veen, R.N.; RODEO Collaborator Group; Goslings, J.C.; Schepers, T. Functional outcome of routine versus on-demand removal of the syndesmotic screw: A multicentre randomized controlled trial. *Bone Joint J.* **2021**, *103*, 1709–1716. [CrossRef] [PubMed]
28. Schepers, T.; van der Linden, H.; van Lieshout, E.M.; Niesten, D.D.; van der Elst, M. Technical aspects of the syndesmotic screw and their effect on functional outcome following acute distal tibiofibular syndesmosis injury. *Injury* **2014**, *45*, 775–779. [CrossRef] [PubMed]
29. Tucker, A.; Street, J.; Kealey, D.; McDonald, S.; Stevenson, M. Functional outcomes following syndesmotic fixation: A comparison of screws retained in situ versus routine removal—Is it really necessary? *Injury* **2013**, *44*, 1880–1884. [CrossRef] [PubMed]
30. Weening, B.; Bhandari, M. Predictors of functional outcome following transsyndesmotic screw fixation of ankle fractures. *J. Orthop. Trauma* **2005**, *19*, 102–108. [CrossRef] [PubMed]
31. Manjoo, A.; Sanders, D.W.; Tieszer, C.; MacLeod, M.D. Functional and radiographic results of patients with syndesmotic screw fixation: Implications for screw removal. *J. Orthop. Trauma* **2010**, *24*, 2–6. [CrossRef]
32. Sanda, I.I.; Hosin, S.; Vermesan, D.; Deleanu, B.; Pop, D.; Crisan, D.; Al-Qatawneh, M.; Mioc, M.; Prejbeanu, R.; Rosca, O. Impact of Syndesmotic Screw Removal on Quality of Life, Mobility, and Daily Living Activities in Patients Post Distal Tibiofibular Diastasis Repair. *Medicina* **2023**, *59*, 2048. [CrossRef] [PubMed] [PubMed Central]
33. Song, D.J.; Lanzi, J.T.; Groth, A.T.; Drake, M.; Orchowski, J.R.; Shaha, S.H.; Lindell, K.K. The Effect of Syndesmosis Screw Removal on the Reduction of the Distal Tibiofibular Joint: A Prospective Radiographic Study. *Foot Ankle Int.* **2014**, *35*, 543–548. [CrossRef] [PubMed]
34. Yang, T.C.; Tzeng, Y.H.; Wang, C.S.; Lin, C.C.; Chang, M.C.; Chiang, C.C. Untreated small posterior fragment of ankle fracture with early removal of syndesmotic screw is associated with recurrent syndesmotic instability. *Injury* **2021**, *52*, 638–643. [CrossRef] [PubMed]
35. Andersen, M.R.; Frihagen, F.; Madsen, J.E.; Figved, W. High complication rate after syndesmotic screw removal. *Injury* **2015**, *46*, 2283–2287. [CrossRef]
36. Juárez-Jiménez, H.G.; Garibay-Cervantes, A.; Rosas-Medina, J.A.; Salas-Morales, G.A.; Rodríguez-Reyes, E.J. Prevalencia de las complicaciones relacionadas con el retiro del tornillo de situación [Prevalence of complications related to the removal of the syndesmotic screw]. *Acta Ortop. Mex.* **2018**, *32*, 76–81. (In Spanish)
37. Jordan, T.H.; Talarico, R.H.; Schuberth, J.M. The radiographic fate of the syndesmosis after trans-syndesmotic screw removal in displaced ankle fractures. *J. Foot Ankle Surg.* **2011**, *50*, 407–412. [CrossRef] [PubMed]

38. Ibrahim, I.O.; Velasco, B.T.; Ye, M.Y.; Miller, C.P.; Kwon, J.Y. Syndesmotic Screw Breakage May Be More Problematic Than Previously Reported: Increased Rates of Hardware Removal Secondary to Pain With Intraosseous Screw Breakage. *Foot Ankle Spec.* **2022**, *15*, 27–35. [CrossRef]
39. Hsu, Y.T.; Wu, C.C.; Lee, W.C.; Fan, K.F.; Tseng, I.C.; Lee, P.C. Surgical treatment of syndesmotic diastasis: Emphasis on effect of syndesmotic screw on ankle function. *Int. Orthop.* **2011**, *35*, 359–364. [CrossRef]
40. Dingemans, S.A.; Birnie, M.F.N.; Sanders, F.R.K.; van den Bekerom, M.P.J.; Backes, M.; van Beeck, E.; Bloemers, F.W.; van Dijkman, B.; Flikweert, E.; Haverkamp, D.; et al. Routine versus on demand removal of the syndesmotic screw; a protocol for an international randomised controlled trial (RODEO-trial). *BMC Musculoskelet. Disord.* **2018**, *19*, 35. [CrossRef] [PubMed] [PubMed Central]

Journal of
Clinical Medicine

MDPI

Article

Anatomical Posterior Acetabular Plate Versus Conventional Reconstruction Plates for Acetabular Posterior Wall Fractures: A Comparative Study

Chang-Han Chuang [1,2,3], Hao-Chun Chuang [4], Jou-Hua Wang [4], Jui-Ming Yang [5], Po-Ting Wu [4,6], Ming-Hsien Hu [3], Hong-Lin Su [1,2,*] and Pei-Yuan Lee [3,*]

1 Department of Life Sciences, National Chung Hsing University, 402 Taichung, Taiwan; skyman889@gmail.com
2 Doctor Program in Translational Medicine, National Chung Hsing University, 402 Taichung, Taiwan
3 Department of Orthopaedic Surgery, Show Chwan Memorial Hospital, 500 Changhua, Taiwan; minghsienhu@gmail.com
4 Department of Orthopaedic Surgery, National Cheng Kung University Hospital, College of Medicine, National Cheng Kung University, 704 Tainan, Taiwan; ajhwang15@gmail.com (J.-H.W.); anotherme500@gmail.com (P.-T.W.)
5 Department of Orthopaedic Surgery, Tainan Sin Lau Hospital, 701 Tainan, Taiwan; jmyang25@gmail.com
6 Department of Biomedical Engineering, National Cheng Kung University, 704 Tainan, Taiwan
* Correspondence: suhonglin@nchu.edu.tw (H.-L.S.); b1208b@ms26.hinet.net (P.-Y.L.)

Abstract: Background: Functional recovery following the surgical fixation of acetabular posterior wall fractures remains a challenge. This study compares outcomes of posterior wall fracture reconstruction using an anatomical posterior acetabular plate (APAP) versus conventional reconstruction plates. **Methods:** Forty patients with acetabular fractures involving the posterior wall or column underwent surgery, with 20 treated using APAPs (APAP group) and 20 with conventional pelvic reconstruction plates (control group). Baseline patient characteristics, intraoperative blood loss and time, reduction quality, postoperative function, and postoperative complications were compared using appropriate non-parametric statistical tests. A general linear model for repeated measures analysis of variance was employed to analyze trends in functional recovery. **Results:** No significant differences were observed in baseline characteristics. APAP significantly reduced surgical time by 40 min (186.5 ± 51.0 versus 225.0 ± 47.7, p =0.004) and blood loss (695 ± 393 versus 930 ± 609, $p = 0.049$) compared to conventional plates. At 3 and 6 months following surgery, the APAP group exhibited higher functional scores (modified Merle d'Aubigné scores 10 ± 1.8 versus 7.8 ± 1.4, $p < 0.001$; 13.4 ± 2.8 versus 10.1 ± 2.1, $p = 0.001$), converging with the control group by 12 months (modified Merle d'Aubigné scores 14.2 ± 2.6 versus 12.7 ± 2.6, $p = 0.072$; OHS 31.6 ± 12.3 versus 30.3 ± 10.1, $p = 0.398$). Radiologically, the APAP group demonstrated superior outcomes ($p = 0.047$). Complication and conversion rates to hip arthroplasty did not significantly differ between groups (10% versus 15%, $p = 0.633$). **Conclusions**: The use of an APAP in reconstructing the posterior acetabulum significantly reduces surgical time, decreases intraoperative blood loss, and leads to earlier functional recovery compared to conventional reconstruction plates. The APAP provides stable fixation of the posterior wall and ensures the durable maintenance of reduction, ultimately yielding favorable surgical outcomes.

Keywords: acetabular fracture; posterior wall fracture; posterior column fracture; internal fixation; anatomical locking plate; plate osteosynthesis

1. Introduction

Fractures of the posterior wall are the most common type of acetabular fractures, accounting for nearly a third of all fractures of the acetabulum [1,2]. Plate osteosynthesis is widely acknowledged as the preferred method for treating specific types of acetabular fractures involving the posterior column or posterior wall [3,4]. Achieving anatomical reduction and ensuring stable fixation are imperative to prevent posttraumatic osteoarthritis (PTOA), osteonecrosis of the femoral head (ONFH), and potential progression to total hip arthroplasty (THA) [5–7]. While restoring acetabular congruence is essential for functional recovery [8], managing fractures of the posterior column or wall presents significant challenges, particularly for less experienced surgeons, due to the complex anatomy of the acetabulum and the frequent occurrence of concomitant hip dislocation [9,10]. A user-friendly internal fixation device would be immensely beneficial in these cases.

Numerous fixation techniques have been proposed, including single plating, dual plating, and fragment-specific fixation [11–13]. However, the complex bone structure often necessitates the manual contouring of plates to conform to the curvature. The intraoperative bending and shaping of plates can be time-intensive and imprecise, potentially compromising their mechanical integrity [14]. Additionally, addressing comminuted wall fractures poses another obstacle. While Ritcher et al. introduced the concept of spring plates beneath a buttress plate, the technique is intricate and carries a risk of articular surface damage and challenges in plate positioning [15]. The previous literature has described a few anatomical plates, including W-shaped and H-shaped acetabular angular plates, designed to reconstruct posterior wall fractures and reduce intra-articular screw penetration [16,17]. While these plates demonstrated a lower penetration rate on immediate postoperative radiographs, their impact on functional recovery compared to that in a control group was not thoroughly explored [16].

This study aims to investigate the efficacy of using an anatomical posterior acetabular plate (APAP, produced by INTAI Technology Corp., Taichung, Taiwan) in promoting functional recovery, reducing surgical time, and preventing complications. To quantitatively assess the clinical utility of the APAP, we compared the outcomes of a patient cohort treated with APAPs to those of a separate group treated with conventional reconstruction plates.

2. Materials and Methods

2.1. Population

From January 2015 to December 2018, acetabular fractures treated by the senior author at a single level-I trauma center were retrospectively reviewed. Patients with posterior wall or posterior column fractures of the acetabulum requiring open reduction and internal fixation (ORIF) were included. Surgical indications encompassed hip instability, hip joint incongruity with an articular step-off exceeding 2 mm, inadequate secondary congruence, the presence of intra-articular fragments, and posterior column displacement exceeding 2 mm. Patients underwent treatment with either the APAP or a pelvic reconstruction plate. All implants used were FDA approved. Exclusion criteria comprised pathological acetabular fractures, neuropathic arthropathy, coagulopathy, dementia, and other conditions affecting postoperative compliance. (see Figure 1)

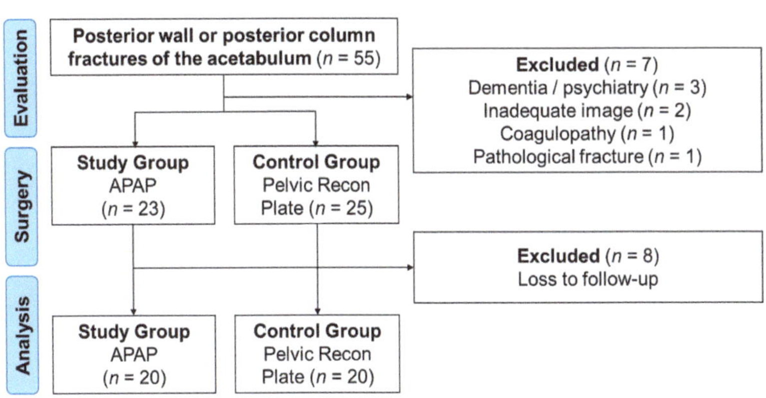

Figure 1. Patient inclusion flow chart.

2.2. Radiographic Evaluation

A standardized preoperative radiographic imaging protocol included standard anteroposterior pelvic films, two 45° oblique Judet views, and pelvic inlet and outlet views. Three-dimensional (3D) computed tomography (CT) images (slice thickness: 3 mm) and reconstructed pelvic images were obtained to enhance surgical planning. For patients with dislocation, attempted closed reduction and skin traction preceded the radiographic protocol.

2.3. Implant Design

The APAP (see Figure 2) was tailored to fit the structure of the posterior column of the acetabulum in the Taiwanese population. Utilizing a series of non-contrast pelvic CT images from our hospital's database, a 3D pelvic reconstruction model was created through segmentation using the marching cubes algorithm. The APAP was made from 18Chromium-14Nickel-2.5Molybdenum stainless steel, also known as AISI 316LVM. This stainless steel is vacuum melted to achieve the high levels of purity and cleanliness required for surgical implants. The plate is manufactured in accordance with the ASTM F139-19 Standard Specification for Wrought 18Chromium-14Nickel-2.5Molybdenum Stainless Steel Sheet and Strip for Surgical Implants (UNS S31673). The APAP was produced by INTAI Technology Corp., Taichung, Taiwan.

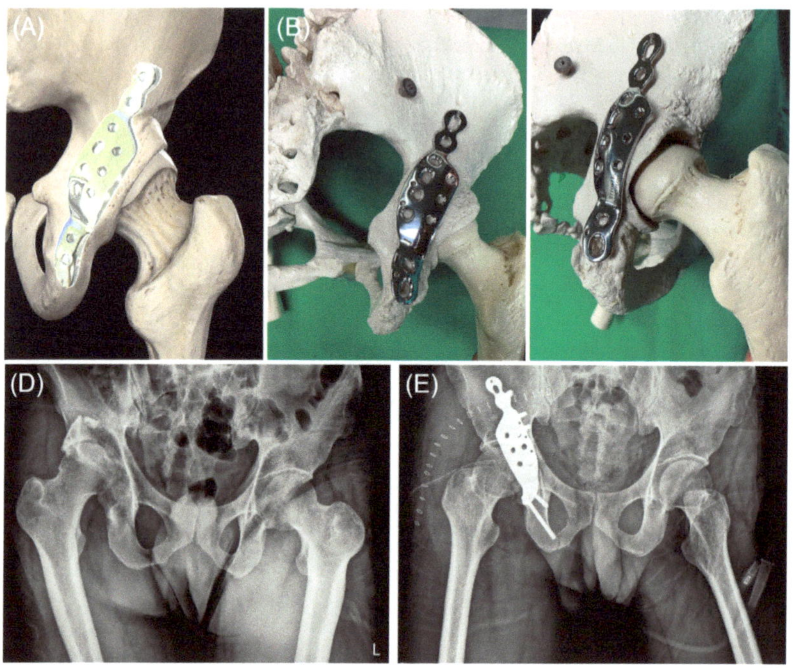

Figure 2. Design and application of the anatomical posterior acetabular plate (APAP). (**A**) A 3D reconstruction of the right hip joint demonstrates the APAP's design and optimal positioning for plating the posterior wall of the acetabulum. (**B**,**C**) Application of the APAP on a sawbone model in posteroanterior and iliac oblique views, respectively. (**D**) Radiograph displaying a case with a posterior wall fracture and concurrent posterior hip dislocation. (**E**) Postoperative radiograph illustrates the case after open reduction and internal fixation with the APAP, achieving anatomical reduction and concentric alignment of the hip joint.

The APAP comprises three components: the iliac, acetabular, and ischial components. The iliac and ischial components feature one locking hole and one compression hole (Figure 2A). The acetabular component incorporates anterior and posterior rows for addressing the posterior column and posterior wall, respectively. The anterior row accommodates either a 4.5 mm compression screw or a 4.5 mm locking screw. The posterior row has a fixed angle and utilizes 3.5 mm locking screws to prevent intra-articular screw penetration. The contour of the APAP is derived from 3D pelvic reconstructions. The acetabular component is slightly underbent to induce a tension band effect. Two sizes, standard and narrow, are available to accommodate variations in the distance between the sciatic notch and the rim of the posterior wall.

2.4. Surgical Procedure

All patients underwent general anesthesia and were positioned prone on a radiolucent table. The standard Kocher–Langenbeck approach was employed to visualize the fracture site, with the hip extended and the knee flexed beyond 90 degrees to facilitate sciatic nerve retraction. A Schanz screw was positioned over the trochanteric region to aid in manual distraction for hip distraction and improved joint visualization. The articular surface was exposed, and incarcerated fragments were elevated until flush with the articular surface. In fractures involving both the posterior column and posterior wall, posterior column reduction preceded posterior wall reduction. Farabeuf clamps or reduction clamps were utilized for fracture reduction, and a Schanz screw was inserted into the ischial tuberosity to serve as a joystick. Preliminary fixation was achieved using Kirschner wires (K-wires) or lag screws following posterior column reduction. Marginal impaction was corrected and temporarily fixed with K-wires.

Patients in the study group were treated with the APAP, applied along the curvature of the ilium, acetabulum, and ischium. Patients in the control group received treatment with a pelvic reconstruction plate. After provisionally fixing the appropriate plate holes, the quality of fracture reduction and implant positioning were assessed under fluoroscopic guidance. Intraoperative fluoroscopic checks included anteroposterior and obturator oblique views of the hip, axial views of the screws, and tangential views of the screws.

2.5. Postoperative Follow-Up and Rehabilitation Protocol

All patients received routine intravenous antibiotics, initiated during anesthesia induction and continued for one day post-surgery. Passive hip mobilization was encouraged on the first postoperative day, with active hip movement encouraged on the second postoperative day. Hip precautions, restricting flexion to less than 90° and preventing adduction, were implemented for the first 6 weeks. Non-weight-bearing ambulation was advised for 4–6 weeks to prevent the early loss of reduction. Patients progressed to full weight bearing only after radiographic and clinical confirmation of fracture union.

2.6. Outcome Measurements

Preoperative patient characteristics, encompassing age, gender, fracture pattern, presence of sciatic nerve injury, marginal impaction, and hip fracture/dislocation, were documented. Surgical details, such as intraoperative blood loss and duration of surgery, were also recorded. After surgery, patients underwent regular follow-ups at the outpatient department at intervals of 1, 2, 3, 6, and 12 months, followed by annual visits. All patients were followed up for a minimum of 2 years. During each follow-up, clinical functional recovery was semi-quantitatively assessed using the modified Merle d'Aubigné scoring system. At the final follow-up, clinical evaluation was conducted using the Oxford Hip Score (OHS) questionnaire [18], while radiological evaluation was performed according to Matta's criteria [1,19]. Utilizing posteroanterior and oblique pelvic X-rays, displacement was categorized as anatomical (0–1 mm), successful (2–3 mm), or poor (>3 mm). Recorded complications included postoperative sciatic nerve palsy, infection, heterotopic ossification (HO), osteonecrosis of the femoral head (ONFH), hip redislocation, implant failure, and the necessity for conversion to total hip arthroplasty (THA).

2.7. Statistical Analysis

To compare baseline characteristics between the study group and the control group, the non-parametric Mann–Whitney U test was utilized for continuous variables, while the Chi-squared test was employed for categorical variables. Functional recovery over time was examined using a general linear model for repeated measures analysis of variance. The cohort was divided based on the implants utilized, and measurements were taken at postoperative intervals of 1, 2, 3, 6, and 12 months. Differences in trends over the year between subgroups was assessed using between-subject effects. The Mann–Whitney U test was employed for the comparison of functional scores at specific time points. All statistical analyses were conducted using SPSS software (version 17.0; IBM, Armonk, NY, USA), with the significance level set at $p < 0.05$.

3. Results

3.1. Patient Characteristics

A total of 40 patients meeting the inclusion criteria were enrolled, with an average follow-up duration of 27.8 months (range, 24–60 months). The study group comprised 20 patients treated with APAP, while the control group consisted of 20 patients treated with a pelvic reconstruction plate. There were no statistically significant differences between the two groups in terms of gender distribution, acetabular fracture pattern based on Judet and Letournel classification, preoperative dislocation rate, time to definitive ORIF, and duration of final follow-up ($p = 0.212$) (Table 1). Motor vehicle accidents were the leading cause of injury, accounting for 90% (36 patients), while falls from height constituted the remaining 10% (4 patients) of cases.

Table 1. Patient characteristics.

		Study Group ($n = 20$)		Control Group ($n = 20$)		
Category	Subcategory	Count	Percentage	Count	Percentage	p Value
Gender	Male	18	90%	15	75%	0.212
	Female	2	10%	5	25%	
Fracture pattern	PW	7	35%	13	65%	0.088
	PCPW	4	20%	3	15%	
	TPW	4	20%	0	0%	
	BC	3	15%	4	20%	
	ACPH	2	10%	0	0%	
Preoperative dislocation	Present	8	40%	6	30%	0.504
	Absent	12	60%	14	70%	
Age		45.7	16.7	45.3	19.8	0.947
BMI		22.7	2.4	23.3	3.4	0.574
Time to ORIF (days)		4.2	3.2	4.1	2.5	0.820
Operative time (minutes)		186.5	51.0	225.0	47.7	0.004
Blood loss (mL)		695	393	930	609	0.049
Follow-up period (months)		40.6	11.7	34.9	8.8	0.121

The study group comprised 20 patients treated with an anatomical posterior acetabular plate (APAP), while the control group consisted of 20 patients treated with pelvic reconstruction plates. The p value was calculated using the Mann–Whitney U test for continuous variables and Chi-squared tests for categorical variables. (SD, standard deviation; PW, posterior wall; PCPW, posterior column and posterior wall; TPW, transverse and posterior wall; BC, both column; ACPH, anterior column and posterior hemi-transverse; BMI, body mass index; ORIF, open reduction and internal fixation).

A comparison of operative times between the two groups revealed a statistically significant difference (186.5 min versus 225 min, $p = 0.004$), indicating that APAP saved approximately 40 min of surgical time. Additionally, blood loss was significantly lower in the study group compared to that in the control group (695 mL versus 930 mL, $p = 0.049$).

3.2. Functional and Radiological Outcomes

Upon stratifying the patients into two groups based on the implants used, notable trends in functional recovery emerged, with a statistically significant difference observed ($p = 0.007$, determined through tests of between-subjects effects of repeated measure ANOVA) (see Figure 3). At 3 and 6 months following surgery, the modified Merle d'Aubigné scores in the two groups showed statistically significant differences (10 ± 1.8 versus 7.8 ± 1.4, $p < 0.001$; 13.4 ± 2.8 versus 10.1 ± 2.1, $p = 0.001$, determined through Mann–Whitney U tests). However, by the 12-month mark, functional recovery appeared to converge once again, with no statistically significant differences observed in the modified Merle d'Aubigné scores (14.2 ± 2.6 versus 12.7 ± 2.6, $p = 0.072$) or the OHS (31.6 ± 12.3 versus 30.3 ± 10.1, $p = 0.398$).

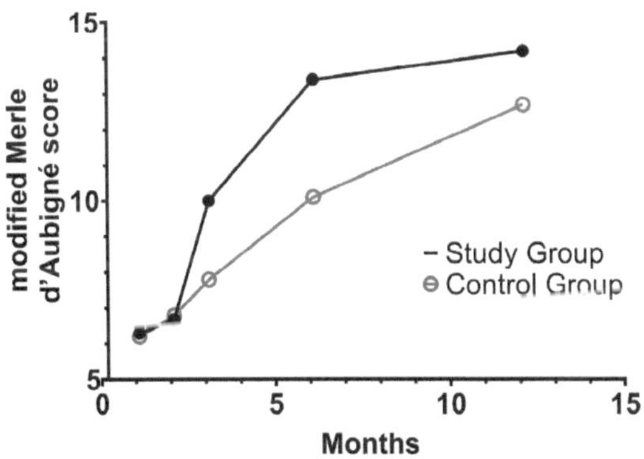

Figure 3. Functional recovery following open reduction and internal fixation of acetabular fractures involving the posterior wall. Patients treated with the anatomical posterior acetabular plate were placed into the study group (black dots), while those with conventional pelvic reconstruction formed the control group (hollow circles). A statistically significant difference in functional recovery emerged ($p = 0.007$, determined through tests of between-subjects effects of repeated measures ANOVA). At 3 and 6 months following surgery, the modified Merle d'Aubigné scores were significantly higher in the study group ($p < 0.001$ and $p = 0.001$, respectively; determined through Mann–Whitney U tests). However, by the 12-month mark, there was no statistically significant difference between the two groups ($p = 0.072$).

Likewise, the radiological outcomes assessed using Matta's criteria at 12 months after surgery did not demonstrate significant differences between the study and control groups ($p = 0.204$, determined through Chi-squared analysis). The radiological outcomes were significantly superior in the study group ($p = 0.047$). Anatomical reduction was sustained in 70% of the study group compared to 35% of the control group, while successful reduction was maintained in 15% of the study group and 50% of the control group (Table 2).

Table 2. Radiological outcomes of acetabular treatment.

Matta Criteria	Study Group	Control Group	*p* Value
Anatomical	14	7	0.047
Successful	3	10	
Poor	3	3	

The study group comprised 20 patients treated with an anatomical posterior acetabular plate (APAP), while the control group consisted of 20 patients treated with pelvic reconstruction plates. *p* value was generated using a Chi-squared test.

3.3. Complications

Postoperative complications are outlined in Table 3. Among patients treated with APAP (the study group), foot drop was noted in two cases: one had preoperative foot drop, which resolved by 3 months after surgery, while the other experienced transient postoperative foot drop, spontaneously resolving within 2 months after surgery. Similarly, two patients in the control group developed postoperative foot drop, with both cases resolving by 6 months after surgery. One patient treated with a conventional pelvic reconstruction plate (the control group) experienced recurrent hip dislocation, resulting in the fracture and fragmentation of the osteonecrotic femoral head, ultimately necessitating conversion to hip arthroplasty (see Figure 4). Notably, none of the three patients in the study group who suffered from postoperative recurrent dislocation experienced femoral head fracture. The rate of conversion to hip arthroplasty did not differ significantly between the study and control groups (10% versus 15%, $p = 0.633$). Postoperative infection rates did not differ significantly between the two groups (5% vs. 10%, $p = 0.548$). Among the patients treated with the conventional pelvic reconstruction plate, one developed a deep infection requiring debridement and implant retention, while the other two experienced superficial infections and cellulitis, both of which were successfully managed with intravenous antibiotics. Additionally, the prevalence of other complications, including osteoarthritis, osteonecrosis of the femoral head, and heterotopic ossification, did not vary between the two groups. (Table 3)

Table 3. Complications rates after open reduction and internal fixation of acetabular fracture.

	Study Group	Control Group	*p* Value
Foot drop	10% (2/20)	10% (2/20)	1.00
Recurrent dislocation	15% (3/20)	10% (2/20)	0.633
Infection	5% (1/20)	10% (2/20)	0.548
Osteoarthritis	35% (7/20)	30% (6/20)	0.736
Osteonecrosis of femoral head	25% (5/20)	20% (4/20)	0.705
Heterotopic ossification	5% (1/20)	10% (2/20)	0.548

The study group comprised 20 patients treated with an anatomical posterior acetabular plate (APAP), while the control group consisted of 20 patients treated with pelvic reconstruction plates. The *p* value was generated using Chi-squared analysis.

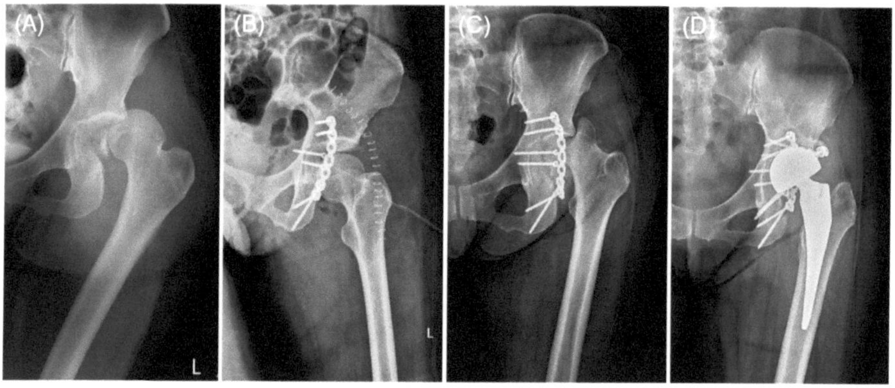

Figure 4. A case of acetabular fracture treated with conventional pelvic reconstruction plate complicated by recurrent dislocation. (**A**) The patient sustained concurrent left acetabular posterior wall fracture and posterior dislocation of the left hip joint. (**B**) The patient underwent open reduction and internal fixation with a conventional pelvic reconstruction plate. (**C**) Eight months after the index surgery, the patient experienced recurrent hip dislocation, accompanied by a concurrent femoral head fracture. (**D**) Eventually, the patient underwent secondary surgery and conversion to bipolar hemiarthroplasty.

4. Discussion

The management of posterior wall or posterior column fractures presents significant challenges due to the critical need for achieving both anatomical reduction and stable fixation, which is inherently difficult to accomplish [20]. This study introduces a novel APAP, which not only eliminates the need for custom bending and reduces intraoperative blood loss but also enhances stability, leading to expedited functional recovery compared to conventional pelvic reconstruction plates. The design of the APAP provides orthopedic trauma surgeons with a durable and time-efficient alternative, paving the way for future advancements in anatomical acetabular plates.

Traditionally, posterior plating for acetabular fractures involved the utilization of rim plates, buttress plates, or spring plates, either individually or in various combinations [12,13,15]. However, these methods are time-consuming and technically demanding. Additionally, repeated contouring of the reconstruction plate could potentially compromise its inherent mechanical strength [14,21]. The past literature has introduced a few anatomical acetabular locking plates, highlighting the biomechanical advantages of such plates over conventional reconstruction plates [22]. For instance, Zhang et al. developed a W-shaped acetabular angular plate (WAAP) for reconstructing acetabular posterior wall fractures [16]. In a retrospective comparison with conventional reconstruction plates, the WAAP effectively reduced intra-articular screw penetration under intraoperative fluoroscopy. However, functional recovery trends between the WAAP group and the conventional reconstruction plate group were not compared. Similarly, Huang et al. proposed an H-shaped anatomical titanium plate for posterior plating in acetabular fractures [17]. Although the authors reported satisfactory radiological and functional outcomes with low complication rates, the study was descriptive and lacked a control group. Other studies have explored the use of 3D printed patient-specific plates [23–25]. Despite promising outcomes, 3D printing technology remains costly and may not be readily available in general hospitals. In contrast, the APAP is a commercialized anatomical locking plate, proven to be a cost-effective and safe alternative to conventional reconstruction plates in the current study. Moreover, the APAP offers an additional ischial component for fixation compared to the plates designed by Zhang et al. and Huang et al. [16,17]. The design of the APAP was intended to replicate the biomechanical advantages of a double plate by incorporating two rows of holes for locking screws. This, combined with the broader width and increased screw count, enhances the rigidity and stability of the construct. These features may explain the slight advantage observed in terms of improved reduction after 12 months. The APAP costs approximately $2500, compared to around $2000 for the low-profile pelvic system. In cases where dual pelvic reconstruction plates are required for treating posterior wall or posterior column fractures, the APAP proves to be economically advantageous, as it requires only a single plate. In summary, the APAP is demonstrated to be a safe, effective, and more versatile option in managing comminuted posterior wall fractures.

Safety and efficacy are the primary goals in the internal fixation of posterior acetabular fractures. Early (<48 h) and delayed surgeries have been extensively studied, with earlier intervention recommended for relatively simple fracture patterns [26], while the timing for complex fractures remains controversial [27]. Complex fracture patterns also tend to result in greater blood loss during surgery compared to posterior wall fractures [27]. Some studies have suggested that combining epidural and general anesthesia can help reduce blood loss [28]. A positive correlation between surgical time and blood loss has been consistently observed in the literature [27,29,30]. In the current study, the use of the anatomical posterior acetabular plate (APAP) shortened surgical time by eliminating the need for bending the plate and simplifying the templating process. Additionally, the anatomical design of the APAP reduced the likelihood of intra-articular screw penetration, thereby minimizing the need for screw adjustments [16]. Less adjustment and less extensive soft tissue dissection, which is possible with a plate that conforms more closely to the native anatomy, thereby reduced the surgical time and associated bleeding. These advantages are particularly beneficial for managing complex posterior acetabular fractures and for surgeons who are in the early stages of treating these fractures.

Acetabular fractures often result in long-term morbidity, with variable trajectories of functional recovery. Letournel reported that despite achieving 94% perfect reductions of posterior wall fractures, only 79.5% of cases attained at least a very good result [10]. This discrepancy was attributed by Letournel et al. to associated osteonecrosis and comminution of the posterior wall [10,31]. Similarly, Matta et al. found slightly inferior outcomes in acetabular fractures involving the posterior wall in their investigation of 20-year survivorship in 816 patients following open reduction and internal fixation of displaced acetabular fractures [32]. The 20-year survivorship of simple posterior wall fractures was 76%, while that of associated posterior column and posterior wall fractures was 85% [32]. Recently, Tucker et al. discussed the recovery trajectory of surgically treated acetabular fractures [33]. Between six months and one year postoperatively, only 37.3% of patients reached the minimal clinically important difference (MCID), and a significant proportion (38.1%) failed to achieve the MCID even after five years [33]. The ratio of anatomical reduction was 70%, or 85% if acceptable alignment was also included, consistent with previous literature. In the current study, the APAP facilitated short-term functional recovery by approximately three months compared with conventional pelvic reconstruction plates. Remarkably, most patients in our study presented with posterior wall involvement, which typically carries a poorer prognosis. The improved functional outcomes in the APAP group may be attributed to several factors. The anatomical design of the plate likely resulted in less soft tissue dissection, reducing surgical trauma and promoting quicker recovery. Additionally, the precise anatomical fit of the APAP provided more stable fixation and better initial alignment, creating a more favorable environment for healing and rehabilitation. The locking screws in the specially designed ischial limb also contributed to enhanced stability. In summary, the APAP shows promise in the treatment of complex acetabular fractures involving the posterior wall and has the potential to hasten postoperative functional recovery.

Late complications of posterior acetabular fractures, such as end-stage hip osteoarthritis, osteonecrosis of the femoral head, or heterotopic ossification, often necessitate conversion to total hip arthroplasty [20]. The conversion rate to hip arthroplasty varies widely. The anatomical restoration of the acetabulum is considered the most critical step in preventing these late complications and eventual conversion to hip arthroplasty [34]. Maintaining anatomical reduction has been linked to favorable functional and radiological outcomes, with reported rates of 71–86.4% and 17–95% in patients, respectively [3,35–38]. Dunet et al. reported a conversion rate of 34.7% over a 10-year period [5], while Cichos et al. reported a conversion rate of 16%, with 52% of conversions occurring within 1 year post-surgery [39]. Similarly, Firoozabadi et al. evaluated 65 patients with posterior wall acetabular fractures treated with ORIF, reporting a 17% conversion rate after 9 years [40]. In our study, the conversion rate to total hip arthroplasty was 15% in patients treated with conventional pelvic reconstruction plates after 4 years of follow-up, consistent with the previous literature. Among patients treated with APAP, the conversion rate was approximately 10%. The relatively low mid-term conversion rate in the APAP group may be attributed to the more stable fixation of the plate and better maintenance of anatomical reduction due to its anatomical design after 4 years.

Several limitations of this study should be acknowledged. First, the sample size was relatively small, as this was a single-institution study, which may limit the statistical power and generalizability of the findings. Additionally, patients who did not complete at least 2 years of follow-up were excluded. Second, the study design was retrospective, which may have introduced bias despite efforts to control for baseline characteristics between the study group and the control group. Third, biomechanical features and fatigue analyses were not included in the current study; thus, a quantitative assessment of the rigidity and efficacy of buttressing was not possible. Fourth, the medium-term follow-up period (mean of 27.8 months) may not fully capture long-term differences in functional recovery and complications. We plan to conduct further analysis after the patients complete a 5-year follow-up. Finally, the potential influence of surgical experience is another limitation, as the learning effect could not be fully accounted for in this retrospective design. More experienced surgeons may achieve shorter surgical times, which could influence the study outcomes. The APAP was not applicable for some more complex acetabular fractures. In other words, the benefits of the APAP may be more pronounced for less experienced surgeons compared to their more experienced counterparts. These limitations warrant cautious interpretation of the study findings and highlight areas for further research.

5. Conclusions

The use of an APAP in reconstructing the posterior acetabulum significantly reduces surgical time, decreases intraoperative blood loss, and leads to earlier functional recovery compared to conventional reconstruction plates. The APAP provides stable fixation of the posterior wall and ensures the durable maintenance of reduction, ultimately yielding favorable surgical outcomes.

Author Contributions: C.-H.C., M.-H.H. and P.-Y.L. contributed to conceptualization and methodology. C.-H.C., J.-H.W. and H.-C.C. performed formal analysis and investigation. C.-H.C. was a major contributor to writing the manuscript. Writing—review and editing were performed by J.-M.Y., P.-T.W., M.-H.H., H.-L.S. and P.-Y.L. All authors have read and agreed to the published version of the manuscript.

Funding: The publication fee was supported by Show Chwan Memorial Hospital, Changhua, Taiwan (SRD-112025, SRD-112027).

Institutional Review Board Statement: The study protocol received approval from the institutional review board of Show Chwan Memorial Hospital (IRB number 1110802) on 10 July 2023, and informed consent was obtained from all patients. The clinical investigations were conducted following the principles expressed in the Declaration of Helsinki.

Informed Consent Statement: Informed consent was obtained from all subjects involved in the study.

Data Availability Statement: The data are available on reasonable request.

Acknowledgments: We are grateful to the Skeleton Materials and Bio-Compatibility Core Lab, Research Center of Clinical Medicine, National Cheng Kung University Hospital for their assistance with this study.

Conflicts of Interest: The authors declare no conflicts of interest.

References

1. Matta, J.M. Fractures of the acetabulum: Accuracy of reduction and clinical results in patients managed operatively within three weeks after the injury. *J. Bone Jt. Surg. Am.* **1996**, *78*, 1632–1645. [CrossRef]
2. Porter, S.E.; Schroeder, A.C.; Dzugan, S.S.; Graves, M.L.; Zhang, L.; Russell, G.V. Acetabular Fracture Patterns and Their Associated Injuries. *J. Orthop. Trauma* **2008**, *22*, 165–170. [CrossRef] [PubMed]
3. Pascarella, R.; Cerbasi, S.; Politano, R.; Balato, G.; Fantasia, R.; Orabona, G.; Mariconda, M. Surgical results and factors influencing outcome in patients with posterior wall acetabular fracture. *Injury* **2017**, *48*, 1819–1824. [CrossRef] [PubMed]
4. Morison, Z.; Moojen, D.J.; Nauth, A.; Hall, J.; McKee, M.D.; Waddell, J.P.; Schemitsch, E.H. Total Hip Arthroplasty After Acetabular Fracture Is Associated With Lower Survivorship and More Complications. *Clin. Orthop. Relat. Res.* **2016**, *474*, 392–398. [CrossRef]
5. Dunet, B.; Tournier, C.; Billaud, A.; Lavoinne, N.; Fabre, T.; Durandeau, A. Acetabular fracture: Long-term follow-up and factors associated with secondary implantation of total hip arthroplasty. *Orthop. Traumatol. Surg. Res.* **2013**, *99*, 281–290. [CrossRef]
6. Schnaser, E.; Scarcella, N.R.; Vallier, H.A. Acetabular fractures converted to total hip arthroplasties in the elderly: How does function compare to primary total hip arthroplasty? *J. Orthop. Trauma* **2014**, *28*, 694–699. [CrossRef]
7. Weber, M.; Berry, D.J.; Harmsen, W.S. Total Hip Arthroplasty after Operative Treatment of an Acetabular Fracture*. *J. Bone Jt. Surg.* **1998**, *80*, 1295–1305. [CrossRef]
8. de Palma, L.; Santucci, A.; Verdenelli, A.; Bugatti, M.G.; Meco, L.; Marinelli, M. Outcome of unstable isolated fractures of the posterior acetabular wall associated with hip dislocation. *Eur. J. Orthop. Surg. Traumatol.* **2013**, *24*, 341–346. [CrossRef]
9. Giannoudis, P.; Nikolaou, V. Surgical techniques—How do I do it?: Open reduction and internal fixation of posterior wall fractures of the acetabulum. *Injury* **2008**, *39*, 1113–1118. [CrossRef]

10. D'Aubigne, R.M.; Postel, M. Functional results of hip arthroplasty with acrylic prosthesis. *J. Bone Jt. Surg. Am.* **1954**, *36*, 451–475. [CrossRef]
11. Li, H.; Yang, H.; Wang, D.; Xu, Y.; Min, J.; Xu, X.; Li, Z.; Yuan, Y. Fractures of the posterior wall of the acetabulum: Treatment using internal fixation of two parallel reconstruction plates. *Injury* **2014**, *45*, 709–714. [CrossRef] [PubMed]
12. Yu, J.K.; Chiu, F.-Y.; Feng, C.-K.; Chung, T.-Y.; Chen, T.-H. Surgical treatment of displaced fractures of posterior column and posterior wall of the acetabulum. *Injury* **2004**, *35*, 766–770. [CrossRef] [PubMed]
13. Chen, M.J.; Hollyer, I.; Wadhwa, H.; Tigchelaar, S.S.; Van Rysselberghe, N.L.; Bishop, J.A.; Bellino, M.J.; Gardner, M.J. Management of the posterior wall fracture in associated both column fractures of the acetabulum. *Eur. J. Orthop. Surg. Traumatol.* **2021**, *31*, 1047–1054. [CrossRef]
14. Liu, P.-C.; Yang, Y.-J.; Liu, R.; Shu, H.-X.; Gong, J.-P.; Yang, Y.; Sun, Q.; Wu, X.; Cai, M. A study on the mechanical characteristics of the EBM-printed Ti-6Al-4V LCP plates in vitro. *J. Orthop. Surg. Res.* **2014**, *9*, 106. [CrossRef]
15. Richter, H.; Hutson, J.J.; Zych, G. The Use of Spring Plates in the Internal Fixation of Acetabular Fractures. *J. Orthop. Trauma* **2004**, *18*, 179–181. [CrossRef] [PubMed]
16. Zhang, Q.; Chen, W.; Wu, X.; Su, Y.; Hou, Z.; Zhang, Y. Comparative Study of W-Shaped Angular Plate and Reconstruction Plate in Treating Posterior Wall Fractures of the Acetabulum. *PLoS ONE* **2014**, *9*, e92210. [CrossRef]
17. Huang, J.; Liao, M.; Chen, X. Application of new H-shaped anatomical titanium plate for posterior wall/posterior column acetabular fractures. *Chin. J. Reparative Reconstr. Surg.* **2021**, *35*, 64–69.
18. Ovre, S.; Sandvik, L.; Madsen, J.E.; Røise, O. Comparison of distribution, agreement and correlation between the original and modified Merle d'Aubig-ne-Postel Score and the Harris Hip Score after acetabular fracture treatment: Moderate agreement, high ceiling effect and ex-cellent correlation in 450 patients. *Acta Orthop.* **2005**, *76*, 796–802.
19. Yu, Y.-H.; Liu, C.-H.; Hsu, Y.-H.; Chou, Y.-C.; Chen, I.-J.; Wu, C.-C. Matta's criteria may be useful for evaluating and predicting the reduction quality of simultaneous acetabular and ipsilateral pelvic ring fractures. *BMC Musculoskelet. Disord.* **2021**, *22*, 1–7. [CrossRef]
20. Bastian, J.; Savic, M.; Cullmann, J.; Zech, W.; Djonov, V.; Keel, M. Surgical exposures and options for instrumentation in acetabular fracture fixation: Pararectus approach versus the modified Stoppa. *Injury* **2016**, *47*, 695–701. [CrossRef]
21. Kim, H.; Jung, Y.; Song, H.S. Plate prebending using a three-dimensional-printed model affords effective anatomical reduction in clavicular shaft fractures. *Clin. Shoulder Elb.* **2023**, *26*, 397–405. [CrossRef] [PubMed]
22. Su, K.; Liu, S.; Wu, T.; Yin, Y.; Zhang, R.; Li, S.; Zhang, Y. Posterior column acetabular fracture fixation using a W-shaped angular plate: A biomechanical analysis. *PLoS ONE* **2017**, *12*, e0187886. [CrossRef]
23. Liu, Z.-J.; Jia, J.; Zhang, Y.-G.; Tian, W.; Jin, X.; Hu, Y.-C. Internal Fixation of Complicated Acetabular Fractures Directed by Preoperative Surgery with 3D Printing Models. *Orthop. Surg.* **2017**, *9*, 257–260. [CrossRef] [PubMed]
24. Wan, L.; Zhang, X.; Zhang, S.; Li, K.; Cao, P.; Li, J.; Wu, G. Clinical feasibility and application value of computer virtual reduction combined with 3D printing technique in complex acetabular fractures. *Exp. Ther. Med.* **2019**, *17*, 3630–3636. [CrossRef]
25. Hsu, C.-L.; Chou, Y.-C.; Li, Y.-T.; Chen, J.-E.; Hung, C.-C.; Wu, C.-C.; Shen, H.-C.; Yeh, T.-T. Pre-operative virtual simulation and three-dimensional printing techniques for the surgical management of acetabular fractures. *Int. Orthop.* **2018**, *43*, 1969–1976. [CrossRef] [PubMed]
26. Furey, A.J.; Karp, J.; O'Toole, R.V. Does early fixation of posterior wall acetabular fractures lead to increased blood loss? *J. Orthop. Trauma* **2013**, *27*, 2–5. [CrossRef]
27. Dailey, S.K.; Archdeacon, M.T. Open reduction and internal fixation of acetabulum fractures: Does timing of surgery affect blood loss and OR time? *J. Orthop. Trauma* **2014**, *28*, 497–501. [CrossRef] [PubMed]
28. Acan, A.E. Effects of different anesthesia techniques on intraoperative blood loss in acetabular fractures undergoing the Modified Stoppa approach. *Ulus Travma Acil. Cerrahi. Derg.* **2020**, *26*, 445–452. [CrossRef]
29. Wójcicki, R.; Pielak, T.; Walus, P.M.; Jaworski, P.; Małkowski, B.; Jasiewicz, P.; Gagat, M.; Łapaj, Ł.; Zabrzyński, J. The Association of Acetabulum Fracture and Mechanism of Injury with BMI, Days Spent in Hospital, Blood Loss, and Surgery Time: A Retrospective Analysis of 67 Patients. *Medicina* **2024**, *60*, 455. [CrossRef]
30. Yang, Y.; Sun, J.; Xiang, Z. The Short- and Mid-term Follow-Up of Single-Column Fixation in Transverse and Posterior Wall Acetabular Fractures. *Orthop. Surg.* **2022**, *14*, 65–72. [CrossRef]
31. Ziran, N.; Soles, G.L.S.; Matta, J.M. Outcomes after surgical treatment of acetabular fractures: A review. *Patient Saf. Surg.* **2019**, *13*, 1–19. [CrossRef] [PubMed]
32. Tannast, M.; Najibi, S.; Matta, J.M. Two to Twenty-Year Survivorship of the Hip in 810 Patients with Operatively Treated Acetabular Fractures. *J. Bone Jt. Surg.* **2012**, *94*, 1559–1567. [CrossRef] [PubMed]
33. Tucker, A.; Roffey, D.M.; Guy, P.; Potter, J.M.; Broekhuyse, H.M.; Lefaivre, K.A. Evaluation of the trajectory of recovery following surgically treated acetabular fractures. *Bone Jt. J.* **2024**, *106-B*, 69–76. [CrossRef]
34. Meena, U.; Tripathy, S.; Sen, R.; Aggarwal, S.; Behera, P. Predictors of postoperative outcome for acetabular fractures. *Orthop. Traumatol. Surg. Res.* **2013**, *99*, 929–935. [CrossRef] [PubMed]
35. Verbeek, D.O.; van der List, J.P.; Villa, J.C.; Wellman, D.S.; Helfet, D.L. Postoperative CT Is Superior for Acetabular Fracture Reduction Assessment and Reliably Predicts Hip Survivorship. *J. Bone Jt. Surg.* **2017**, *99*, 1745–1752. [CrossRef]
36. Long, H.-T.; Deng, Z.-H.; Zou, M.; Lin, Z.-Y.; Zhu, J.-X.; Zhu, Y. Effects of the acetabular fracture index and other factors of posterior wall acetabular fracture on functional outcome. *J. Int. Med. Res.* **2017**, *45*, 1394–1405. [CrossRef]

37. Verbeek, D.O.; van der List, J.P.; Tissue, C.M.; Helfet, D.L. Long-term patient reported outcomes following acetabular fracture fixation. *Injury* **2018**, *49*, 1131–1136. [CrossRef]
38. Briffa, N.; Pearce, R.; Hill, A.M.; Bircher, M. Outcomes of acetabular fracture fixation with ten years' follow-up. *J. Bone Jt. Surg. Br. Vol.* **2011**, *93-B*, 229–236. [CrossRef]
39. Cichos, K.H.; Spitler, C.A.; Quade, J.H.; McGwin, G., Jr.; Ghanem, E.S. Fracture and Patient Characteristics Associated With Early Conversion Total Hip Arthroplasty After Ace-tabular Fracture Fixation. *J. Orthop. Trauma* **2021**, *35*, 599–605. [CrossRef]
40. Firoozabadi, R.M.; Hamilton, B.; Toogood, P.; Routt, M.; Shearer, D. Risk Factors for Conversion to Total Hip Arthroplasty After Acetabular Fractures Involving the Posterior Wall. *J. Orthop. Trauma* **2018**, *32*, 607–611. [CrossRef]

Journal of
Clinical Medicine

MDPI

Article

Management Options for Traumatic Posterior Sternoclavicular Joint Dislocation: A Narrative Review with a Single Institution's Experience

Corrado Ciatti [1,2,*], Virginia Masoni [3], Pietro Maniscalco [1,2], Chiara Asti [1,4], Calogero Puma Pagliarello [1], Gianfilippo Caggiari [4], Marco Pes [4], Fabrizio Rivera [5] and Fabrizio Quattrini [1,2]

1 Department of Orthopedics and Traumatology, Guglielmo da Saliceto Hospital, AUSL Piacenza, 29121 Piacenza, Italy; p.maniscalco@ausl.pc.it (P.M.); c.asti@studenti.uniss.it (C.A.); c.pumapagliarello@ausl.pc.it (C.P.P.); fabrizioquattrini@yahoo.it (F.Q.)
2 Department of Orthopedics and Traumatology, University of Parma, 43121 Parma, Italy
3 Department of Orthopedics and Traumatology, University of Turin, Via Zuretti, 29, 10126 Turin, Italy; virginia.masoni@unito.it
4 Department of Orthopedics and Traumatology, University of Sassari, 07100 Sassari, Italy; gianfilippocaggiari@gmail.com (G.C.); marco92pes@gmail.com (M.P.)
5 Department of Orthopedics and Traumatology, Ospedale SS Annunziata, ASL CN1, Via Ospedali, 9, 12038 Savigliano, Italy; rivgio@libero.it
* Correspondence: dadociatti@icloud.com

Abstract: Background: Posterior sternoclavicular joint (SCJ) dislocations are rare events that can evolve into real emergencies due to the vital structures in the mediastinum. When closed reduction maneuvers fail, open SCJ reconstruction becomes mandatory, with literature proposing several stabilization techniques that either preserve or remove the SCJ's mobility. This study is a narrative review of the most recent literature regarding posterior trauma to the SCJ along with a single institution's experience of this pathology, managed either conservatively or surgically, with a figure-of-eight autologous semitendinosus graft in case of closed reduction failure. **Methods:** This article provides an overview of posterior traumatic SCJ dislocation, and it describes five cases of patients managed for traumatic posterior SCJ dislocation treated either conservatively or surgically with a figure-of-eight semitendinosus tendon autograft reinforced with high-strength suture tape. A comparison with the most recent literature is performed, focusing on biomechanics. **Results:** The demographics, the mechanism of injury, the management algorithm and the surgical strategy align with the most recent literature. Despite the final treatment, at one year of follow-up, the ROM was restored with full strength throughout the range of motion of the shoulder with no neurological deficits. The reduced joint successfully healed in imaging, and patients returned to their daily lives. The surgical site wounds and donor harvest sites were perfectly healed. **Conclusions:** Although recent recommendations for treating posterior traumatic SCJ dislocation have advanced, no universally accepted method of stabilization exists, and the surgical strategy is generally entrusted to the surgeon's experience. The literature still increasingly supports figure-of-eight ligament reconstruction with a biological or synthetic graft. This work further implements the literature by reporting good outcomes at follow-up.

Keywords: SCJ; posterior dislocation; biomechanics; figure-of-eight; semitendinosus

1. Introduction

Sternoclavicular joint (SCJ) injuries represent 3% of all shoulder-girdle lesions and less than 1% of all dislocations [1–4]. Traumatic dislocations are more likely to occur in young, active men after high-energy trauma, such as sports injuries, road traffic accidents and falls [1–3,5–7].

Dislocations most commonly occur anteriorly due to the SCJ's anatomy, which includes a stout posterior capsular ligament and the costoclavicular ligament [1,8]. Nonetheless, posterior SCJ dislocation may lead to life-threatening consequences due to vital structures in the mediastinum [7–9].

For this reason, a high index of suspicion and immediate identification is necessary, with a missing rate of 25% at initial presentation [1–3,7–13]. The patient most often complains of neck and shoulder pain, which increases with movement of the ipsilateral girdle, with a possible palpable defect and deformity of the SCJ [1,3].

While radiography, in a serendipity view, is used, a CT scan is the preferred imaging modality to diagnose dislocation and assess the mediastinal structures [2,14].

Another classification is acute or chronic SCJ dislocation, with the chronic ones resulting from missed initial diagnosis, delayed clinical presentation and recurrent dislocation after closed reduction performed in the acute setting [14–16].

Despite the normal range of motion (ROM) of SCJ being narrow, this joint impacts the scapulothoracic, the glenohumeral rhythm, and the ROM of the shoulder girdle, being the only true connection between the axial skeleton and the upper limb [1–3].

The literature has developed several recommendations concerning the management of posterior SCJ dislocations [1–3]. A closed reduction is attempted in the first 48 h, followed by a subsequent imaging re-evaluation [1–3]. In case of failure or recurrent chronic instability, an open reduction is necessary, and, in this case, SCJ reconstruction is suggested [1,17]. However, no universal guidelines exist concerning the surgical strategy that should be adopted to stabilize this joint [3,18]. The review by Kendal et al. [2] and the most recent literature [1,3], based on the biomechanical study by Spencer and Kuhn in 2004 [19], support reconstruction with tendon grafts, especially with a figure-of-eight configuration [1–3]. Pins and Kirschner wires should be avoided due to possible migration in the vital structures of the mediastinum, as well as ORIF with plates and screws due to the necessity of their removal to restore motion [1–3].

This study provides a comprehensive overview on posterior traumatic SCJ dislocation. Management algorithms and outcomes are described. Moreover, it reports the experience from a single institution by describing five cases of this rare pathology managed either conservatively or surgically. Specifically, it focuses on the adopted surgical strategy, which consists of the reconstruction with a figure-of-eight autologous semitendinosus graft. Preoperative and intraoperative details are reported. A comparison with the most recent literature concerning the management methods is performed, with a complete explanation of the importance of the anatomy and biomechanics as the leading factors guiding authors to adopt this surgical technique.

2. Methods, Study Design and Surgical Technique

A comprehensive narrative review of the current literature on posterior traumatic SCJ dislocations was conducted taking into account the epidemiology, the management and the adopted surgical strategy for this pathology.

A retrospective analysis of all orthopedic consults occurring at the Emergency Department (ED) of the Guglielmo da Saliceto Hospital in Piacenza in Italy was performed to identify episodes of posterior sternoclavicular joint dislocation. Patient data were extracted from the database of the ED. The analyzed time frame was from January 2020 to December 2023.

All patients who were older than eighteen years old and presented with a traumatic posterior SCJ dislocation were included in the study, with no other exclusion criteria except for the follow-up. Indeed, patients who did not complete a minimum follow-up of 12 months and who had atraumatic posterior SCJ dislocation were excluded. This last group was excluded since the atraumatic dislocations follow other management pathways, and, as reported in the literature, they tend to occur in patients with different baseline characteristics, as in patients with trapezius palsy or generalized hyperlaxity [1]. Inclusion and exclusion criteria are summarized in Scheme 1.

ED
January 2020 - December 2023
Posterior SCJ dislocation

Inclusion Criteria

- > 18 years old
- Traumatic Posterior SCJ dislocation
- Minimum Follow-up 12 months

Total 6 patients (1 refused the management)

5 patients included

Exclusion Criteria

- ≤ 18 years old
- Atraumatic Posterior SCJ dislocation
- Follow-up < 12 months

Scheme 1. Inclusion and Exclusion Criteria.

Six patients who met the inclusion criteria were detected (five males and one female), but one of them was excluded because the patient refused the proposed treatment. Consequently, five patients, all males, were included in the study. The mean age was 34.4 years old (range 28–43 years old). All patients underwent a complete physical examination of the other near joints; three patients had not sustained any other injuries, two patients reported other fractures (one of them an ipsilateral distal fibular fracture, and the other a contralateral distal radial fracture, respectively). Three of them had a fall from a height, one patient reported a motor-bike accident and one had a trauma during sports activity, specifically during a rugby match. All of them reported indirect trauma, with a blow on the posterolateral side of the shoulder without loss of consciousness.

They were all subjected to X-ray examinations when they arrived at the ED. Moreover, a CT scan was requested for all cases to have a definitive diagnosis and for the potential involvement of thoracic essential organs. However, no systemic symptoms, such as cough, hoarseness, shortness of breath or venous congestion were present. At the CT scan, complete posterior dislocation of the SCJ was always confirmed (Figure 1). In addition, fractures and infractions of the ribs, lung parenchymal contusions and apical subpleural hematomas were detected.

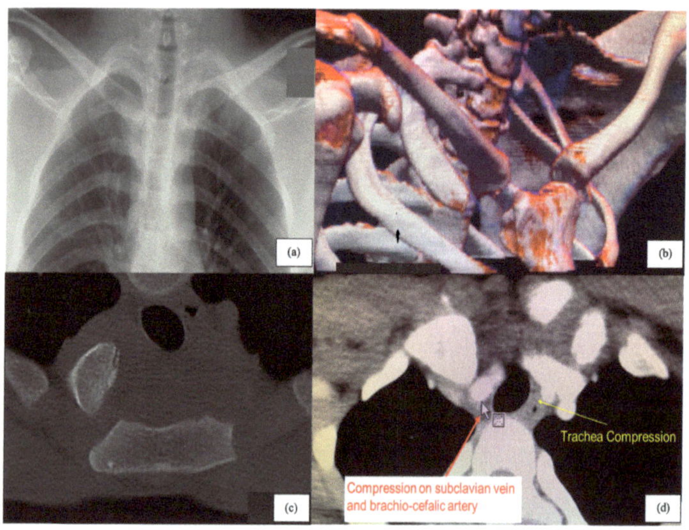

Figure 1. Preoperative evaluation of posterior SCJ dislocation: (**a**) chest X-ray; (**b**) 3D reconstruction; (**c**) axial CT scan bone view; (**d**) axial CT scan.

A closed reduction maneuver was performed acutely in all cases in the ED under sedation and local anesthesia with the presence of the anesthesiologist and the vascular surgeon. After the trial maneuver, a CT scan was performed to assess the reduction. The reduction was fruitless in two cases, while in three patients it led to a reduction of the dislocation.

2.1. Conservative Treatment

For the three successful cases, once a CT scan verified the reduction, the patients were discharged home, and four outpatient visits were scheduled at 1–3–6–12 months after the trauma. At the follow-ups, X-rays were usually performed along with clinical examination, except for the third month where a CT scan was used to assess the maintenance of the reduction. A CT scan was also employed in cases of inconclusive X-rays. No recurrences were recorded in imaging, and, at the last follow-up, all patients had successfully recovered complete range of motion of the shoulder (in abduction/adduction, rotation and flexion/extension) and muscle strength, were pain-free while moving their arms and were back to their daily lives.

2.2. Surgical Treatment with a Figure-of-Eight Semitendinosus Tendon Autograft Reinforced with High-Strength Suture Tape

Regarding the two closely irreducible dislocations, the patients were admitted to the hospital for open surgical reduction and SCJ reconstruction. After the exclusion of SARS-CoV-2 infection through a nasopharyngeal swab in accordance with the COVID-19 protocol rules [20,21], the patients underwent surgery. The subsequent described procedure was the same for both patients.

A second closed reduction was attempted in the operating room, in the hopes anesthesia would simplify the procedure. The anesthesiologist was present throughout the procedure, and the thoracic surgeon and vascular surgeon were on standby in the operating room. Once the anesthesia was performed, we attempted the maneuvers described by Rockwood and Buckerfield maneuvers, without obtaining a successful reduction [1,14,22]. We tried, without success, to clamp the proximal end of the clavicle with bone forceps and pull and rotate it upwards. Consequently, an open reduction was needed. Given the detected instability, SCJ reconstruction with an autologous tendon graft in a figure-of-eight was selected. The medical team was made up of orthopedic surgeons, a thoracic surgeon and an anesthesiologist.

The first surgical step was the harvest of the tendon graft. The semitendinosus tendon was preferred. The patients were positioned supine with a tourniquet to the thigh, and 2 g of cefazoline were administered preoperatively (Figure 2). For both surgeries, after setting up the sterile field, the tendon was harvested, tubularized with a non-absorbable suture on a workstation and then stored in a compound made of 500 mL of saline solution 0.9% + 1 g of vancomycin, similar to the hamstring harvest for anterior cruciate ligament reconstruction. The first surgical step ended with tourniquet removal, adequate hemostasis, surgical site washing, drain-positioning, suturing and dressing.

In the second surgical stage, open reduction of the SCJ and subsequent stabilization with the autologous semitendinosus tendon graft in a figure-of-eight reinforced with high-strength suture tape was accomplished according to the preoperative planning (Figure 3).

With the patient still supine in the sterile field, the SCJ was exposed with a straight incision extending from the center of the medial clavicle to the mid-superior aspect of the sternal manubrium (Figure 2a). The posterior SCJ dislocation was found. After releasing the medial part of the clavicle and the corresponding articular facet of the sternum, four bone tunnels of 5.0 mm in diameter were drilled, two in the clavicle and two in the sternum in parallel, adequately protecting the noble structures underlying these bones. After the reduction of the clavicle with blunt forceps, the joint was stabilized, with the semitendinosus tendon graft being passed through the holes in a figure-of-eight configuration and then reinforced with high-strength suture tape (Figure 4).

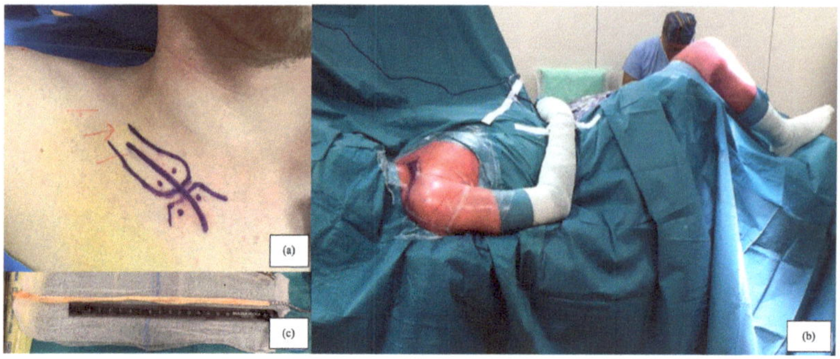

Figure 2. Surgical setting: (**a**) anatomical landmarks for identification of SCJ and drill hole planning; (**b**) double sterile field for SCJ access and tendon harvest; (**c**) tubularized autologous semitendinosus tendon graft.

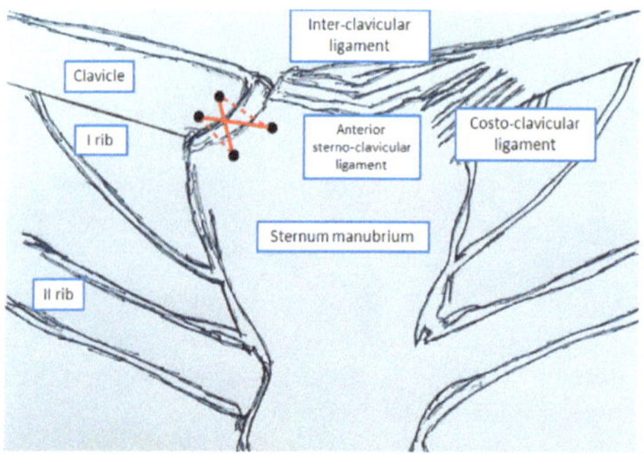

Figure 3. Preoperative planning.

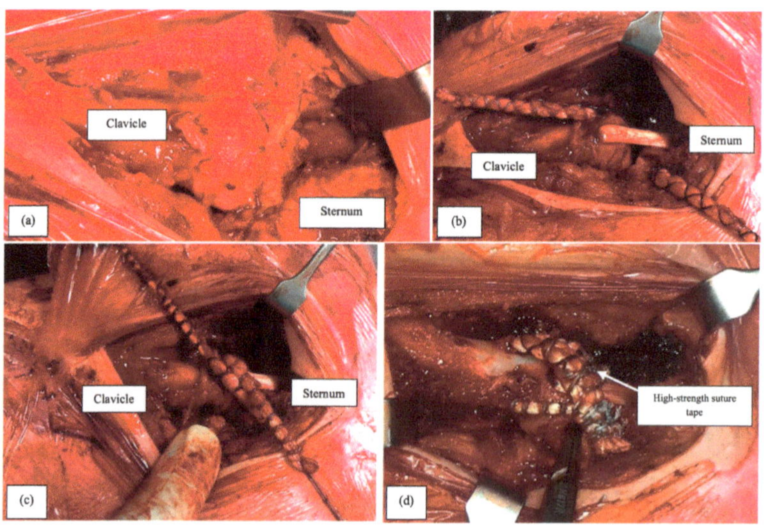

Figure 4. Intraoperative details of reconstruction with autologous semitendinosus tendon graft augmented with high-strength suture tape: (**a**) clavicle and sternum exposure; (**b**) graft passage in the drilled holes in the clavicle and sternum; (**c**) graft realization in the figure-of-eight; (**d**) figure-of-eight repair augmented with high-strength suture tape.

The post-operative protocol includes a neutral arm sling for the first three weeks after surgery, with active and passive movements forbidden. Elbow, wrist and hand mobilization were allowed and suggested from day one after surgery. The stitches were removed fifteen days after surgery. At three weeks, the patient started the rehabilitation of the shoulder with passive pendular movements first, and then with active motion in the fourth/fifth weeks. A return to sport was allowed six months after surgery. Both patients were followed up for one year postoperatively, specifically at 1–3–6–12 months after surgery. As for the conservative group, X-rays, along with clinical examination were usually performed at the follow-ups, except for the third month where a CT scan was used to assess the maintenance of the reduction. A CT scan was also employed in cases of inconclusive X-rays.

3. Results

All five patients, both the conservatively treated and the surgically managed, had returned to their daily lives by 12 months of follow-up.

For those conservatively managed no recurrences were recorded on imaging, and all the patients had successfully recovered their range of motion and muscle strength and were pain-free while moving their arms.

For those surgically treated, at three months the CT scan showed a complete reduction of the SCJ, both in the axial and the coronal views (Figure 5). At the end of the follow-up, ROM was restored, with an optimal strength recovery and no neurological deficits; in both cases, the healing was successful; no recurrences were recorded, and the patients returned to their daily lives without pain while moving their shoulder girdles (Figure 6).

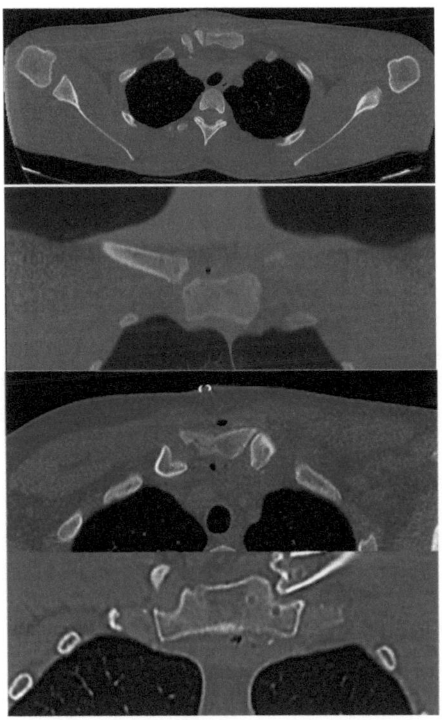

Figure 5. CT scan at 3 months post operation: reduction confirmed on axial and coronal scan on both patients.

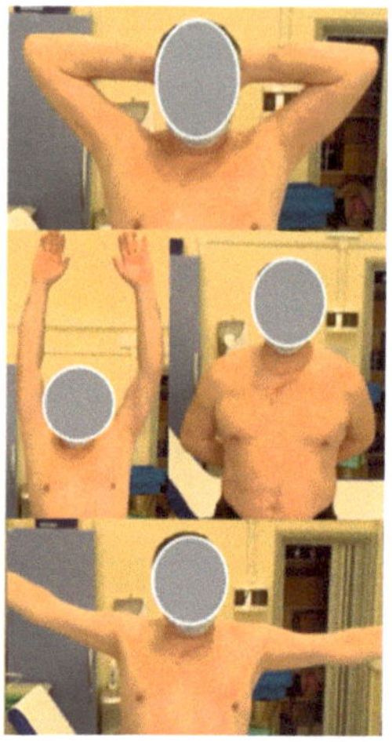

Figure 6. Clinical evaluation, 1 year follow-up, ROM restored and wound healed.

A comprehensive comparison with the most recent literature will be provided in Section 4.

4. Discussion

This paper describes five cases of posterior traumatic SCJ dislocation handled according to the most recent recommendations, implementing the literature in this rare but potentially life-threatening pathology [1–3]. The diagnostic algorithm with the initial management and the surgical strategy adopted for the failed closed reduction cases align with the literature since SCJ reconstruction with tendon autograft and allograft is increasingly promoted due to biomechanical studies [1–3,19]. Indeed, reconstruction without fusion allows restoration of the ROM without the increased risk of developing degenerative changes or osteoarthritis of the distal joints that would otherwise need to compensate.

However, SCJ dislocation remains a rare pathology and the scientific literature about this topic is still poor, with the introduction of recommendations and systematic review only occurring in recent years [1–3].

The demographic characteristics, as well as the mechanism of trauma reported, are in line with the literature [1–3]. Kendal et al., in their systematic review, reported a mean age of 25.3 years old, with most patients being males [2]. Trauma is the most common cause of posterior SCJ dislocation, with high-energy processes in contact sports such as rugby and motor-vehicle collisions being the most common culprits [5,6,12].

They result either from indirect trauma when a posterolateral compressive force is applied to the shoulder and transmitted to the SCJ as a vector force or as direct anteroposterior trauma to the SCJ [1–3]. Atraumatic SCJ dislocations exist, but they tend to occur in patients with generalized hyperlaxity or trapezius palsy [1,2].

Due to the anatomy of the SCJ, which has a robust posterior capsular ligament and the costoclavicular ligament, anterior dislocation occurs more frequently, with posterior SCJ dislocations comprising 5% to 27% of all SCJ dislocations [15,22].

From a clinical point of view, posterior SCJ dislocation is often characterized by neck and shoulder pain increased by ipsilateral shoulder movement [1,3,9]. A deformity of the SCJ can be present even if swelling of the joint gives the illusion of an anterior dislocation in the case of a posterior dislocation [1,14]. As reported by Ingoe et al. it is advisable to examine the nearby joints, such as the acromioclavicular joint (ACJ), in order to detect other injuries which could lead to a floating clavicle [3,23,24]. Posterior SCJ dislocation should be suspected and identified since it can lead to life-threatening complications due to the presence of noble structures near the joint: disorders of the neurological structures (brachial plexus, phrenic and vagus nerves) and/or vascular ones (compression or laceration of the subclavians, internal jugulars, internal thoracic or brachiocephalic vessels), pneumothorax, myocardial conduction abnormalities, esophageal or tracheal rupture, mediastinal compression and thoracic outlet syndrome could occur [2]. In case of complications, wider symptomatology, such as the presence of cyanosis, choking, cervical bruit, tracheal hematoma, stridor, dyspnea and respiratory distress, dysphagia, hoarseness, odynophagia, compromised circulation to the arm, diaphragmatic paralysis and even death could occur [7–10]. Overlapping adjacent structures make assessing and interpreting SCJ dislocation on routine chest radiographs difficult [1–3]. SCJ dislocation may not be so immediate to diagnose, even with dedicated radiographic views, such as the serendipity view [2,7,14]. Moreover, the literature agrees about distinguishing between SCJ dislocation and physeal fractures, since the medial clavicular physis is the last to close around 23–25 years of age [9,12,15]. Consequently, a computed tomography (CT) scan is the imaging modality of choice for definitive diagnosis and a three-dimensional understanding of the SCJ [1–3,9]. When vascular injuries are suspected, intravenous contrast can be administered [1–3]. In the cases described, a CT scan was performed pre- and post- operatively and post-reduction maneuvers to assess the maintenance of the reduction. MRI can be helpful in physeal injuries and in case of chronic instability to assess the ligament status [1,3,9]. In MRI the articular surfaces and the intra-articular disc are better visualized in coronal sequences, whereas axial sequences depict anterior and posterior capsules and ligaments [9]. The sagittal sequences are useful in assessing the costoclavicular ligament [9].

Recommendations from the literature agree that posterior dislocation needs to be reduced when diagnosed [1–3,22].

A closed reduction should be attempted in the first 48 h, with a success rate reported in adults by Ingoe et al. between 38% and 50% [3,24]. If this maneuver is effective, a follow-up CT scan can be indicated to detect any recurrent dislocations [1–3]. On the other hand, both the failure of closed reduction maneuvers and the frequent presentation over 48 h, due to the aforementioned difficulties in diagnosis, require an open reduction [1–3,22]. Indeed, a closed reduction after 48 h has a high probability of being unsuccessful [2,18]. The five cases described in this study underwent this management algorithm, with a first closed reduction acutely attempted.

Moreover, the literature suggests that when closed reduction is successful, the SCJ is usually stable without additional intervention, while in case of failure and open reduction, the SCJ needs to be reconstructed [1–3]. However, a universally accepted stabilization method for posterior SCJ dislocation does not exist, and various techniques have been described depending on several features, such as biomechanics, the patient's future expectation goals, surgical expertise and degree of instability [1–3].

4.1. Anatomy and Biomechanics of the SCJ

The SCJ is the only true connection between the upper limb and the axial skeleton, representing one of the most stable joints in the human body [1–3,9]. It is a diarthrodial joint with a saddle-like shape where only the lower 2/3 of the medial clavicle is wrapped by articular cartilage [1,2,25]. Due to the limited osseous congruence, SCJ stability lies on strong ligament structures and a fibrocartilaginous intra-articular disk, which has mobility along the anteroposterior and vertical axes [9,25]. The ligaments of the SCJ are represented by the anterior and the posterior sternoclavicular capsular ligament, the costoclavicular ligament and the interclavicular ligament [1,2,9,13,25]. The thicker posterior capsular ligament was considered in a biomechanical study by Spencer et al. to be the most crucial structure to avoid anterior and posterior translation, with the anterior capsular ligament impeding only anterior translation [1,9,25]. This is the main reason why most dislocations occur anteriorly since posterior SCJ dislocations require higher forces [1,2,25].

However, the costoclavicular ligament has recently received more attention [1,9,25]. It is a stout, short, flattened, inverted cone with two laminae on the anterior and posterior aspects of the clavicle [9,25]. Raising and lowering movements occur between the articular disk and the clavicle, whereas protraction and retraction occur between the articular disc and the sternum [1–3,9].

SCJ injury impacts the scapulothoracic and glenohumeral rhythm [1–3,9]. Most of the motion of the SCJ occurs in the anteroposterior direction with protraction and retraction of approximately 35° in either direction [1–3,26]. The SCJ can elevate up to 35°, and other essential movements are anterior and posterior rotation concerning the lateral axis of the clavicle [1–3,26].

For these reasons, the reconstruction procedure of the SCJ is essential to restoring the ROM of the shoulder girdle [1–3]. Recent literature suggests avoiding open reduction and internal fixation with plates and screws since this could limit glenohumeral motion and usually necessitate implant removal to restore function and avoid chronic degenerative changes [1–3].

Apart from the anatomy of the SCJ, it is important to mention the "safe zone" avascular plane behind the joint and anterior to the muscle belly, especially when reconstruction techniques requiring drilling holes are performed, since protective retractors could be placed in this location [1–3]. Finally, as mentioned above, since the medial clavicle is the last ossification center to fuse between the ages of 22 and 25, proximal clavicle physeal fracture-separation in young patients could mimic a sternoclavicular dislocation in up to 50% of cases [1–3,10,12]. As a result, these two entities should be distinguished [1–3].

4.2. Open Reduction and SCJ Stabilization and Reconstruction Options

Open reduction is needed when closed reduction fails and in cases of recurrent dislocation or chronic instability, and the literature advocates stabilization with SCJ reconstruction [1–3,19]. Indeed, as reported by Ingoe et al. direct repair of the ligaments is usually not achievable and reconstruction with sutures or tendons is advisable [3].

SCJ dislocation can be further classified as acute or chronic [1,2,14–16]. Kendal et al. reported in their systematic review that most are chronic dislocations resulting from missed injuries, delayed clinical presentation or recurrent dislocations following a closed acute reduction maneuver [1,2,14–16]. Moreover, Glass et al. stated that the effectiveness of the surgery is not adversely affected by failure of conservative treatment [27].

The presence in the operating theater of a vascular or cardiothoracic surgeon and an anesthesiologist is usually endorsed since teamwork and a shared approach leads to safer surgery [1–3]. The two reported cases were managed according to the abovementioned suggestions, and the equipped specialized surgical team was present in the operating room.

A universally accepted stabilization method does not exist, and the literature reports many options [1–3,22,28]. However, recently, recommendations have been developed [1–3]. Still, results are hard to compare because studies are often characterized by small numbers of patients and different treatment options (such as internal fixation with plates and screws, cannulated screws, trans-osseous suture, reconstruction with hamstring tendons or LARS, and tension bands) and by a short follow-up. In addition, few of them differentiate acute from chronic SCJ dislocation; therefore, advantages and disadvantages for each technique are reported [1–3,28].

The literature agrees that open reduction and internal fixation with screws and plates should be avoided unless in the case of comminuted fracture-dislocations [1–3]. This is because implants usually need to be removed since they lead to an arthrodesis, thus limiting motion on the ipsilateral shoulder girdle with the possibility of degenerative changes [1–3]. Moreover, usually, a bi-cortical fixation is necessary, with the risk of screw thread protrusion posterior to the clavicle, where the vessels are located [3].

Pins or Kirschner wires should be avoided due to their possible migration, which can damage noble structures [29]. In particular, a risk of death of up to 40% has been estimated when using Kirschner wires due to potential vascular complications [9,19]. The most striking case in this regard was reported by Ballas et al. concerning a posterior SCJ dislocation treated with three wires: the first was removed after a short time since it was protruding below the skin; the second protruded vertically in front of the sternum after two years, giving symptoms similar to myocardial infarction; the last one migrated into the pelvic cavity giving abdominal symptoms, and multiple surgical interventions were necessary to extract it [29]. In the same paper, the authors also carried out a literature review, reporting 88 cases of wire migration, of which 18 followed sternoclavicular joint dislocation [29].

Another surgical solution is medial clavicular resection with soft tissue reconstruction [1,2]. This is usually reserved for cases with degenerative changes, medial clavicle fractures or irreducible locked dislocations [1,2].

Thus, the literature conveys that SCJ reconstruction should be adopted with biological (such as allograft or autograft) or synthetic grafts [1–3,28]. Indeed, both Provencher et al. [1] and Kendal et al. [2] suggested the use of a figure-of-eight tendon autograft or allograft. This configuration has gained popularity after the biomechanical study by Spencer and Kuhn which evaluated three different reconstruction techniques with cadaveric models [19]. They assessed (1) the intramedullary ligament reconstruction, (2) the subclavius tendon reconstruction and (3) the use of a figure-of-eight of a semitendinosus graft through drill holes in the clavicle and the sternum's manubrium [19]. They demonstrated that the figure-of-eight graft's stiffness and load to failure were greater than the other two techniques, especially in the posterior direction [19].

However, this procedure is not without complications and tips are given by several authors [1–3,19]. The drill holes in the bones should be spaced 1.0 to 1.5 cm apart to allow for adequate bone ridge and 1.0 to 2.0 cm away from the end of the clavicle to avoid stress fracture [1,2,19]. The graft type usually guides the size of the holes [1].

Several grafts are used, such as the palmaris, the semitendinosus and the gracilis, with overall good outcomes and a low revision rate [1–3].

The authors of this paper, in agreement with the literature, chose the figure-of-eight configurations for one crucial reason: despite the SCJ having a limited range of motion, this joint is fundamental for the physiology of the shoulder girdle and the resulting stabilization with ORIF would fix and limit its ROM. Subsequently, stress concentration may occur during functional exercises, and the surgical fusion of the joint could induce the patient to compensate for any movement by using the downstream joints [1–3,9]. Indeed, the paper's authors believe that SCJ ROM should be re-established in order to avoid chronic degenerative changes to it or to the downstream joints.

In this regard, Tytherleigh-Strong et al. evaluated a series of 19 patients with acute traumatic posterior SCJ dislocation treated with hamstring tendon autograft reconstruction technique within 14 days from the injury [30]. After a minimum follow-up of three years, they reported a high survivorship grade (96%), good clinical outcomes and a high rate of return to sports, since 86% of patients who practiced sports were able to return to their pre-injury level [30]. In addition, Provencher et al. analyzed patients operated with a figure-of-eight technique, reporting a revision rate of 8.3% for recurrent or persistent instability [1].

Using autologous tendons increases the risk of morbidity at the graft-harvest site as well as infection associated with the use of the graft tissue, which, however, are rarely reported [1–3]; conversely, it removes the intolerance to osteosynthesis devices and graft rejection [1–3]. The authors did not report complications, neither at the graft site nor at the SCJ surgical site.

Artificial ligaments are another similar surgical way to stabilize the SCJ in young and active patients [28]. The employment of the LARS (Ligament Augmentation and Reconstruction System) technique has been demonstrated to be a feasible option, able to address both the costoclavicular and capsular ligaments [28]. Quayle et al. reported 5 cases of SCJ dislocations treated with LARS and interference screws, with promising short- and mid-term outcomes with lowering of pain and improvement of joint function [28]. However, in all these reconstruction procedures, fusion of the joint is avoided, and SCJ motion is restored [1–3].

Lastly, even if repair is usually not achievable [3], Kendal et al. proposed in acute cases the use of synthetic material such as sutures passed through uni-cortical holes to repair and augment the SC ligament, avoiding damage to the mediastinal structures and preventing iatrogenic physeal injuries in children [2].

In the cases presented in this work, a high-strength suture tape was used as an internal brace as described by Ingoe et al. [3].

This study, with its strengths and limitations, is significant in that it aligns with the current literature. It does so by following the recommendations and adopting the most suggested surgical technique.

However, it includes few patients and a one-year follow-up.

Moreover, since the number of participants is limited, a descriptive analysis of both the surgical technique and the results with a comparison with the current literature was mainly performed. A statistical analysis was not accomplished.

As mentioned, this is a common limitation in the literature since this pathology is rare, and it is difficult for a single center to have a huge cohort of patients.

Consequently, for future research, higher-quality studies, especially multicenter studies with control groups or RCTs, will be necessary to determine the best surgical technique.

5. Conclusions

Traumatic posterior SCJ dislocation can lead to life-threatening consequences due to its proximity to vital structures. After diagnosis, a closed reduction in the first 48 h is suggested, and, in case of failure, open reduction and SCJ reconstruction are indicated. No universal guidelines for the stabilization method exist, but the recent literature suggests a figure-of-eight reconstruction with a tendon allograft or autograft. A series of posterior traumatic SCJ dislocations is reported, managed according to the recent recommendations either conservatively or surgically with a figure-of-eight semitendinosus tendon autograft augmented with high-strength suture tape. Given the importance of SCJ motion for the shoulder girdle, the authors of this paper adopted this technique, and they reported, at one year of follow-up, a complete shoulder ROM with full strength throughout.

Author Contributions: Conceptualization, C.C. and F.Q.; methodology, C.C., V.M. and F.Q.; validation, P.M. and F.R.; investigation, C.C. and F.Q.; writing—original draft preparation, C.C., V.M., C.A., C.P.P., M.P., G.C. and F.Q.; writing—review and editing, C.C., V.M., M.P. and F.Q., visualization, P.M., G.C. and F.R.; supervision, P.M. and F.R. All authors have read and agreed to the published version of the manuscript.

Funding: This research received no external funding.

Institutional Review Board Statement: This retrospective chart review study was in accordance with the ethical standards of the institutional and national research committee and with the 1964 Helsinki Declaration and its later amendments or comparable ethical standards. Ethical approval was waived by the local Ethics Committee as authors solely analyzed pre-existing and anonymous data in a retrospective manner; moreover, all the procedures performed were part of the routine standard care.

Informed Consent Statement: Written informed consent has been obtained from the patients to publish this paper in anonymous form.

Data Availability Statement: The original data presented in this study are available under request to the corresponding author.

Conflicts of Interest: The authors declare no conflicts of interest relevant to this paper.

Abbreviations

SCJ	sternoclavicular joint
ROM	range of motion
g	gram

ED Emergency department
CT computed tomography
MRI magnetic resonance imaging
LARS ligament augmentation and reconstruction system
ORIF open reduction and internal fixation
RCTs randomized controlled trials
mm millimeters
ml milliliters
ACJ acromioclavicular joint

References

1. Provencher, M.T.; Bernholt, D.L.; Peebles, L.A.; Millett, P.J. Sternoclavicular Joint Instability and Reconstruction. *J. Am. Acad. Orthop. Surg.* **2022**, *30*, e1076–e1083. [CrossRef]
2. Kendal, J.K.; Thomas, K.; Lo, I.K.Y.; Bois, A.J. Clinical Outcomes and Complications Following Surgical Management of Traumatic Posterior Sternoclavicular Joint Dislocations: A Systematic Review. *JBJS Rev.* **2018**, *6*, e2. [CrossRef]
3. Ingoe, H.M.A.; Mohammed, K.; Malone, A.A.; Beadle, G.; Sharpe, T.; Cockfield, A.; Lloyd, R.; Singh, H.; Colgan, F. Traumatic posterior sternoclavicular joint dislocation—Current aspects of management. *Injury* **2023**, *54*, 110983. [CrossRef] [PubMed]
4. Boesmueller, S.; Wech, M.; Tiefenboeck, T.M.; Popp, D.; Bukaty, A.; Huf, W.; Fialka, C.; Greitbauer, M.; Platzer, P. Incidence, characteristics, and long-term follow-up of sternoclavicular injuries: An epidemiologic analysis of 92 cases. *J. Trauma Acute Care Surg.* **2016**, *80*, 289–295. [CrossRef]
5. Singer, G.; Ferlic, P.; Kraus, T.; Eberl, R. Reconstruction of the sternoclavicular joint in active patients with the figure-of-eight technique using hamstrings. *J. Shoulder Elb. Surg.* **2013**, *22*, 64–69. [CrossRef]
6. Helfen, T.; Jansen, S.; Fleischhacker, E.; Böcker, W.; Wirth, S.; Ockert, B. Injuries of the sternoclavicular region indicate concomitant lesions and need distinguished imaging. *Eur. J. Trauma. Emerg. Surg.* **2021**, *47*, 1399–1406. [CrossRef]
7. Philipson, M.R.; Wallwork, N. Traumatic dislocation of the sternoclavicular joint. *Orthop. Trauma.* **2012**, *26*, 380–384. [CrossRef]
8. Edwin, J.; Ahmed, S.; Verma, S.; Tytherleigh-Strong, G.; Karuppaiah, K.; Sinha, J. Swellings of the sternoclavicular joint: Review of traumatic and non-traumatic pathologies. *EFORT Open Rev.* **2018**, *3*, 471–484. [CrossRef]
9. Dhawan, R.; Singh, R.A.; Tins, B.; Hay, S.M. Sternoclavicular joint. *Shoulder Elb.* **2018**, *10*, 296–305. [CrossRef] [PubMed]
10. Lee, J.T.; Nasreddine, A.Y.; Black, E.M.; Bae, D.S.; Kocher, M.S. Posterior Sternoclavicular Joint Injuries in Skeletally Immature Patients. *J. Pediatr. Orthop.* **2014**, *34*, 369–375. [CrossRef] [PubMed]
11. Chaudhry, S. Pediatric Posterior Sternoclavicular Joint Injuries. *J. Am. Acad. Orthop. Surg.* **2015**, *23*, 468–475.
12. Tepolt, F.; Carry, P.M.; Heyn, P.C.; Miller, N.H. Posterior Sternoclavicular Joint Injuries in the Adolescent Population: A Meta-analysis. *Am. J. Sports Med.* **2014**, *42*, 2517–2524. [CrossRef] [PubMed]
13. Negri, J.H.; Malavolta, E.A.; Assunção, J.H.; Gracitelli, M.E.C.; Pereira, C.A.M.; Neto, R.B.; Croci, A.T.; Neto, A.A.F. Assessment of the function and resistance of sternoclavicular ligaments: A biomechanical study in cadavers. *Orthop. Traumatol. Surg. Res.* **2014**, *100*, 727–731. [CrossRef] [PubMed]
14. Groh, G.I.; Wirth, M.A. Management of traumatic sternoclavicular joint injuries. *J. Am. Acad. Orthop. Surg.* **2011**, *19*, 1–7. [CrossRef] [PubMed]
15. Wirth, M.A.; Rockwood, C.A., Jr. Acute and Chronic Traumatic Injuries of the Sternoclavicular Joint. *J. Am. Acad. Orthop. Surg.* **1996**, *4*, 268–278. [CrossRef] [PubMed]
16. Hellwinkel, J.E.; McCarty, E.C.; Khodaee, M. Sports-related sternoclavicular joint injuries. *Phys. Sportsmed.* **2019**, *47*, 253–261. [CrossRef] [PubMed]
17. Lacheta, L.; Dekker, T.J.; Goldenberg, B.T.; Horan, M.P.; Rosenberg, S.I.; Pogorzelski, J.; Millett, P.J. Minimum 5-Year Clinical Outcomes, Survivorship, and Return to Sports After Hamstring Tendon Autograft Reconstruction for Sternoclavicular Joint Instability. *Am. J. Sports Med.* **2020**, *48*, 939–946. [CrossRef] [PubMed]
18. Laffosse, J.-M.; Espié, A.; Bonnevialle, N.; Mansat, P.; Tricoire, J.-L.; Bonnevialle, P.; Chiron, P.; Puget, J. Posterior dislocation of the sternoclavicular joint and epiphyseal disruption of the medial clavicle with posterior displacement in sports participants. *J. Bone Jt. Surg. Br. Vol.* **2010**, *92*, 103–109. [CrossRef]
19. Spencer, E.E., Jr.; Kuhn, J.E. Biomechanical analysis of reconstructions for sternoclavicular joint instability. *J. Bone Jt. Surg. Am.* **2004**, *86*, 98–105. [CrossRef] [PubMed]
20. Maniscalco, P.; Ciatti, C.; Gattoni, S.; Quattrini, F.; Pagliarello, C.P.; Patane, A.C.; Capelli, P.; Banchini, F.; Rivera, F.; Sanna, F.; et al. Proximal humerus fractures in COVID-19 lockdown: The experience of three orthopedics and traumatology departments in the first ten weeks of the Italian epidemic. *Acta Biomed.* **2021**, *92*, e2021104. [CrossRef] [PubMed] [PubMed Central]
21. COVIDSurg Collaborative. Machine learning risk prediction of mortality for patients undergoing surgery with perioperative SARS-CoV-2: The COVIDSurg mortality score. *Br. J. Surg.* **2021**, *108*, 1274–1292.
22. Iwai, T.; Tanaka, K.; Okubo, M. Closed reduction of a posterior sternoclavicular joint dislocation: A case report. *Trauma. Case Rep.* **2018**, *17*, 1–4. [CrossRef] [PubMed] [PubMed Central]

23. Oladeji, L.O.; Vivace, B.; Kelly, S.; Wiesemann, S.; DeFroda, S.F. The Floating Clavicle: Surgical Technique for Management of an Ipsilateral Acromioclavicular and Sternoclavicular Joint Dislocation. *Arthrosc. Tech.* **2023**, *12*, e697–e702. [CrossRef] [PubMed] [PubMed Central]
24. Groh, G.I.; Wirth, M.A.; Rockwood, C.A. Treatment of traumatic posterior sternoclavicular dislocations. *J. Shoulder Elb. Surg* **2011**, *20*, 107–113. [CrossRef] [PubMed]
25. Spencer, E.E.; Kuhn, J.E.; Huston, L.J.; Carpenter, J.E.; Hughes, R.E. Ligamentous restraints to anterior and posterior translation of the sternoclavicular joint. *J. Shoulder Elb. Surg.* **2002**, *11*, 43–47. [CrossRef] [PubMed]
26. Ludewig, P.M.; Phadke, V.; Braman, J.P.; Hassett, D.R.; Cieminski, C.J.; LaPrade, R.F. Motion of the shoulder complex during multiplanar humeral elevation. *J. Bone Jt. Surg. Am.* **2009**, *91*, 378–389. [CrossRef] [PubMed] [PubMed Central]
27. Glass, E.R.; Thompson, J.D.; Cole, P.A.; Gause, T.M.; Altman, G.T. Treatment of Sternoclavicular Joint Dislocations: A Systematic Review of 251 Dislocations in 24 Case Series. *J. Trauma Acute Care Surg.* **2011**, *70*, 1294–1298. [CrossRef]
28. Quayle, J.M.; Arnander, M.W.; Pennington, R.G.; Rosell, L.P. Artificial ligament reconstruction of sternoclavicular joint instability. Report of a novel surgical technique with early results. *Tech. Hand Up. Extrem. Surg.* **2014**, *18*, 31–35. [CrossRef] [PubMed]
29. Ballas, R.; Bonnel, F. Endopelvic migration of a sternoclavicular K-wire. Case report and review of literature. *Orthop. Traumatol. Surg. Res.* **2012**, *98*, 118–121. [CrossRef] [PubMed]
30. Tytherleigh-Strong, G.; Sabharwal, S.; Peryt, A. Clinical Outcomes and Return to Sports after Open Reduction and Hamstring Tendon Autograft Reconstruction in Patients with Acute Traumatic First-Time Posterior Dislocation of the Sternoclavicular Joint. *Am. J. Sports Med.* **2022**, *50*, 3635–3642. [CrossRef]

Journal of
Clinical Medicine

MDPI

Article

Trends and Changes in Treating Proximal Humeral Fractures in Italy: Is Arthroplasty an Increasingly Preferred Option? A Nation-Wide, Population-Based Study over a Period of 22 Years

Enrico Ciminello [1,*], Andrea Modesti [2], Emilio Romanini [3,4], Stefano Lepore [5], Gabriele Tucci [3,6], Stefano Di Gennaro [4], Giandomenico Logroscino [2,7], Paola Ciccarelli [1], Tiziana Falcone [1] and Marina Torre [1]

1 Italian Implantable Prostheses Registry, Italian National Institute of Health, 00161 Rome, Italy; paola.ciccarelli@iss.it (P.C.); tiziana.falcone@iss.it (T.F.); marina.torre@iss.it (M.T.)
2 Department of Life, Health and Environmental Sciences, University of L'Aquila, 67100 L'Aquila, Italy; andrea.modesti@graduate.univaq.it (A.M.); giandomenico.logroscino@univaq.it (G.L.)
3 GLOBE, Italian Working Group on Evidence Based Orthopaedics, 00197 Rome, Italy; emilio.romanini@gmail.com (E.R.); tuccigab@yahoo.it (G.T.)
4 Polo Sanitario San Feliciano, 00166 Rome, Italy; stefanodige1@gmail.com
5 I Orthopaedic Unit, A. Cardarelli Hospital, 80131 Naples, Italy; stefano.lepore@aocardarelli.it
6 Ospedale dei Castelli, Ariccia, 00040 Rome, Italy
7 Department of Minimally Invasive and Computer-Assisted Orthopaedic Surgery, University of L'Aquila, 67100 L'Aquila, Italy
* Correspondence: enrico.ciminello@iss.it; Tel.: +39-3385721611

Abstract: Background: Proximal humeral fractures (PHFs) are common, especially in the elderly, and account for 4% to 10% of all fractures, with women more often affected than men. Treatments include conservative methods, internal fixation and arthroplasty, with surgical approaches increasingly being used due to technological advancements. This study analyzes the evolution of PHF treatments in Italy from 2001 to 2022, using data from the Italian Hospital Discharge Records (HDRs) Database, and includes a stratified analysis by age and sex. **Methods**: Using HDR data from 2001 to 2022, records with ICD9-CM codes for proximal humeral fractures (812.0 and 812.1) among diagnoses were selected and categorized into three treatment groups: arthroplasty, fixation and conservative. Time series were analyzed with stratification by sex and age. **Results**: The extracted data included 486,368 records of PHFs, with 223,742 cases treated surgically (arthroplasty or internal fixation) and 262,626 treated conservatively; the average patient age was 66.6 years, with a higher proportion of women, especially among arthroplasty patients. Over time, the use of fixation and arthroplasty increased from 20% of treatments in 2001 to over 60% in 2022, with fixation becoming the most common treatment method by 2014 and arthroplasty significantly increasing among women, particularly in the 65–74 and 75–84 age groups. **Conclusions**: The study shows that in Italy, over the past two decades, treatment for PHFs has shifted from conservative methods to a preference for internal fixation and increasingly for arthroplasty, particularly among women and patients aged 65–84, reflecting evolving trends and technological improvements.

Keywords: proximal humeral fractures; arthroplasty; shoulder; administrative data; epidemiology; registries; public health

1. Introduction

Proximal humeral fractures (PHFs) are very common and represent a serious health problem [1]. They are among the most frequent fractures in adults [2] and one of the most common age-related fractures in the elderly, with women more often affected than men. According to several studies conducted in different populations, prevalence ranges from 4 to 10% of all fractures [3]. PHFs account for about 80% of all humeral fractures. In general, they mostly occur after the age of 50 with low-energy trauma, whereas for patients younger than 50, high-energy trauma is involved, mainly in male patients [1]. It has been suggested that this rate increases as the average population age rises [4,5]. The incidence rate of these fractures varies considerably depending on the geographical area and the year of the study [6,7]. The treatment is sometimes controversial, and some cases may be technically challenging. Numerous studies have attempted to determine the optimal treatment for PHFs, but no definitive guidelines have been established, particularly in three- and four-part fractures and in the elderly population [8]. The difficulty lies mainly in finding the most appropriate treatment depending on the number of bone fragments and the involved areas of epiphysis [9,10]. The controversy between conservative and surgical treatment has intensified after the publication of the ProFHER trial [11]. Moreover, there is still considerable debate around comparisons of various operative modalities, mainly between intramedullary nailing, open reduction with internal fixation and arthroplasty, as to which is the best method to achieve better functional outcomes [12,13]. Indeed, several variables influence the choice of treatment, including age, bone quality, daily activities and other factors. Even the classification system for PHFs lacks consensus: while the Neer classification is globally the most widely used, other systems, such as those by Hertel or the AO system, are also applied [14,15]. Furthermore, for the same type of fracture, various fixation techniques and systems are frequently employed, leading to some confusion regarding the gold standard to be adopted [16]. Anyway, in recent years, the operative approaches seem to be increasingly used in many countries due to surgical and technological innovation.

The aim of this study is to describe how the approach to treating PHFs has evolved in the last two decades in Italy, with a particular focus on the differences in time trends of conservative treatment, fixation and arthroplasty, using population data from the Italian Hospital Discharge Records (HDRs) Database between 2001 and 2022. A stratified analysis by patient age and sex is also provided.

2. Materials and Methods

The Italian Ministry of Health consolidates the National Hospital Discharge Records (HDRs) Database annually and provides the Italian National Institute of Health with it. This data source allows the collection of administrative, demographic and clinical information on almost every hospitalization in the country, with coverage increasing from 94.2% in 2001 to 99% in 2019 [17]. Medical procedures performed during hospitalization and related diagnoses are reported in HDRs by using the ICD9-CM international classification coding system.

HDRs for the years from 2001 to 2022 were browsed, and only those records where at least one ICD9-CM code for diagnoses with the first four digits equal to 812.0 (Fracture of upper end of humerus closed) or 812.1 (Fracture of upper end of humerus open) appeared in one or more field of main or secondary diagnosis were selected. Records were then divided into three groups, based on ICD9-CM codes appearing in any of the main or secondary procedure fields, according to the procedure performed during hospitalization. If the code 81.80 (Total shoulder replacement) or 81.81 (Partial shoulder replacement) appeared, the patients were considered as treated via "Arthroplasty". If the code 79.10 (Closed reduction of fracture with internal fixation), or 79.11 (Closed reduction of humeral fracture with internal fixation), or 79.30 (Open reduction of fracture with internal fixation), or 79.31 (Open reduction of humeral fracture with internal fixation) appeared, the patient was considered as treated with internal "Fixation". If none of the above-mentioned codes appeared, the performed treatment was considered as "Conservative".

The operative flow reporting the data extraction process is the following:

IF (812.0 OR 812.1) IN diagnoses (first four digits) THEN keep the record
IF (80.80 OR 80.81) IN procedures THEN record is arthroplasty
IF (79.10 OR 79.11 OR 79.30 OR 79.31) IN procedures AND (81.80 OR 81.81) NOT IN procedures THEN record is fixation

IF (79.10 AND 79.11 AND 79.30 AND 79.31 AND 81.80 AND 81.81) NOT IN procedures THEN record is conservative

This operative flow introduces by construct a hierarchy in the group assignment. Arthroplasty is at the highest level of the hierarchy, while conservative treatment is at the lowest one and fixation is in between. This respects the burden of the treatment on patients, with arthroplasty being the most invasive and definitive treatment, used when the others would have no or little efficacy, while conservative is the one with the lowest impact and fixation represents an intermediate approach. This hierarchy implies that, for instance, a record for which both arthroplasty and fixation codes appear would be labeled as arthroplasty, assuming that it was necessary after an ineffective fixation.

Once the records of interest were extracted, the time series were analyzed on an annual basis for overall surgical volume and stratified by sex and age class, according to the partition used by the Italian Arthroplasty Registry: Age < 45; 45 ≤ Age < 55; 55 ≤ Age < 65; 65 ≤ Age < 75; 75 ≤ Age < 85; Age ≥ 85 [18]. Both absolute counts and proportions were taken into account. The series were decomposed and variations in trends and proportions were investigated via the Cox–Stuart test and the Proportion Trend test, respectively. The threshold for statistical significance was fixed to 0.05. Statistical analysis was performed via software R version 4.2.3 (2023-03-15 ucrt)—"Shortstop Beagle".

3. Results

The HDR Database included 231,601,523 records from 2001 to 2022. Out of these, 486,368 records were extracted as satisfying the condition on diagnoses involving fractures of the upper end of the humerus. In total, 223,742 cases were treated via invasive surgery (either arthroplasty or internal fixation) and 262,626 were treated with a conservative approach. The data extraction process is summarized in the flowchart in Figure 1.

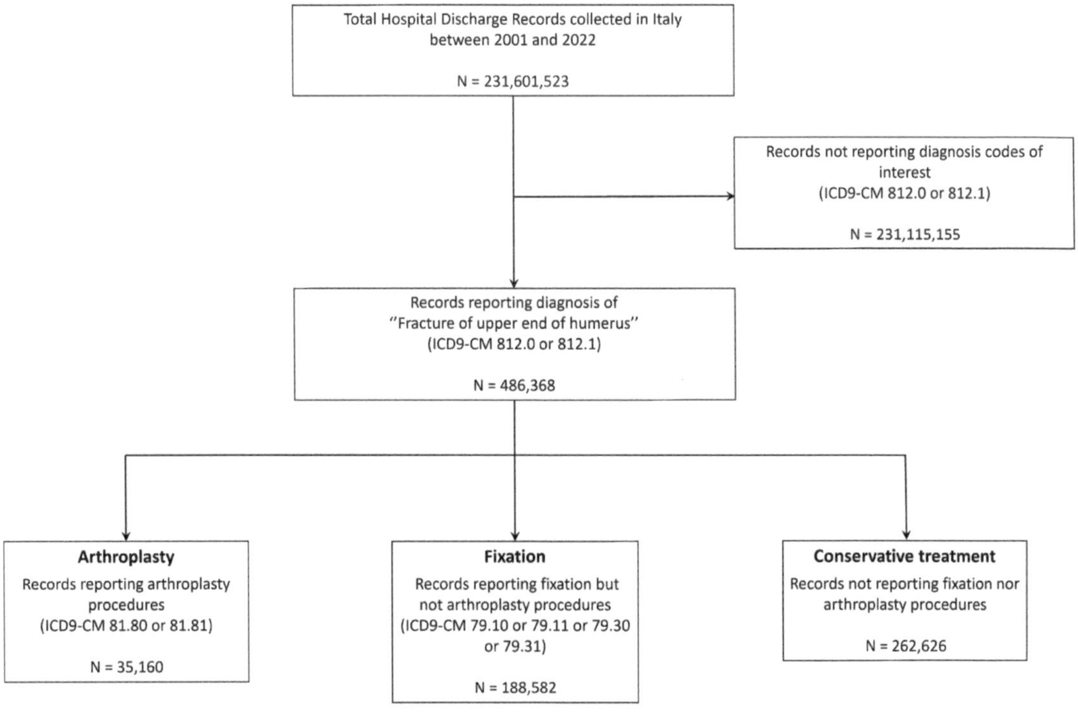

Figure 1. Data extraction flowchart.

The overall average age was 66.6 (21) years, with patients treated by arthroplasty being generally older than the other groups, with an average age of 73.5 (11.2) years. Patients were mainly females (70.3%), in particular among those treated with arthroplasty (82.5%). Patient distribution over sex and age classes is reported in Table 1.

Table 1. Patients' features by treatment group.

	Arthroplasty	Fixation	Conservative	Total
N	35,160	188,582	262,626	486,368
Age	73.5 (11.2)	63 (19.2)	68.3 (22.8)	66.6 (21)
Females	29,001 (82.5%)	128,213 (68%)	184,694 (70.3%)	341,908 (70.3%)
Males	6159 (17.5%)	60,369 (32%)	77,932 (29.7%)	144,460 (29.7%)
Age < 45	219 (0.6%)	27,629 (14.7%)	33,900 (12.9%)	61,748 (12.7%)
44 < Age < 55	881 (2.5%)	20,941 (11.1%)	16,541 (6.3%)	38,363 (7.9%)
54 < Age < 65	3925 (11.2%)	35,796 (19.0%)	30,324 (11.5%)	70,045 (14.4%)
64 < Age < 75	12,468 (35.5%)	48,448 (25.7%)	53,497 (20.4%)	114,413 (23.5%)
74 < Age < 85	15,055 (42.8%)	43,143 (22.9%)	79,388 (30.2%)	137,586 (28.3%)
Age > 84	2612 (7.4%)	12,625 (6.7%)	48,976 (18.6%)	64,213 (13.2%)

The number of hospital admissions considering the ICD9 codes of interest significantly decreased in the observed period ($p < 0.01$). The number of fractures treated with fixation and arthroplasty increased over time, both in absolute terms and proportion, shifting from 20% of the total treatments in 2001 to over 60% in 2022 ($p < 0.01$). The number of internal fixations increased until it exceeded the number of conservative treatments in 2014, and it remained the most used way to treat PHFs until 2022. When stratifying by sex, fixation became the most used technique for males in 2013 and for females in 2014. Moreover, arthroplasty strongly increased in females, accounting for 20% of the total choices for females (Figure 2 and Supplementary Materials).

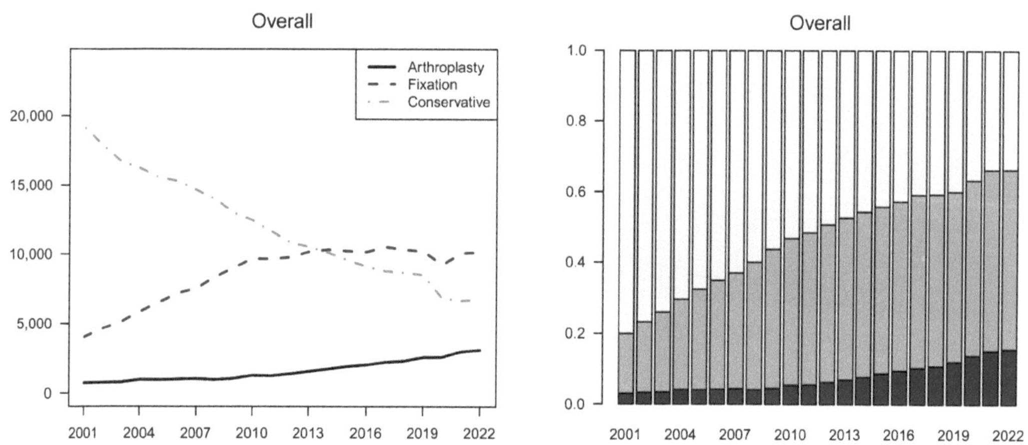

Figure 2. *Cont.*

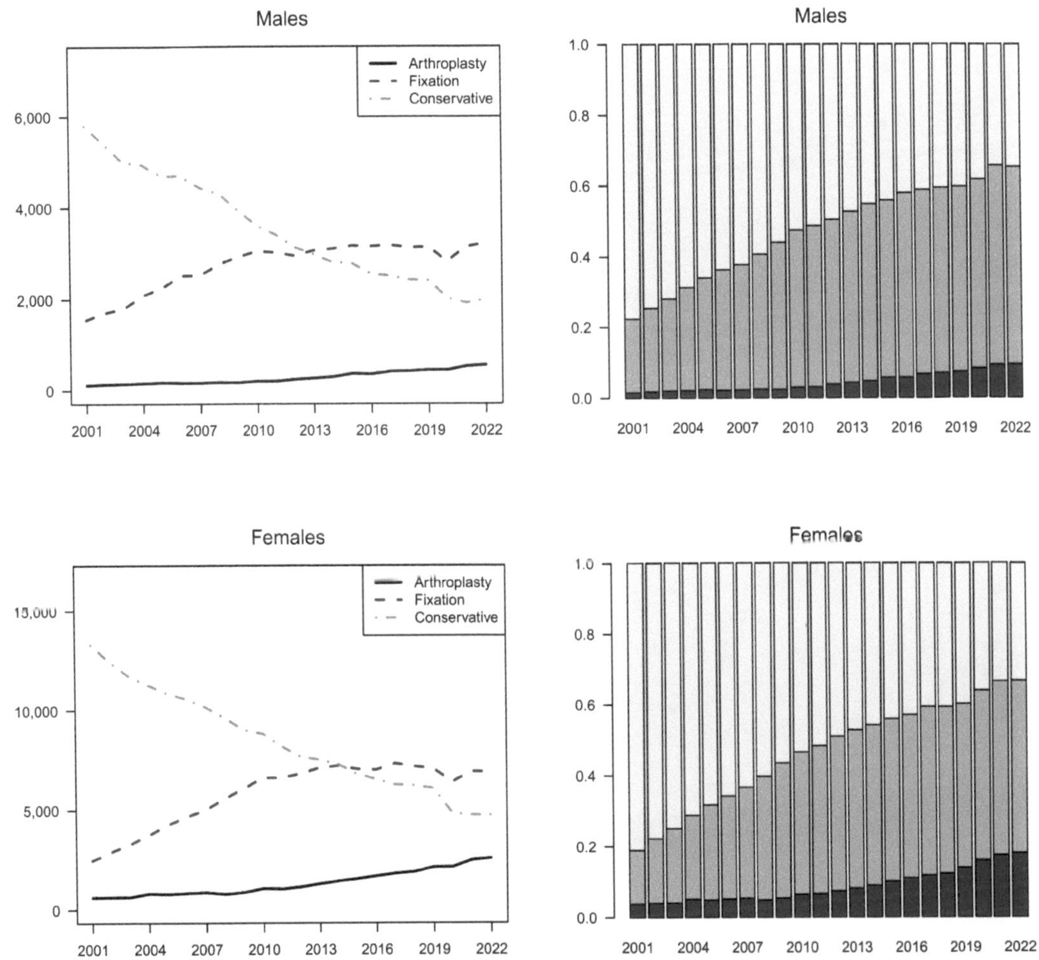

Figure 2. Trends by treatment group (2001–2022). Counts (**left** column) and proportions (**right** column), overall and by sex. Dark gray: arthroplasty; gray: fixation; light gray: conservative.

The age class analysis highlighted that the increase in preference towards arthroplasty was stronger in age classes 65–74 and 75–84 (Figures 3 and 4 and Supplementary Materials). In general, this approach increased only slightly and is usually avoided in the youngest and oldest patients.

Fixation became the most performed treatment in all age classes except for the elderly, more precisely in the age class over 84 years, where the conservative approach was always the most preferred option (Figures 3 and 4 and Supplementary Materials).

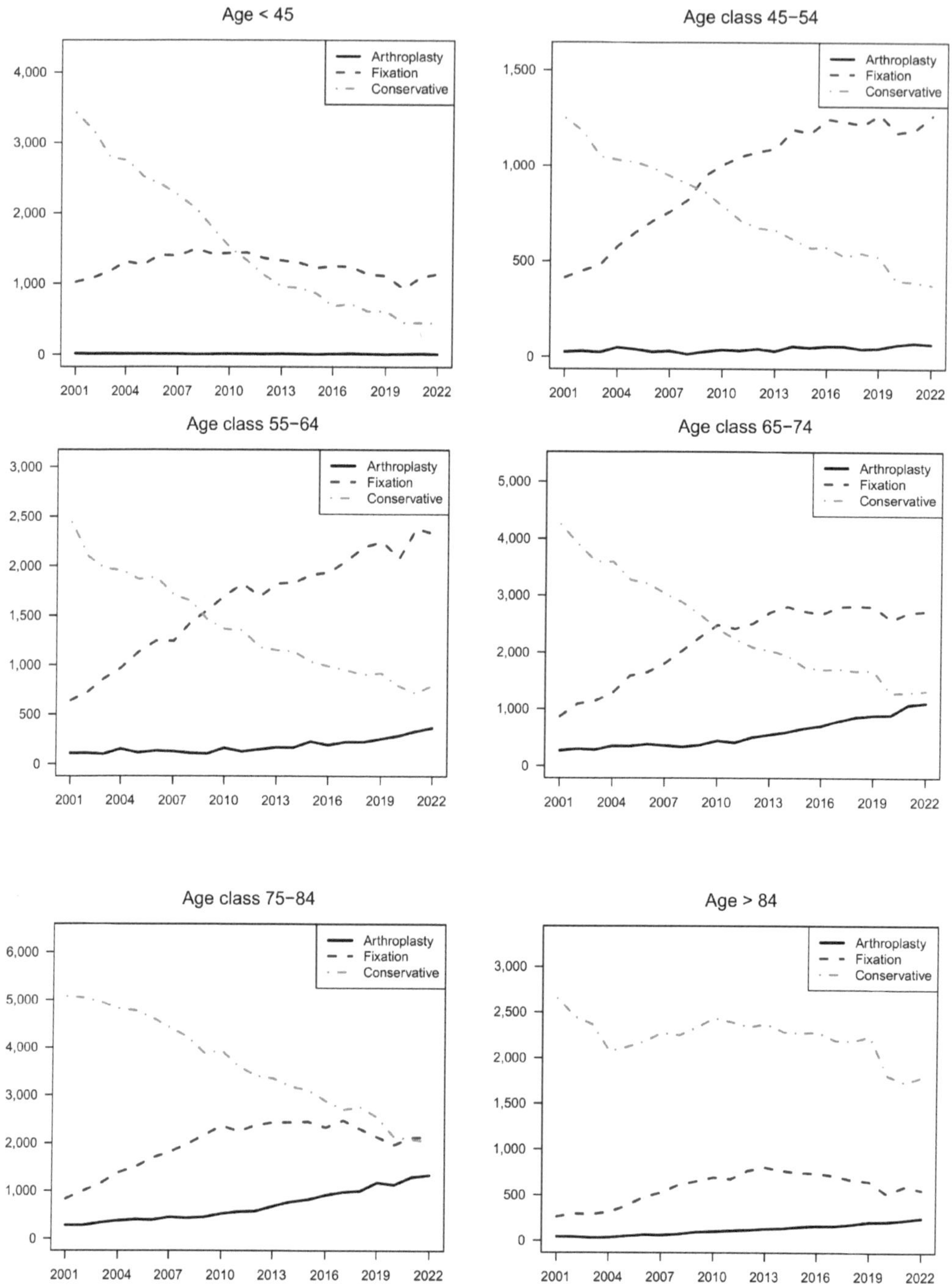

Figure 3. Trends by treatment group (2001–2022). Counts by age class.

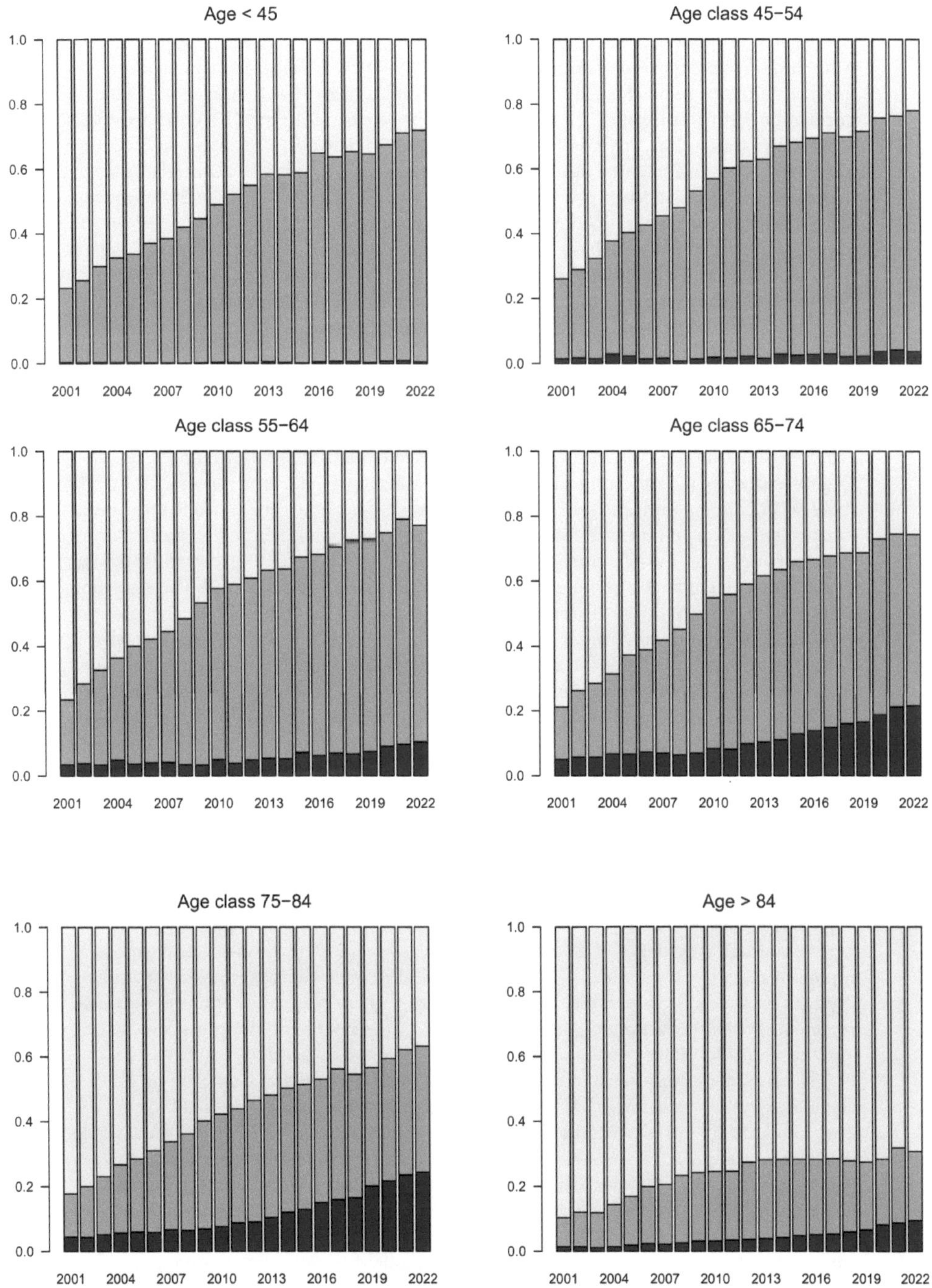

Figure 4. Trends by treatment group (2001–2022). Proportions by age class. Dark gray: arthroplasty; gray: fixation; light gray: conservative.

4. Discussion

This study targeted the analysis of the evolution of PHF treatment approaches in hospitalized patients over a period of 22 years (2001–2022) in Italy, mainly observing the differences in time trends for arthroplasty, fixation and conservative treatment in the Italian population with stratification by age and sex. The work highlighted how the approach to treating PHFs in Italy has changed over the last two decades. The use of arthroplasty has increased over time, and although it was the less used approach during the 22 years under consideration, it accounted for almost 20% of all treatment choices in 2022. Fixation has increased over time, remaining the preferred treatment during the observed period. Conservative treatment, which was the most used approach in 2001, has been decreasingly used over time and was overtaken by fixation in 2014. Arthroplasty is an increasingly selected option for females and for patients between 65 and 84 years of age. On the other hand, the choice of fixation spikes among the youngest, while a conservative approach is the preferred option for the elderly.

In recent years, there have been considerable improvements in surgical options for PHF treatment. Open reduction internal fixation with angular stability systems, minimally invasive plate osteosynthesis surgical approaches, 3D reconstruction models, computerized planning software, jig cutting guides, patient-specific instrumentation, robotic-assisted surgery and, more recently, artificial intelligence are the most notable advancements in PHF surgery [19,20]. The introduction of locking plates has broadened the possible indications for open reduction and internal fixation. This treatment option is favored, in particular for younger patients, for most fracture configurations, as it is suitable for four-part fractures and allows direct visualization of the reduction and grafting techniques [21,22]. The evolution of reverse total shoulder arthroplasty design [23] and the continuous improvement of the surgical technique have led to better and more reproducible outcomes, especially in complex fractures and in older patients [24]. Indeed, studies have shown that arthroplasty might provide a benefit for patients, even if more invasive and expensive than fixation. Nowadays, this surgical option may allow for a shorter recovery time and a better functional restoration [13], especially in the 64–75 age group where the use of this technique has significantly increased. Furthermore, arthroplasty is preferred in women over 65 years of age compared to men, probably due to the higher bone fragility that would cause less successful fixation [25]. On the other hand, arthroplasty is less used in younger patients because of the naturally limited device survival, which could potentially lead to multiple revisions during the lifespan of the patients. At the same time, for patients over 85, this surgical procedure may have a higher impact on their general health because of the high surgical risk. However, based on the recent results of a Cochrane Systematic Review [26], it seems that there is evidence of no differences between surgical and non-surgical treatment in patient-reported function and quality of life. Moreover, there is no clear indication of which treatment is preferable, considering that surgery compared with non-surgical treatment showed high or moderate evidence that it does not have a better outcome at one and two years after injury.

The results of the current study confirm the trend observed in Germany until 2016, where the operative treatment of PHFs by fixation and arthroplasty increased [27]. On the other hand, they contrast with the findings in Australia, Finland and the USA, where the non-operative approach is increasingly preferred together with arthroplasty, in particular in patients over 65 and in females, whereas the fixation approach is decreasingly used because of the risk of postoperative complications [28–31]. Further studies at the international level, providing population data and a wide variety of metrics (socioeconomics, health, sport and diet habits, environmental), may investigate differences in incidence between countries, injury patterns and reasons behind the choices of treatment. At present, the lack of evidence may lead to different approaches and clinical practices being followed in different countries.

To our knowledge, this is the first population study performed in Italy on PHFs and related treatments at the population level and over such a long period of time. This study therefore offers a global view of the PHF phenomenon and shows how its treatment has evolved over 22 years. Furthermore, the analysis by sex and age gives a clear picture of the evolution of this issue in the population by its characteristics.

The main limitation of this study lies in the administrative nature of the data used. The diagnosis and related treatment procedure were identified by using the ICD-9 ICM coding, which could be subject to error due to the incorrect compilation of the source data and the lack of an audit on the accuracy and clinical significance of the codes reported. Indeed, the ICD9-CM codes for arthroplasty only distinguish between total and partial shoulder replacement and cannot identify revisions. This may result in a bias of analyzed counts and does not allow for further studies on device survival and the subsequent efficacy and safety of arthroplasty in the treatment of PHF. Moreover, ICD9-CM codes do not provide technical information on the device, like the design (anatomical or inverse), making any discrimination impossible in such sense. Therefore, the use of such administrative data is useful to provide an overview of the epidemiological patterns in hospitalized patients, but caution should be recommended when drawing a conclusion of clinical relevance. A further possible limitation of this study is related to the fact that, due to the intrinsic nature of the data collected, we only evaluated patients with PHFs requiring hospitalization, excluding from the analysis those treated conservatively in outpatient care. As only a small percentage of patients intended for conservative treatment are admitted to hospital, this introduces a potential bias regarding the real number of surgical and conservatively treated patients. Another limitation is that this system lacks a classification of fractures and does not provide information on the severity of fractures, which certainly influences the indication to treatment.

HDRs do not report any information on design, materials of the devices or perioperative information (e.g., operated side and approach), which makes it difficult to carry out a complete assessment of arthroplasties. For this reason, given the increasing trend in arthroplasty, in particular for patients between 65 and 84 years of age, a dedicated tool for data collection, focusing on meaningful information about the devices and the procedures, is of primary importance. To this purpose, the Italian Arthroplasty Registry (Registro Italiano Artroprotesi, RIAP [32]), established by law at the Italian National Institute of Health (Istituto Superiore di Sanità, ISS, Rome, Italy), has been collecting records about shoulder replacements with a specifically implemented data collection flow since 2017. The RIAP registry, like all medical device registries, is an extremely powerful and important tool for monitoring the long-term safety and efficacy of devices, thereby contributing to the protection of patient health. As proved by arthroplasty registries worldwide, such tools allow the long-term tracking of devices, enabling the early identification of potential safety problems, subsequently enhancing product recalls if necessary, and allow studies with high detail on important clinical issues. For instance, registries make it possible to perform dedicated studies analyzing devices' design and technical information, which is essential for deriving epidemiological and clinical conclusions to improve patients' health and decision-making. However, registries need to be continuously fed with complete and representative data on the phenomenon, which is not yet possible for RIAP, given the current voluntary nature of its feeding [33,34].

5. Conclusions

The study highlights that over the past two decades in Italy, there has been a significant shift in the treatment of PHFs in hospitalized patients, with a marked increase in the use of surgical methods, particularly fixation and arthroplasty, which has increased from 20% to over 60% of treatments. This trend is especially evident among older patients and women, with fixation becoming the leading treatment method since 2014. The preference for arthroplasty has grown notably in the 65–84 age groups, indicating an evolving approach towards more invasive treatments over time due to technological advancements and improved outcomes.

The significant increase in the number of joint replacements worldwide and the lack of evidence for the treatment of PHFs highlight the crucial need to promote the establishment of topic-specific registries to collect data prospectively on shoulder arthroplasty revision surgery [24]. Indeed, the development of new technologies brings new prostheses with new designs onto the market, and registries should be able to record as many features as possible to properly monitor devices and produce reliable assessments.

To achieve this aim, the International Society of Arthroplasty Registries (ISAR [35]) paved the way to forge common agreements at the international level within the arthroplasty registry community [36]. The Orthopaedic Data Evaluation Panel (ODEP), an independent panel of experts, provides objective evaluation of the evidence reliability of medical implants performance. It has developed a system to assess shoulder prostheses up to 10 years survival and has already evaluated 154 items related to shoulder replacement [37].

A synergic interaction between these different infrastructures may provide sound evidence for a better and safer treatment of patients, which should be reflected in an improvement in patient safety.

Supplementary Materials: The following supporting information can be downloaded at https://www.mdpi.com/article/10.3390/jcm13195780/s1. Supplementary_File_S1.xlsx contains the counts of the following time series by year on which figures in this manuscript are built: total Proximal Humeral Fractures (PHFs); PHFs treated by arthroplasty, fixation and conservative approach; PHFs by sex; PHFs by age class.

Author Contributions: Conceptualization, E.C. and A.M.; methodology, E.C. and M.T.; validation, E.R. and M.T.; formal analysis, E.C.; investigation, E.C., A.M. and M.T.; resources, M.T.; data curation, E.C.; writing—original draft preparation, E.C., A.M., E.R. and T.F.; writing—review and editing, E.C., T.F., P.C., S.L., G.T., G.L. and M.T.; visualization, E.C.; supervision, E.R. and M.T.; project administration, M.T.; funding acquisition, M.T.; clinical expertise: A.M., E.R., S.L., G.T., S.D.G. and G.L. All authors have read and agreed to the published version of the manuscript.

Funding: This research received no external funding.

Institutional Review Board Statement: Data were anonymized and aggregated from an administrative database, and no Ethics Committee approval was needed under national law to conduct this study. Based on the large numbers used, identification of procedures undergone by individuals was assumed to be extremely low. The study was conducted following the principles of the Declaration of Helsinki.

Informed Consent Statement: Not applicable.

Data Availability Statement: The data presented in this study are available in aggregated form on request from the corresponding author.

Acknowledgments: This study was carried out within the project "Italian National Registry of Implantable Prostheses (RIPI): maintaining and updating specific registries already included, strengthening national and international cooperation, and establishing methods to compare registry data with other data sources available at the Ministry of Health", coordinated by the Italian National Institute of Health and supported by the General Directorate of Medical Devices and Pharmaceutical Service of the Italian Ministry of Health, and within the "Project ECS 0000024 Rome Technopole—CUP B83C22002820006, NRP Mission 4 Component 2 Investment 1.5, Funded by the European Union—NextGenerationEU", Partner Italian National Institute of Health, Spoke 2 (Technology transfer, new entrepreneurship, business incubation and acceleration) and Flagship project FP4 (Development, innovation and certification of medical and non-medical devices for health). We acknowledge Mascia Masciocchi, Attanasio Cornacchia, Alessia Biondi, Eugenio Carrani, Paola Laricchiuta and Stefania Ceccarelli for their management support of the RIPI and RIAP projects).

Conflicts of Interest: The authors declare no conflicts of interest.

References

1. Bergdahl, C.; Ekholm, C.; Wennergren, D.; Nilsson, F.; Möller, M. Epidemiology and patho-anatomical pattern of 2,011 humeral fractures: Data from the Swedish Fracture Register. *BMC Musculoskelet. Disord.* **2016**, *17*, 159. [CrossRef] [PubMed]
2. Roux, A.; Decroocq, L.; El Batti, S.; Bonnevialle, N.; Moineau, G.; Trojani, C.; Boileau, P.; de Peretti, F. Epidemiology of proximal humerus fractures managed in a trauma center. *Orthop. Traumatol. Surg. Res.* **2012**, *98*, 715–719. [CrossRef] [PubMed]
3. Passaretti, D.; Candela, V.; Sessa, P.; Gumina, S. Epidemiology of proximal humeral fractures: A detailed survey of 711 patients in a metropolitan area. *J. Shoulder Elb. Surg.* **2017**, *26*, 2117–2124. [CrossRef] [PubMed]
4. Kannus, P.; Palvanen, M.; Niemi, S.; Sievanen, H.; Parkkari, J. Rate of proximal humeral fractures in older Finnish women between 1970 and 2007. *Bone* **2009**, *44*, 656–659. [CrossRef]
5. Bell, J.E.; Leung, B.C.; Spratt, K.F.; Koval, K.J.; Weinstein, J.D.; Goodman, D.C.; Tosteson, A.N.A. Trends and variation in incidence, surgical treatment, and repeat surgery of proximal humeral fractures in the elderly. *J. Bone Jt. Surg.* **2011**, *93*, 121–131. [CrossRef] [PubMed]
6. Court-Brown, C.M.; Caesar, B. Epidemiology of adult fractures: A review. *Injury* **2006**, *37*, 691–697. [CrossRef]
7. Launonen, A.P.; Lepola, V.; Saranko, A.; Flinkkilä, T.; Laitinen, M.; Mattila, V.M. Epidemiology of proximal humerus fractures. *Arch. Osteoporos.* **2015**, *10*, 2. [CrossRef]
8. Mease, S.J.; Kraeutler, M.J.; Gonzales-Luna, D.C.; Gregory, J.M.; Gardner, M.J.; Choo, A.M. Current Controversies in the Treatment of Geriatric Proximal Humeral Fractures. *J. Bone Jt. Surg.* **2021**, *103*, 829–836. [CrossRef]
9. Neer, C.S., II. Displaced proximal humeral fractures. I. Classification and evaluation. *J. Bone Jt. Surg.* **1970**, *52*, 1077–1089. [CrossRef]
10. Meinberg, E.G.; Agel, J.; Roberts, C.S.; Karam, M.D.; Kellam, J.F. Fracture and dislocation classification compendium-2018. *J. Orthop. Trauma* **2018**, *32*, S1–S170. [CrossRef]
11. Handoll, H.H.; Brealey, S.; Rangan, A.; Keding, A.; Corbacho, B.; Jefferson, L.; Chuang, L.H.; Goodchild, L.; Hewitt, C.; Torgerson, D. The ProFHER (PROximal Fracture of the Humerus: Evaluation by Randomisation) trial—A pragmatic multicentre randomised controlled trial evaluating the clinical effectiveness and cost-effectiveness of surgical compared with non-surgical treatment for proximal fracture of the humerus in adults. *Health Technol. Assess.* **2015**, *19*, 1–280. [CrossRef] [PubMed]
12. Pandey, R.; Raval, P.; Manibanakar, N.; Nanjayan, S.; McDonald, C.; Singh, H. Proximal humerus fractures: A review of current practice. *J. Clin. Orthop. Trauma* **2023**, *43*, 102233. [CrossRef] [PubMed]
13. Davey, M.S.; Hurley, E.T.; Anil, U.; Condren, S.; Kearney, J.; O'Tuile, C.; Gaafar, M.; Mullett, H.; Pauzenberger, L. Management options for proximal humerus fractures—A systematic review & network meta-analysis of randomized control trials. *Injury* **2022**, *53*, 244–249. [CrossRef] [PubMed]
14. Majed, A.; Macleod, I.; Bull, A.M.; Zyto, K.; Resch, H.; Hertel, R.; Reilly, P.; Emery, R.J. Proximal humeral fracture classification systems revisited. *J. Shoulder Elb. Surg.* **2011**, *20*, 1125–1132. [CrossRef]
15. Marmor, M.T.; Agel, J.; Dumpe, J.; Kellam, J.F.; Marecek, G.S.; Meinberg, E.; Nguyen, M.P.; Sims, S.; Soles, G.L.; Karam, M.D. Comparison of the Neer classification to the 2018 update of the Orthopedic Trauma Association/AO fracture classification for classifying proximal humerus fractures. *OTA Int.* **2022**, *5*, e200. [CrossRef]
16. Lanting, B.; MacDermid, J.; Drosdowech, D.; Faber, K.J. Proximal humeral fractures: A systematic review of treatment modalities. *J. Shoulder Elb. Surg.* **2008**, *17*, 42–54. [CrossRef]
17. Direzione Generale Della Programmazione Sanitaria—Ufficio 6 Ministero della Salute. Rapporto Annuale Sull'attività di Ricovero Ospedaliero. Dati SDO 2019. Roma: 2020. Available online: https://www.salute.gov.it/portale/documentazione/p6_2_2_1.jsp?lingua=italiano&id=3002 (accessed on 2 May 2024).
18. Ciminello, E.; Madi, S.A.; Laricchiuta, P.; Torre, M. Interventi di artroprotesi: Analisi dei dati SDO nazionali 2020 e 2021 (Appendix 2A). In *Registro Italiano ArtroProtesi*; Torre, M., Ceccarelli, S., Biondi, A., Ciccarelli, P., Masciocchi, M., Eds.; Report Annuale 2022; Il Pensiero Scientifico Editore: Roma, Italy, 2023; pp. 65–108.
19. Fidanza, A.; Caggiari, G.; Di Petrillo, F.; Fiori, E.; Momoli, A.; Logroscino, G. Three-dimensional printed models can reduce costs and surgical time for complex proximal humeral fractures: Preoperative planning, patient satisfaction, and improved resident skills. *J. Orthop. Traumatol.* **2024**, *25*, 11. [CrossRef]
20. Twomey-Kozak, J.; Hurley, E.; Levin, J.; Anakwenze, O.; Klifto, C. Technological innovations in shoulder replacement: Current concepts and the future of robotics in total shoulder arthroplasty. *J. Shoulder Elb. Surg.* **2023**, *32*, 2161–2171. [CrossRef]
21. Fletcher, J.W.; Windolf, M.; Richards, R.G.; Gueorguiev, B.; Buschbaum, J.; Varga, P. Importance of locking plate positioning in proximal humeral fractures as predicted by computer simulations. *J. Orthop. Res.* **2019**, *37*, 957–964. [CrossRef]
22. Omid, R.; Trasolini, N.A.; Stone, M.A.; Namdari, S. Principles of Locking Plate Fixation of Proximal Humerus Fractures. *J. Am. Acad. Orthop. Surg.* **2021**, *29*, e523–e535. [CrossRef]
23. Flatow, E.L.; Harrison, A.K. A history of reverse total shoulder arthroplasty. *Clin. Orthop. Relat. Res.* **2011**, *469*, 2432–2439. [CrossRef] [PubMed]
24. Larose, G.; Virk, M.S. The Evolution of Reverse Total Shoulder Arthroplasty and Its Current Use in the Treatment of Proximal Humerus Fractures in the Older Population. *J. Clin. Med.* **2022**, *11*, 5832. [CrossRef]
25. Patel, A.H.; Wilder, J.H.; Ofa, S.A.; Lee, O.C.; Iloanya, M.C.; Savoie III, F.H., II; Sherman, W.F. How age and gender influence proximal humerus fracture management in patients older than fifty years. *JSES Int.* **2022**, *6*, 253–258. [CrossRef] [PubMed]

26. Handoll, H.H.; Elliott, J.; Thillemann, T.M.; Aluko, P.; Brorson, S. Interventions for treating proximal humeral fractures in adults. *Cochrane Database Syst. Rev.* **2022**, *2022*, CD000434. [CrossRef]
27. Klug, A.; Gramlich, Y.; Wincheringer, D.; Schmidt-Horlohé, K.; Hoffmann, R. Trends in surgical management of proximal humeral fractures in adults: A nationwide study of records in Germany from 2007 to 2016. *Arch. Orthop. Trauma Surg.* **2019**, *139*, 1713–1721. [CrossRef] [PubMed]
28. Papalia, A.G.; Romeo, P.V.; Kingery, M.T.; Alben, M.G.; Lin, C.C.; Simcox, T.G.; Virk, M.S. Trends in the treatment of proximal humerus fractures from 2010 to 2020. *J. Shoulder Elb. Surg.* **2024**, *33*, e49–e57. [CrossRef]
29. Alrabaa, R.G.; Ma, G.; Truong, N.M.; Lansdown, D.A.; Feeley, B.T.; Zhang, A.L.; Ma, C.B. Trends in surgical treatment of proximal humeral fractures and analysis of postoperative complications over a decade in 384,158 patients. *JBJS Open Access* **2022**, *7*, e22. [CrossRef] [PubMed]
30. McLean, A.S.; Price, N.; Graves, S.; Hatton, A.; Taylor, F.J. Nationwide trends in management of proximal humeral fractures: An analysis of 77,966 cases from 2008 to 2017. *J. Shoulder Elb. Surg.* **2019**, *28*, 2072–2078. [CrossRef] [PubMed]
31. Leino, O.K.; Lehtimäki, K.K.; Mäkelä, K.; Äärimaa, V.; Ekman, E. Proximal humeral fractures in Finland: Trends in the incidence and methods of treatment between 1997 and 2019. *Bone Jt. J.* **2022**, *104*, 150–156. [CrossRef]
32. Italian Arthroplasty Registry. 2024. Available online: https://riap.iss.it/riap/en/ (accessed on 30 July 2024).
33. Valentini, R.; Ciminello, E.; Mari, V.; Pascucci, S.; Cornacchia, A.; Lepore, S.; Boniforti, F.; Tornago, S.; Alfieri Montrasio, U.; Zanoli, G.; et al. *Capitolo 2. Analisi dei dati RIAP 2007–2021 In Registro Italiano ArtroProtesi*; Torre, M., Ceccarelli, S., Biondi, A., Ciccarelli, P., Masciocchi, M., Eds.; Report Annuale 2022; Il Pensiero Scientifico Editore: Roma, Italy, 2023; pp. 14–55.
34. Torre, M.; Carrani, E.; Franzò, M.; Ciminello, E.; Urakcheeva, I.; Bacocco, D.L.; Valentini, R.; Pascucci, S.; Madi, S.; Ferrara, C.; et al. Il Registro Italiano delle Protesi Impiantabili: Una nuova realtà per la sicurezza del paziente. *Boll. Epidemiol. Naz.* **2021**, *2*, 16–23. [CrossRef]
35. International Society of Arthroplasty Registries. Available online: https://www.isarhome.org/home (accessed on 30 July 2024).
36. Malchau, H.; Porter, M.L. Editorial Comment: 2014 Meeting of The International Society of Arthroplasty Registers. *Clin. Orthop. Relat. Res.* **2015**, *473*, 3368–3369. [CrossRef] [PubMed]
37. ODEP Orthopaedic Data Evaluation Panel. Available online: https://www.odep.org.uk/ (accessed on 29 July 2024).

Journal of
Clinical Medicine

MDPI

Article

Distal Triceps Tendon Rupture—First Retrospective Study in Central Europe

Jaroslav Sekáč [1], Peter Šagát [2,*], Peter Bartík [2], Miroslav Kilián [3], Dragoş Ioan Tohănean [4], Jason Perez [3], Veronika Vasilcova [2,5] and Štefan Durdík [6]

1 Faculty of Medicine, Comenius University, 81372 Bratislava, Slovakia; jaroslavsekac@yahoo.com
2 GSD/Health and Physical Education Department, Sport Sciences and Diagnostic Research Group, Prince Sultan University, Riyadh 11586, Saudi Arabia; pbartik@psu.edu.sa (P.B.); vasilcovave@mngha.med.sa (V.V.)
3 Department of Trauma Surgery, Slovak Medical University and University Hospital, 82606 Bratislava, Slovakia; miroslav.kilian@szu.sk (M.K.); jperez@psu.edu.sa (J.P.)
4 Faculty of Physical Education and Mountain Sports, Transilvania University of Brasov, 500019 Braşov, Romania; dragos.tohanean@unitbv.ro
5 King Abdulaziz Medical City, Riyadh 11426, Saudi Arabia
6 Clinic of Oncology and Surgery, Faculty of Medecine, Comenius University, 81250 Bratislava, Slovakia; stefan.durdik@ousa.sk
* Correspondence: sagat@psu.edu.sa

Abstract: Background: This retrospective study is the only one in the last 10 years from central Europe and provides a current picture of prevalence, new diagnostic modalities, new methods of surgical treatment, and also offers new insights into post-operative care. Triceps tendon rupture is the least reported among all the tendon injuries in the literature. In general, effective treatments for tendon injuries are lacking because the understanding of tendon biology lags behind that of the other components of the musculoskeletal system. Tendon tissue has a low number of cells and growth hormones and thus a lack of natural healing ability. Understanding the links between the mechanical and biological parameters involved in tendon development, homeostasis, and repair is a prerequisite for the identification of effective treatments for chronic and acute tendon injuries. **Methods:** The authors statistically evaluated the set of patients with this diagnosis in the largest University Hospital in Slovakia over the last 10 years. **Results:** Between 2014 and 2023, 23 patients with distal triceps tendon ruptures (DTTR) were treated at University Hospital. In some years not a single patient with this diagnosis underwent surgery, reinforcing the idea that DTTR may be either rare or underdiagnosed. The incidence in our region is 0.46 cases per 100,000 inhabitants. The average age of patients was 57.7 years, with a male predominance of 90%. Less than half of the patients (43.5%) underwent surgical intervention, and the median time from injury to surgery was less than 10 days. This rapid timeline indicates a high standard of medical care, given the semi-elective nature of the surgery and the need for MRI (Magnetic Resonance Imaging) confirmation of tendon rupture exceeding 50% of the fibers before proceeding with surgery. The three standard surgical techniques were employed in approximately equal proportions. **Conclusions:** This study suggests that none of the methods is currently preferred, and that the choice of the technique was largely determined by perioperative findings and the surgeon's discretion. Post-operative complications were minimal, with only one patient experiencing any issues after surgery.

Keywords: distal triceps rupture; triceps repair; transosseous; suture anchor; rerupture; range of motion

1. Introduction

The most common tendon injuries are rotator cuff tears of the shoulder, hand flexor injuries, and achilles tendon injuries [1]. Triceps tendon rupture is the least reported among all the tendon injuries in the literature [2,3]. 65 years ago, Anzel evaluated a series of

1014 patients with tendon ruptures in various locations, and triceps tendon ruptures accounted for only 0.8% of this series [4]. Currently the prevalence is increasing, and the prevalence of triceps tendon injuries has been found to be 3.8% [5]. Theoretically, the types of tendon injuries are tendon avulsion or inside the muscle belly. In practice, a rupture almost always occurs in the area of the tendon-bone junction, and the cause is an eccentric contraction of the triceps causing a tendon deformity of more than 8% [6]. Traditionally the triceps tendon has a uniform attachment to the olecranon ulnae. This premise has caused problems in assessing the degree of damage in traumatic triceps tendon ruptures. In 2006, an anatomic study by Madsen confirmed that in most cases the medial head of the triceps has a single attachment to the olecranon ulnae [7]. This insertion is located in a deeper layer and forms a narrower part of the attachment, and very rarely is only this part damaged [8]. The long and lateral head of the triceps has a common attachment that runs more superficially, gradually extending laterally into the surrounding area towards the musculus anconeus, which helps to strengthen the bone-tendon junction. The width of the attachment correlates with the size of the olecranon and ranges from 20 to 40 mm. Paradoxically, the thickness of the tendon is not as pronounced. The attachment itself occupies a large surface area, reaching 400 mm^2 in diameter and is dome-shaped [9]. These current findings are particularly important in partial tendon ruptures when a decision has to be made whether to proceed conservatively or with surgical revision. MRI is an appropriate method of choice to accurately assess the current condition. A schematic representation of the three basic types of partial DTTR rupture can be seen in Figure 1, while the normal anatomic attachment relationships of the triceps tendon in sagittal section to the olecranon ulna and a sub-complete rupture of the triceps tendon of the right hand are shown in Figures 2 and 3. Furthermore, the place of attachment of the individual heads of the triceps to the olecranon ulnae is presented in Figure 4.

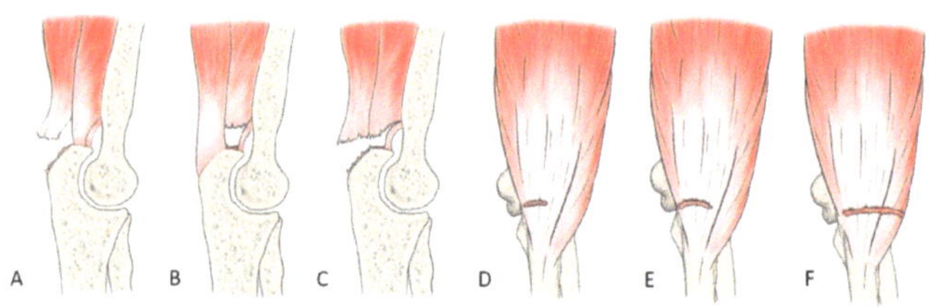

Figure 1. Illustration of the three basic types of DTTR partial rupture. (**A**): "Superficial tear"—the tendinous portion of the lateral and long head of the triceps (**B**): "Deep tear"—the deep muscular portion of the distal triceps involving the medial head of the triceps (**C**): "Full body tear"—a sub complete tear of the DTTR. (**D–F**)—coronal planes showing partial, complete, and lateral involvement [10].

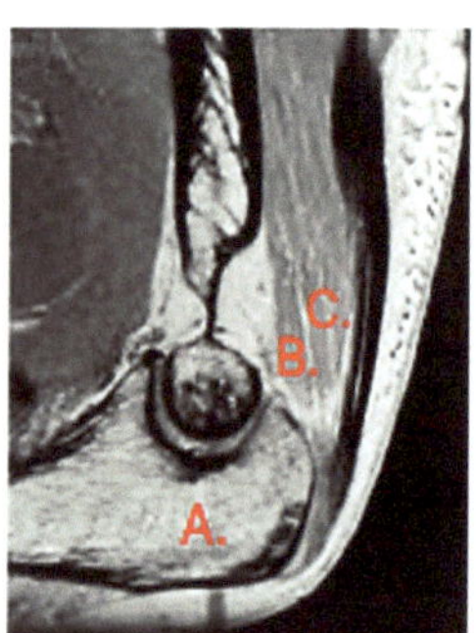

Figure 2. Normal anatomic attachment relationships of the triceps tendon in sagittal section to the olecranon ulnae. MRI: A—olecranon, B—medial head, C—common tendon of lateral and long head (own source).

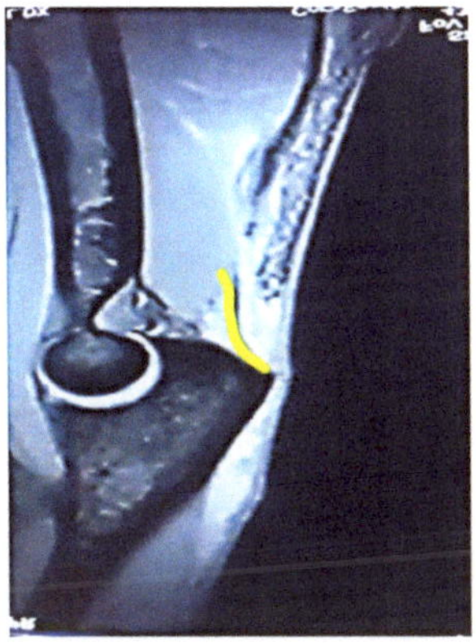

Figure 3. Sub complete rupture of the triceps tendon of the right hand (own source). Yellow line: that is the place of the rupture.

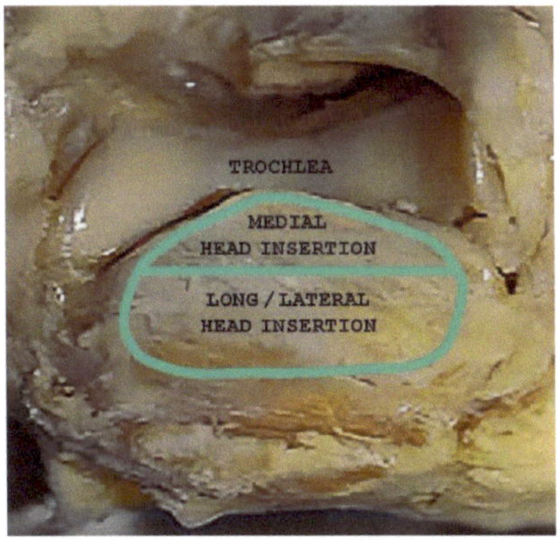

Figure 4. Place of attachment of the individual heads of the triceps to the olecranon ulnae (Own source).

2. Diagnosis and Design of Appropriate Treatment

It is surprising, given the ease of access and palpation of the triceps tendon in a healthy individual, how many incorrect diagnostic conclusions are described in the literature for triceps tendon injuries. Patients presenting with partial tears or complete tears may also have only subtle differences in clinical manifestations. This can lead to difficulty in differential diagnosis and therapeutic decision-making. It is not uncommon for a patient to present to a rehabilitation outpatient clinic with a partial tendon lesion that nevertheless meets the criteria for surgical treatment. Surgically treated acute tendon injuries have a treatment success rate of more than 95%; on the contrary, conservative management always results in a functional deficit, especially in young patients working manually, and studies also indicate an increased risk of re-injury (re-rupture) with a non-operative approach [11]. If more than 50% of the tendon bundles are ruptured and the time since the injury is no more than a few weeks, it is appropriate to refer the patient immediately to an orthopaedic outpatient clinic for consideration of suture and fixation of the tendon to the olecranon ulnae. The examination of the patient begins with taking a medical history with a focus on the mechanism of injury. A fall on an outstretched hand may result in an injury mostly to the lateral and long head of the distal triceps tendon and an intact medial head tendon; however, direct injuries can involve full-thickness ruptures. Clinical examination of the patient alone may not always confirm the diagnosis. Patients typically present with pain, bruising, ecchymosis, swelling, and a decreased active range of motion (Figure 5). Palpable defects are commonly found and present in up to 80% of patients [12]. Provocative tests may be helpful, e.g., the modified Thompson squeeze test: the patient lies prone with the elbow at the end of the table and the forearm hanging down; the triceps muscle is firmly squeezed; and the inability to extend the elbow against gravity suggests complete disruption of the triceps proper and lateral expansion. Incorrect assessment of the extent of the damage results in non-indication of surgical treatment. The second possible scenario points to the risk that more extensive tendon damage (more than 50%) develops into complete damage, and subsequent complete rupture of a chronic nature requires a different surgical procedure. Primary repair of a torn triceps tendon is possible within the first 3 weeks after injury. The management of chronic tendon ruptures is a challenge. Plain radiographs should be presented in every case. The presence of small flakes superior to the olecranon is a tell-tale sign of an avulsion fracture—this picture may not always be present, but on the other hand, its presence confirms the diagnosis. An ultrasonography (US) examination is advantageous in terms of time, cost-effectiveness, and accessibility [13]. Direct patient interaction allows direct correlation with the site of pain through comparison with the contralateral elbow. Dynamic US allows the use of stress maneuvers and visualization of transient conditions that may not otherwise be revealed during static examination. MRI is the method of choice in the indication of surgical treatment for partial tendon lesions. An MRI best evaluates isolated medial head attachment. We then proceed in a non-sodial fashion when evaluating the MRI. On sagittal sections we focus on the olecranon ulnae and see the fat pad overlying it, usually. Next, we look for a hematoma, which confirms that this is a traumatic event. The medial head of the triceps bypasses the fat pad. Its partial rupture is called a deep triceps tendon rupture. Conversely, the remaining two heads of the triceps, when ruptured, are seen retracted several centimeters from the olecranon, superficially deposited and possibly with a small bony fragment detached from the tendon portion of the olecranon. Bursitis, or chronic tendinopathy, is also a frequent concomitant finding.

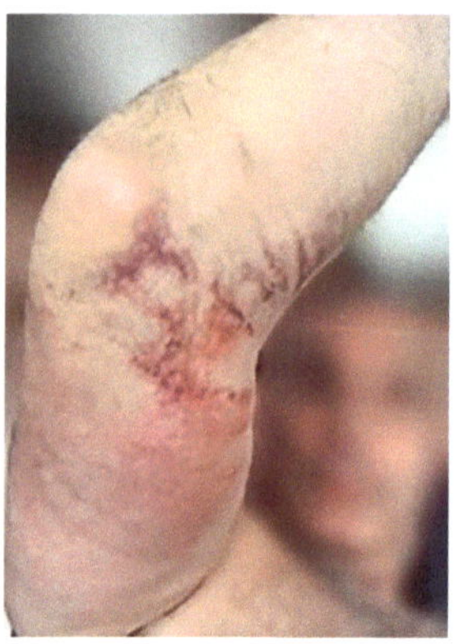

Figure 5. Condition immediately after the injury, mobility in the elbow joint was preserved as it was a partial lesion that gradually expanded with insufficient immobilization. Partial tears may be easily missed, as patients may have a good range of active motion but do typically present with reduced power on extension of the elbow. A palpable "step-off" defect will confirm the diagnosis (own source).

3. Surgical Treatment

In general, any tear that exceeds 50% of the tendon integrity and full-thickness tears are surgically treated. There is consensus that surgical treatment leads to excellent results. Conversely, conservative management can lead to functional deficits, especially in young, active patients performing manual occupations, and studies indicate an increased risk of re-injury (re-tear) with a non-operative approach. There is also a risk of misdiagnostic assessment of the degree of tendon damage in that delayed reconstruction may require a tendon graft. Surgical treatment of the ruptured triceps tendon is currently performed in a day surgery setting. The surgery itself can be performed openly, arthroscopically, or percutaneously. In Slovakia, only the open approach is currently used. Safety at the suture-tendon interface is a critical component of soft tissue fixation. The Krackow suture became a concept after its introduction by Ken Krackow in 1986. Over the next 3 decades, different variants of the Krackow suture technique were developed: the McKeon double Krackow suture (MDK), the Ostrander modified Krackow suture (OMK), and the Wilson double Krackow suture (WDK). Biomechanical testing demonstrated that the MDK had less elongation after cyclic loading than the WDK suture, but no differences in the ultimate load to failure were found between the three groups. No differences in cross-sectional diameter were found between the constructs [14]. The requirements for suture material include good sliding properties, lack of bulkiness, and high tensile strength to maintain tissue approximation. New suture materials with a salt-infused silicone core were designed to minimize laxity and preserve consistent tissue approximation in order to avoid gap formation [15]. Salt attracting the water in a liquid environment and fluid absorption leads to radial expansion of the suture material due to swelling of its core, resulting in shortening of the braid and thus a self-tensioning of the suture material. Also, an important part of surgical technique in tendon suture is the question of how many knots are required to ensure long-term strength in postoperative rehabilitation. The practice of 7 needed knots to achieve knot security is standard for commonly used sewing material [16]. On the other hand, slippage and self-seating of the knots under load are unavoidable even with the highest tying loads. Surgery is preferably performed within the first three weeks of injury. Because of the heterogeneity of types of tears, repair techniques, and outcome measures, it is impossible to determine the superiority of one technique over another. Three basic methods of attaching the tendon to the olecranon are transosseous tunnel only (TT), suture anchor only (SA), and transosseous tunnel plus suture anchor (TTSA) repair techniques. However, given the similarities between the various methods of repair, surgeons can be confident in repairing this type of injury by whichever modality they deem appropriate. Previous data may have encouraged surgeons to perform a more costly procedure in hopes of improved postoperative outcomes. Currently, based on literature sources and our experience, surgical repair of the avulsed tendon has proven to give universally good results irrespective of the technique. There is no consensus among surgeons on the best method of repair. Our surgical technique provides a solid tendon repair without the need for further osteosynthetic removal. Despite the success of operative repair, it is also associated with a relatively high complication rate, with reports as high as 22%. Common complications are re-rupture, infection, and ulnar neuropathy. For chronic ruptures, a primary tendon repair is not possible due to the degenerated tendon quality with significant tendon retraction, and tendon transfers are required. The reconstruction with a graft includes achilles allograft or ipsilateral semitendinous tendon, anconeus, latissimus dorsi, plantaris, or palmaris longus tendon. Partial tears can be treated conservatively with bracing and physio.

Post-Operative Course—Phases of the Healing Process

There is no consensus in the literature regarding the optimal postoperative protocol, the duration of immobilization, and the timing of rehabilitation. We recommend the rehabilitation program be divided into three phases. Common sense is the rule. When setting up the protocol, it is advisable if the physiotherapist has the hospital discharge report and the operative protocol. Age, associated conditions, preoperative extent of tendon damage, and method of tendon fixation are taken into account, and an individual rehabilitation plan is created [17]. One-size-fits-all does not exist. The healing process in the case of a ruptured tendon takes place in three phases [18]. Understanding the healing process of the tendon is the pathway to successful restoration of function.

4. Phase 1

4.1. Histopathologist's View: Phase 1—Inflammation

Every healing process begins with an inflammatory reaction [19]. Initially, a fibrin network is formed at the site of injury, which facilitates the migration of macrophages and neutrophils to the site of injury [20]. Wound macrophages are activated with the help of rPDGF-BB (recombinant platelet-derived growth factor-BB) [21]. We have two main phenotypes—M1 macrophages, which have a pro-inflammatory effect, creating a protective barrier against pathogens and removing waste products of metabolism. The other type is M2 macrophages, which promote healing and tissue remodeling by releasing specific growth factors [1,20,22,23]. At the same time, pro-inflammatory cytokines and other substances are released from these cells to aid the healing process. Another important component is the tenocytes that arrives at the site of damage. Tenocytes are the cells in which the extracellular matrix (ECM) and its most important component, collagen, and growth factors are formed [24]. The inflammation phase lasts only a few days after the injury (or surgery) and ends around the time when the sutures are removed from the surgical wound and the first follow-up by the surgeon is carried out, i.e., week 2. We can also stimulate this phase medially or, on the other hand, dampen it. As an example, Virchenko's findings that systemic administration of non-steroidal anti-inflammatory drugs (NSAIDs) for 7 days after achilles tendon injury in rats produced tendon healing with lower mechanical resistance and reduced cross-sectional area of the healed area [25]. On the other hand, tendon healing was improved when the drug was started only from day 6 post-operatively, which is explained by the cessation of excessive pro-inflammatory activity [26]. Therefore, the early inflammatory cascade is neither to be disrupted nor dampened and is necessary to restore the native properties of the tendon. Whereas in the later period, the persistence of inflammatory activity has, on the contrary, a detrimental effect on healing.

4.2. Rehabilitation Physician's View: Phase 1—Protective

Early mobilization after tendon surgery is crucial to avoid commonly observed post-operative soft tissue adhesions. Today, an individually manufactured dynamic brace is applied directly in the operating room with adjustment of the possible passive flexion according to the extent of damage detected perioperatively. Usually, the elbow is placed in 30–45° elbow flexion with the forearm in a neutral position, and the wrist is often supported. Post-operative position is decided by the surgeon, based on tension and quality of the tendon repair. This position is unique to each patient. The goal is a progressive elbow flexion by weekly advancing the range of motion block. Also, in our series a few years ago, we used the RICE (rest, ice, compression, and elevation) protocol and left the cast splint for the first 2 to 3 weeks. This acronym was first used by Dr. Mirkin [27]. However, Mirkin himself later admitted that rest was not the best way to heal an injury. Ice packs for the first few days after surgery are really effective in controlling pain and helping to reduce swelling. Elevating the limb slightly above body level by supporting the brace acts as a preventive measure against the increase in swelling that occurs for the first 2 weeks in the forearm area, and mild compression prevents unwanted movements. Exercises that can be practiced in the first phase: passive rotation of the forearm, passive later active flexion of the forearm gradually up to 45°. It is not recommended to massage the surgical scar area. It is also important to focus on the PROM (Passive Range of Motion) in the shoulder joint area, which is stiffened when the brace is worn 24 h a day for several weeks, which has its own weight. The long head triceps tendon on the scapula also plays a role.

5. Phase 2

5.1. Histopathologist's View: Phase 2—Proliferative

Tenocytes form new collagen fibers and gradually bridge the defect. The main component of the extracellular matrix (ECM) is type I collagen. Its structure, and thus strength, is not like that of mature collagen fibers, which have developed a precise spatial structure. How the spatial arrangement of collagen is gradually formed is not clear at present.

Tendon stem/progenitor cells called TSPCs also come in and help to repair the damaged site. Transcription of specific genes—scleraxis (Scx), mohawk (Mkx), and Egr1, which induce tenogenesis in stem cells—occurs. Angiogenesis occurs immediately after injury, and the number of vessels/mm^3 gradually increases with a peak on day 3, followed by a gradual decrease during phase 2.

5.2. Rehabilitation Doctor's View: Phase 2—Restoration of Mobility

From the very first days after the operation, the patient performs active flexion in the elbow joint to the extent allowed by the surgeon's adjustment of the dynamic brace. The main goal in phase 2 is to achieve full ROM (range of motion)—the act of moving as far as anatomically possible during a given exercise. In some situations, movements are sometimes restricted for several weeks in order to avoid gap formation between the sutured tendons, jeopardizing their healing. In this phase we can start with early controlled motion (ECM). There is not really a consensus in the literature about the optimal time frame to begin early controlled motion. Currently, we start the exercise phase immediately after suture removal, i.e., on post-operative day 8 to 12. This phase is crucial in terms of range of motion in the elbow joint. The goal is to achieve a normal range of motion—extension 0° to −10°, flexion up to 140–150° and pronation 90°. At the first meeting with the physiotherapist, the range of passive movement will be measured with a goniometer, grip strength will be measured with a dynamometer of both limbs, and the circumference of both limbs will be measured for comparison in the elbow, forearm, and just below the deltoid muscle (most pronounced atrophy in the shoulder area). Gradually increase the range of motion at both the elbow and shoulder—increasing the angle of the elbow ideally 10–15° per week. Painfulness as the tendon heals paradoxically subsides as it is gradually loaded. Leaving the brace on overnight is a prevention of damage to the suture in sleep. In general, it is advisable to exercise independently at least twice a day, and each visit to the rehabilitation clinic is associated with a change of exercises according to the improvement of the range of motion. We can use stick exercises—where the healthy hand provides passive movement at the injured limb—and ball exercises to exercise the forearm muscles. We provide ongoing skin care and massage of the surgical wound to prevent post-operative adhesions to the skin. Properly chosen load increases collagen repair; conversely, overloading or underloading can have negative effects on the tendon. Mechanical stimulation promotes cell proliferation and collagen synthesis, which improves tendon repair and remodeling, increases tendon tensile strength, and reduces adhesion. Mechanical loading in varying degrees has a positive effect during all phases. The combination of Phase I and Phase II takes approximately the first 6 weeks after surgery, and this is exactly the time it takes for the patient to reach full range of motion. Some centers also use supportive therapies such as low-frequency ultrasound [28], pulsed magnetic fields [29], and dry needle technique. Two to three sessions at weekly intervals are usually recommended; the effect occurs relatively quickly within 48 h and is associated with improved blood circulation, stimulation of cellular activity, and pain relief. The term "dry" is intended to emphasize that the needle does not serve to administer any medication [30]. Another method reported in the literature is, e.g., "band flossing"—a method that consists of fixing the affected joint with a special bandage that causes compression, thereby reducing pain during movement and, conversely, after removal, a "sponge effect" improves blood circulation to the affected area [31]. We do not indicate supportive therapy in the patient and rather emphasize exercises. Swimming exercises are recommended about 5 weeks after surgery. All other types of exercises are performed standing or seated, without much involvement of the triceps itself.

6. Phase 3

To achieve effective healing, a balance needs to be struck between too low a load, which leads to increased adhesions, slowed maturation of reparative tissue, and, in particular, stiffness and thus joint soreness, and too high a load, which leads to tearing or rupture at the original site of damage.

6.1. Histopathologist's View: Stage 3—Remodelling

After about 10 weeks, the fibrous tissue gradually changes to scar tissue, and this process continues for the following years. Mature tendons contain predominantly tenocytes and tenoblasts, which account for around 90–95% of the cell population [32]. The healed tissue does not reach the biomechanical properties before injury, and abnormality can be observed even one year after injury [33]. Due to the large difference in mechanical properties between tendon and bone tissue, a large concentration of stress is generated at the junction of the two parts, and the rights of this junction are at the highest risk of damage during postoperative rehabilitation. The attachment of the uninjured tendon to the bone is the so-called "enthesis". This site is exposed to particularly high mechanical forces, and protection from damage is addressed by the condensed structure of the tendon at the junction and the shallow angle of attachment of the tendon to the bone [34]. The extracellular matrix (ECM) remodels and forms a more organized structure through collagen exchange with the formation of collagen cross-links. Cell density and vascularity gradually decrease.

6.2. Physiotherapist's View: Phase 3—Muscle Strengthening

Here comes the main tool for restoring the functional and biomechanical properties of the tendon to pre-injury levels, and that is gradual loading of the tendon. The tendon is a mechanosensitive tissue, and this property allows us to treat it when it is injured based on mechanical loading and deforming it sufficiently [35]. Gradual loading of the triceps muscle starts on an individual basis, usually after 6 to 10 weeks. Here, we have found it very useful to start with the exercise in the prone position, the bent elbow hanging loosely off the edge of the bed, and slowly the patient tries to extend the arm and thus actively engage the triceps muscle itself. Also, in this position it is excellent to practice the shoulder joint, but in a relaxed manner, not trying to forcefully tighten the range of motion. Here, the patient suddenly realizes how greatly the triceps muscle has weakened by its inactivity. At this time, our goal is to gain the strength back. Theories state that our muscles are able to handle 20–50% more load in the eccentric phase of the movement than in the concentric phase of the movement, which implies that we can take advantage of the higher load and create more mechanical tension in eccentric training. Mechanical tension is directly proportional to building muscle mass. This is a logical explanation for why many studies begin with eccentric exercises with the assistance of a second person or machine. Muscles do not use their full potential in the eccentric phase, which in turn happens in the concentric phase of the movement. In the eccentric phase of the movement, we perform a slower movement, with better focus on the range of motion itself, thus preventing injury. Eccentric training, on the other hand, is more demanding for recovery, and therefore we do not perform strength exercises every day. In our case, however, with atrophied muscle, the mere initiation of strength training is such a significant boost that muscle mass grows very quickly in the beginning, regardless of exercise technique. This phase has the main motto: injury healing is driven by applied mechanical loads. Remodeling of the scar tissue itself in the injured area takes at least one year. An example for an eccentric contraction of the triceps, i.e., from the outstretched arm, we go to the elbow flexion by the so-called braking force—leaning both outstretched arms against the wall and gradually bringing the head closer to the wall, or on the pulley, gradually releasing the weight upwards [36]. When exercising with weights, the principle of small weights with a large number of repetitions applies. Characteristically, and usually surprisingly to the patient, the volume of the muscle itself lags visually despite the increase in muscle strength. Usually sixteen weeks after the operation, sports-specific and work-specific activities begin. On the other hand, high loads at the suture site can lead to gaps, microtears, or rupture of the suture site and consequently to poor healing. Of course, we must never exercise against pain during any of the exercises.

7. Materials and Methods

Twenty-three patients with triceps ruptures treated by surgery were included in the retrospective study. All procedures for this retrospective study were approved by our Institutional Review Board for this retrospective clinical study. All procedures followed were in accordance with the ethical standards of the responsible committee on human experimentation (institutional and national) and with the Helsinki Declaration of 1975, as revised in 2008. All patients underwent proper clinical examinations, including preoperatively standardized MRI and, in the majority of cases, ultrasound scanning and then treated by surgery. Physical examination included the assessment of pain at the affected area, a questionnaire for elbow weakness and functionality assessment, and palpation for a palpable defect. Standardized ultrasound scanning examination (ultrasonography) was performed by an experienced ultrasonographer under the supervision of a musculoskeletal fellowship-trained radiologist. Also, MRIs images were read by fellowship-trained musculoskeletal radiologists. The surgical technique does not influence the length of the postoperative follow-up period. The final obligatory follow-up was conducted upon the conclusion of the third phase of rehabilitation. The median follow-up period was 4.2 months, with an interquartile range of 3.3 to 5.4 months. This indicates that the majority of patients have a comparable length of follow-up.

The University Hospital in Bratislava (the capital of the Slovak Republic) serves a catchment area of nearly 500,000 inhabitants and is the largest hospital in the Slovak Republic. This information helps to give an approximate idea of the prevalence of triceps tendon injuries in this region. Between 2014 and 2024, over the past 10 years, 23 patients with triceps tendon injuries were treated at the emergency or surgical outpatient clinic of this hospital. Four distinct types of injuries were identified: acute tears, chronic tears, partial tears (either acute or chronic), and snapping triceps. The study excluded patients under 18 years of age, those with open injuries in the elbow area, patients with associated fractures in the elbow joint, patients with snapping triceps, and patients with chronic ruptures where primary tendon repair was not possible. The data were obtained from hospital records. The issue of obtaining informed consent prior to surgical treatment, which in our hospital always encompasses the potential utilization of documentation for scientific purposes, remains a highly contentious topic in the medical community. In establishing the doctor-patient relationship, it is crucial to recognize that the duty to provide information shifts from what "a reasonable doctor or practitioner" might consider essential for the patient to know to what "a reasonable patient" would need to know in order to make an informed decision. All legal systems in the European Union require informed consent to be obtained before any medical procedure is carried out, and there is a clear regulatory framework. The information and subsequent expression of consent are based on a fiduciary relationship between the doctor and the patient. In Europe today, the requirement for safety and quality of healthcare has long since replaced the 'original' requirement for health, which is fully linked to the direct participation of users in life decisions [37]. In our subgroup of patients, we focused on the patient's ability to engage in informed decision-making in relation to their healthcare. We paid particular attention to the overall benefit and appropriateness of the care provided to ensure that it was tailored to the patient's individual needs. It is essential that patients receive clear and comprehensive information regarding their treatment, available therapeutic options, and potential risks, including in the post-operative period. In the Slovak Republic, only the doctor is responsible for providing instructions to the patient. The question of the actual surgical technique and its alternatives is explicitly delineated in the written consent form, which is provided to the patient prior to the surgical procedure. In this document, the patient confirms in writing that they are aware of the three basic surgical techniques that may be employed and that they consent to the surgeon's discretion in selecting one of these techniques based on the findings of the perioperative evaluation. Conversely, other factors such as the timing of surgery, the maximum waiting period, and the potential for alternative settings, including conservative management, are seldom taken into account, despite their relevance to the patient. It is reasonable to conclude that each health professional is responsible for their own actions that may affect psychophysical integrity and should therefore be required to inform and obtain consent individually. However, when considering consent to treatment in a broader sense, it is an error to break down the organic process into hundreds of micro-activities carried out by individual, isolated professionals with a single act of consent, particularly when this needs to be documented in writing. Out of the 23 cases, based on clinical findings and imaging studies, surgical treatment was recommended for 12 patients. Two patients declined surgery due to their subjective perception of sufficient range of motion, age, and the nature of their work. We conducted this retrospective cohort study on 10 patients with DTTR between 2014 and 2024. The procedure was performed under a supraclavicular block or general anesthesia. The patient was positioned either in the lateral decubitus or prone position, and the use of a tourniquet was left to the surgeon's discretion. A 10 cm posterior incision was made. The surgeon could repair the distal triceps rupture using the technique they deemed appropriate or were most experienced with, as no single method appeared to offer a lower risk of complications or reoperation.

For the data analysis we used Microsoft IBM SPSS software—version 25.

8. Results

Based on the processed data, we can formulate the following conclusions.

1. Incidence

Our findings align with the literature, confirming that, unlike tendon injuries in other locations where incidence is rising for various reasons, triceps tendon ruptures remain a rare injury. University Hospital provides healthcare services in the capital of Slovakia, which has a population of approximately 500,000. Over a 10-year period, we treated 23 patients, averaging 2.3 cases per year. This incidence in our region is 0.46 cases per 100,000 inhabitants. For purposes of comparison, the estimated national incidence of distal biceps tendon rupture is 2.55 per 100,000 patient-years [38].

2. Evaluation of demographic data

Demographics: Triceps tendon ruptures most commonly affect men in the fourth and fifth decades of life. From our pooled results we observed the mean age at rupture to be 57.7 years. There was a 9:1 ratio of males to females (Figure 6).

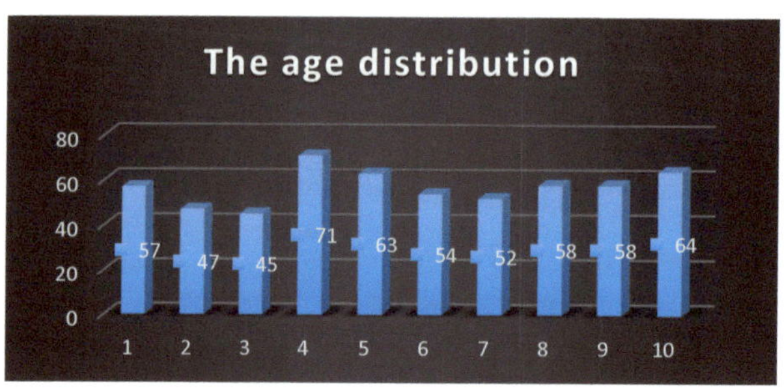

Figure 6. Proportion of unoperated patients with a verified partial triceps lesion.

3. The indication for surgery

Over a 10-year period, 23 patients with confirmed triceps tendon injuries were treated. When determining the indication for surgery, we consider multiple factors (see above). The decisive factor is assessing the extent of tendon damage. As mentioned earlier, any tear involving more than 50% of the tendon's integrity, as well as full-thickness tears, are managed surgically. In borderline cases, MRI plays a key role in the decision-making process. Although this imaging is not available 24/7 in our facility, it can be performed within 24 h for such cases. In our patient group with partial or complete tendon lesions, fewer than 50% were indicated for surgical intervention.

4. Qualitative indicator of health care

In cases of partial tendon rupture, an additional MRI examination is necessary to assess the extent of the damage. Additionally, in patients with comorbidities, especially since these injuries typically affect older individuals, further examinations are required as part of the standard preoperative workup for semi-urgent surgeries. On the other hand, the time between the injury and surgery is crucial for the success of the primary repair. An acute rupture is defined as an injury occurring within 3 weeks of trauma. For chronic ruptures, primary tendon repair is usually not possible, and tendon transfers are required. In our patient group, no tendon transfers were necessary as all surgeries were performed within 3 weeks of injury. According to the literature, the median time from triceps rupture to surgery is 22 days [39]. In our patient group, the time from injury to surgery was from 1 to 21 days (Figure 7).

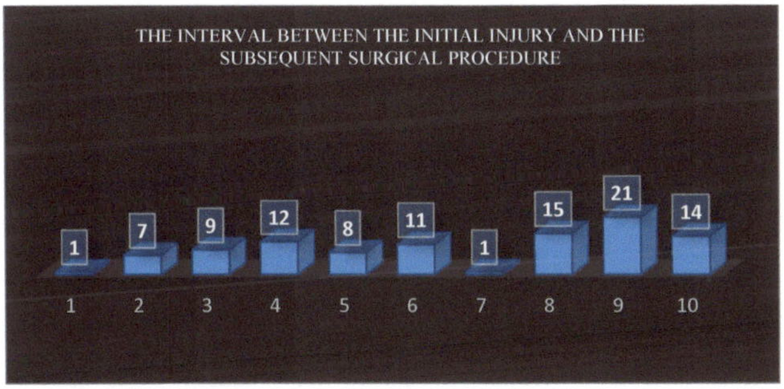

Figure 7. The interval between the initial injury and the subsequent surgical procedure.

5. Preoperative magnetic resonance examination and ultrasound

The first application of ultrasound (US) was performed during World War I for the detection of submarines (sonar) [40]. The main advantages of diagnostic US in medicine include real-time assessment, absence of radiation, reduced cost, and portability [41]. It is erroneous to consider ultrasound as a rival imaging modality; rather, it should be regarded as a supplementary imaging modality. In order to undertake an ultrasound (US) examination of the triceps tendon, it is essential to have direct experience of performing US examinations of the tendon. In this location, due to the more complex anatomical proportions at the site of interest, the phenomenon of anisotropy observed during ultrasound imaging becomes fully apparent. This is a change in the resulting echo of the tendon when the angle of the transducer is changed. If the tendon fiber has a light appearance and the transducer is positioned perpendicular to the tendon, it may appear darker. Conversely, if the transducer is oriented obliquely, it can potentially introduce significant errors. The significance of lesion localization in determining the most appropriate examination method is substantiated by the preference for ultrasound over MRI in the assessment of the rotator cuff. One meta-analysis of rotator cuff imaging has shown that ultrasound has an accuracy of 95% [42]. Dynamic sonography is also instrumental in differentiating partial and full-body tendon tears. The absence of tendon translation through the affected area and retraction of the torn tendon stump are indicative of a full-body tear. Conversely, these techniques are only applicable to the evaluation of an isolated tendon, rendering them ineffective in assessing tendons that converge with other tendons. In conclusion, ultrasound can be regarded as a viable alternative to MRI in instances where MRI is contraindicated or when the patient is unable to tolerate MRI. The findings of all studies comparing MRI and US indicate that MRI is a more precise imaging technique for identifying the type of tear, although US is a more cost-effective option [43]. When using an MRI as a decisive factor in determining the indication for surgery in unclear cases, we were also interested in the percentage of MRI examinations performed pre-operatively. Unfortunately, this number is skewed, as it is not possible to accurately determine for non-operated patients. These patients typically continue treatment and follow-up in outpatient clinics and private rehabilitation facilities outside of our hospital.

6. Technique of surgical procedure

Recently, instrumentation for tendon fixation has significantly become widespread. An ideal suture anchor is easy to handle, maintains sufficient pull-out strength, prevents suture abrasion, and is absorbable without resulting in any reactions as the material dissolves [44]. Currently, biodegradable suture anchors have been developed to help overcome complications associated with metallic anchors [45]. It is essential that surgeons understand key characteristics of a variety of currently available anchors [46]. In our series, all three standard methods of fixation of the triceps tendon to the olecranon were used, and none of the methods is currently dominant. There were 12 surgical procedures performed in 10 patients with triceps tendon lesions. In one patient, two surgical revisions were required because of infection in the surgical wound. Due to the rarity of this occurrence, a special team was not formed to deal with this problem, and patients were operated on by different surgeons. There is no consensus among our surgeons on the best method of repair. The procedure was completed under a supraclavicular block. Approximately 10 cm posterior incision was made (Figure 8).

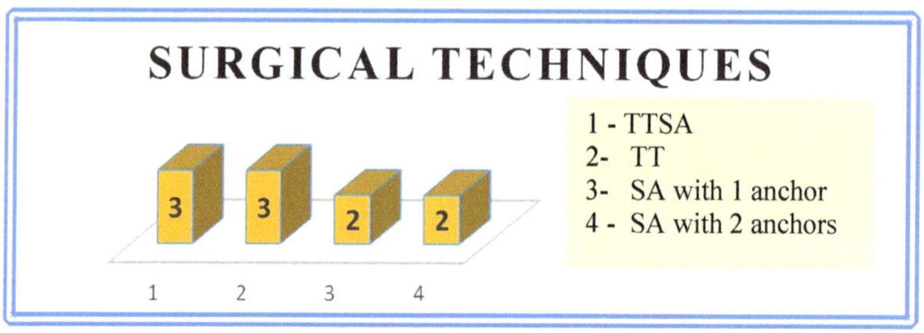

Figure 8. The surgical techniques employed in the patient cohort can be broadly classified into four categories. TTSA—transosseous tunnel plus suture anchor repair; TT—suture-only transosseous tunnel repair. SA—suture anchor repair with one or two anchors.

7. Postoperative complications

The three most common complications with this type of injury include ulnar neuropathies, infections, and pain. These complications are detected in the immediate postoperative period and are therefore accurately evaluated in our series. In our series, one patient was found to have an infection in the wound. Subsequently, the condition was managed with 2 reoperations—the first involved revision, debridement, and loading of a vacuum drain, which we use for secondary wound healing, and then after 7 days the vacuum drain was removed, and a secondary wound suture was performed. The re-rupture rate remains problematic as it can occur several months after the injury, and patients with this injury are not usually dispensed, and efforts to follow up with patients have been unsuccessful. The re-rupture rate is reported to be relatively low, up to 4%, and in our series, it was not necessary to reoperate the patient for this reason.

9. Discussion

This comprehensive study on triceps tendon ruptures conducted over a period of a decade provides several important insights into the nature and treatment of this relatively rare injury. First and foremost, triceps tendon ruptures are infrequent, with only 23 cases treated over the course of 10 years, which averages out to 2.3 cases annually. This equates to an incidence rate of approximately 0.46 per 100,000 people in the capital of Slovakia, which underscores the rarity of this type of injury. The data also reveal that triceps tendon ruptures predominantly affect men between the ages of 40 and 50, with a striking male-to-female ratio of 9:1. The mean age of rupture in the cohort was found to be 57.7 years, further indicating that this injury is more common in middle-aged individuals.

Surgical intervention is the preferred treatment option, particularly in cases where the tendon rupture is extensive—defined as tears involving more than 50% of the tendon or full-thickness ruptures. In many instances, MRI plays a critical role in evaluating partial tears or borderline cases, guiding the decision-making process for surgery. Prompt surgical intervention is crucial, as delays beyond three weeks post-injury are associated with an increased risk of complications related to chronic rupture, such as muscle atrophy and decreased function. Encouragingly, all patients in this study underwent surgery within 21 days of their injury, minimizing the risk of such complications. MRI imaging is especially helpful in assessing the extent of injury in cases of partial tears and is also instrumental in managing patients with comorbid conditions that may complicate recovery.

Advances in surgical techniques, particularly the introduction of biodegradable suture anchors, have improved fixation methods and the overall success of surgeries. Despite this progress, there is still no consensus on a single dominant surgical method, as surgeons often choose techniques based on their individual experience and the specifics of the injury. Common postoperative complications observed in this study include ulnar neuropathies, infections, and persistent pain. However, it is worth noting that only one patient required revision surgery due to an infection, which was managed with a vacuum drain. Although re-ruptures remain a concern, follow-up is often challenging due to the relatively long recovery times associated with these injuries, and no cases of re-rupture required reoperation in this cohort.

The findings of this study highlight the importance of timely and effective treatment for triceps tendon ruptures and the ongoing advancements in surgical materials and techniques. The results also align with previous studies, such as that of Koplas et al. [5], which reported a prevalence of triceps tendon injuries of 3.8%. In their study, 5 women and 23 men were found to have either partial or complete tears, with the mean age of those affected being 46.6 years, a finding similar to ours. Additionally, the gender distribution observed in their study mirrors our own, with middle-aged men being the most commonly affected group. Koplas et al. also noted that triceps brachii ruptures often go clinically undiagnosed, a point that aligns with our own observations.

Supporting our findings, Giannicola et al. [47] confirm that distal triceps tendon ruptures (DTTR) are indeed a rare injury. Anzel et al., in their analysis of 1014 tendon ruptures, reported a prevalence of 0.8% for DTTR. More recent studies, including Giannicola's, have shown a higher prevalence of triceps tendon tears, citing 3.8% of cases found through MRI investigations. Despite these numbers, it remains highly likely that a significant proportion of patients with this injury go undiagnosed. Several factors contribute to this, including the clinical condition immediately following the injury. For instance, if the lateral extension and the functional anconeus remain intact, active elbow extension may still be preserved, making the diagnosis less obvious. Additionally, the swelling and pain that accompany the injury limit the availability of imaging and investigative options. The rarity of the injury itself means that clinicians may be less inclined to consider it as a possibility, further contributing to the likelihood of an undiagnosed rupture.

Another challenge in managing triceps tendon ruptures is the relatively long healing time, which often extends up to a year before patients can return to pre-operative levels of muscle strength. This underscores the potential of telemedicine to enhance the quality of post-operative care in this context. Telemedicine is not a comprehensive substitute for conventional clinical examination. However, it does facilitate the monitoring of patients over extended distances and over prolonged periods, thereby alleviating discomfort. Once the application has been installed on the patient's mobile device, communication with healthcare professionals can commence on a daily basis. At the present time, the potential of telemedicine is still not being fully realized in Europe. That is mostly due to the still high costs of setting up and performing telemedicine services. Also, the limited scope of implementation can be attributed to the deficiencies in the technical infrastructure in EU

Member States, as well as concerns pertaining to confidentiality and privacy in the context of health data management [48].

This protracted recovery period complicates both diagnosis and treatment, as the injury may not become apparent until the muscle strength does not recover as expected. Eighteen different scoring systems are currently available to evaluate elbow disorders, each with its own set of objective and subjective criteria. However, there is no single, universally accepted outcome evaluation system that is both reliable and sensitive enough to detect clinically relevant changes. The variability in patient groups, imaging techniques, and reported outcomes makes it difficult to draw reliable conclusions across different studies, highlighting the need for more consistent and standardized approaches to assessing and treating triceps tendon injuries.

10. Conclusions

Triceps tendon ruptures occurrence is rare, with only 23 cases over 10 years, averaging 2.3 cases per year, equating to an incidence rate of 0.46 per 100,000 people in Slovakia's capital. The injury predominantly affects men aged 40–50, with a 9:1 male-to-female ratio, and the mean age of rupture was 57.7 years. Surgical intervention is primarily considered for tears involving more than 50% of the tendon or full-thickness ruptures, with MRI often guiding borderline cases.

Adult tendons have a limited natural healing capacity, which derives from the nature of the tendon with its poor cellularity, limited vascularization, and low metabolism. Tendon tissue heals by fibrovascular scarring, and current treatment strategies fail to restore the functional, structural, and biochemical properties of the tendon to the level of the original tissue [49–51]. Currently, despite new knowledge gained from studies in animal models and technological advances, tendon tissue restitution and repair remain an ongoing problem [51]. In the near future, randomized trials will have to be designed in order to better handle intermediate results and, most importantly, to evaluate long-term follow-up as well.

Author Contributions: Conceptualization, J.S.; Methodology, J.S.; Validation, J.S. and M.K.; Formal analysis, J.S.; Resources, J.S., D.I.T. and Š.D.; Data curation, P.Š.; Writing—original draft, J.S. and M.K.; Writing—review & editing, P.Š., P.B., D.I.T., J.P. and V.V.; Supervision, M.K. and Š.D. All authors have read and agreed to the published version of the manuscript.

Funding: This research received no external funding.

Institutional Review Board Statement: Ethical Committee University hospital Bratislava, EK 2/11/2024. Approval day the 14 November 2024.

Informed Consent Statement: Informed consent was obtained from all subjects involved in the study.

Data Availability Statement: Due to privacy and ethical reasons we do not wish to share additional data.

Acknowledgments: The authors would like to acknowledge the support of Prince Sultan University.

Conflicts of Interest: The authors declare no conflict of interest.

Abbreviations

TT	suture only transosseous tunnel repair
SA	suture anchor-only repair
TTSA	transosseous tunnel plus suture anchor repair
DTTR	distal triceps tendon ruptures
PROM	passive range of motion

References

1. Zhang, W.; Gong, Y.; Zheng, X.; Qiu, J.; Jiang, T.; Chen, L.; Lu, F.; Wu, X.; Cheng, F.; Hong, Z. Platelet-Derived Growth Factor-BB Inhibits Intervertebral Disc Degeneration via Suppressing Pyroptosis and Activating the MAPK Signaling Pathway. *Front. Pharmacol.* **2021**, *12*, 799130. [CrossRef] [PubMed]
2. Waugh, R.L.; Hathcock, T.A.; Elliott, J.L. Ruptures of muscles and tendons. *Surgery* **1949**, *25*, 370–392. [PubMed]

3. Zacharia, B.; Roy, A. A clinicoradiological classification and a treatment algorithm for traumatic triceps tendon avulsion in adults. *Chin. J. Traumatol.* **2021**, *24*, 266–272. [CrossRef] [PubMed] [PubMed Central]
4. Anzel, S.H.; Covey, K.W.; Weiner, A.D.; Lipscomb, P.R. Disruption of muscles and tendons; an analysis of 1014 cases. *Surgery* **1959**, *45*, 406–414. [PubMed]
5. Koplas, M.C.; Schneider, E.; Sundaram, M. Prevalence of triceps tendon tears on MRI of the elbow and clinical correlation. *Skelet. Radiol.* **2011**, *40*, 587–594. [CrossRef]
6. Thomopoulos, S.; Parks, W.C.; Rifkin, D.B.; Derwin, K.A. Mechanisms of tendon injury and repair. *J. Orthop. Res.* **2015**, *33*, 832–839. [CrossRef]
7. Madsen, M.; Marx, R.G.; Millett, P.J.; Rodeo, S.A.; Sperling, J.W.; Warren, R.F. Surgical anatomy of the triceps brachii tendon: Anatomical study and clinical correlation. *Am. J. Sports Med.* **2006**, *34*, 1839–1843. [CrossRef]
8. Keener, J.D.; Chafik, D.; Kim, H.M.; Galatz, L.M.; Yamaguchi, K. Insertional anatomy of the triceps brachii tendon. *J. Shoulder Elb. Surg.* **2010**, *19*, 399–405. [CrossRef]
9. Yeh, P.C.; Stephens, K.T.; Solovyova, O.; Obopilwe, E.; Smart, L.R.; Mazzocca, A.D.; Sethi, P.M. The Distal Triceps Tendon Footprint and a Biomechanical Analysis of 3 Repair Techniques. *Am. J. Sports Med.* **2010**, *38*, 1025–1033. [CrossRef]
10. Pederzini, L.A.; Eygendaal, D.; Denti, M. *Elbow and Sport*, 1st ed.; Springer: Berlin/Heidelberg, Germany; ISAKOS: New York, NY, USA, 2016.
11. Gajdoš, R.; Kaniansky, M.; Jančiar, M. Parciálne ruptúry distálnej šľachy tricepsu s avulziou špičky olekranonu—Je potrebná operačná liečba? *Ortopedie* **2012**, *6*, 4.
12. Walker, C.M.; Noonan, T.J. Distal Triceps Tendon Injuries. *Clin. Sports Med.* **2020**, *39*, 673–685. [CrossRef] [PubMed]
13. Tagliafico, A.; Gandolfo, N.; Michaud, J.; Perez, M.M.; Palmieri, F.; Martinoli, C. Ultrasound demonstration of distal triceps tendon tears. *Eur. J. Radiol.* **2012**, *81*, 1207–1210. [CrossRef] [PubMed]
14. Hong, C.K.; Lin, C.L.; Kuan, F.C.; Wang, P.H.; Yeh, M.L.; Su, W.R. A Biomechanical Evaluation of Various Double Krackow Suture Techniques for Soft-Tissue Graft Fixation. *Arthroscopy* **2018**, *34*, 663–668. [CrossRef] [PubMed]
15. Pastor, T.; Zderic, I.; Dhillon, M.; Gueorguiev, B.; Richards, R.G.; Pastor, T.; Vögelin, E. New dynamic suture material for tendon transfer surgeries in the upper extremity—A biomechanical comparative analysis. *Arch. Orthop. Trauma Surg.* **2024**, *144*, 2905–2914. [CrossRef]
16. Neuhofer, S.; Wieser, K.; Lajtai, G.; Müller, D.; Gerber, C.; Meyer, D.C. Surgical knot tightening: How much pull is necessary? *Knee Surg. Sports Traumatol. Arthrosc.* **2014**, *22*, 2849–2855. [CrossRef]
17. Agarwalla, A.; Gowd, A.K.; Jan, K.; Liu, J.N.; Garcia, G.H.; Naami, E.; Wysocki, R.W.; Fernandez, J.J.; Cohen, M.S.; Verma, N.N. Return to work following distal triceps repair. *J. Shoulder Elb. Surg.* **2021**, *30*, 906–912. [CrossRef]
18. Liang, W.; Zhou, C.; Deng, Y.; Fu, L.; Zhao, J.; Long, H.; Ming, W.; Shang, J.; Zeng, B. The current status of various preclinical therapeutic approaches for tendon repair. *Ann. Med.* **2024**, *56*, 2337871. [CrossRef]
19. Arvind, V.; Huang, A.H. Reparative and Maladaptive Inflammation in Tendon Healing. *Front. Bioeng. Biotechnol.* **2021**, *9*, 719047. [CrossRef]
20. Dakin, S.G.; Dudhia, J.; Smith, R.K.W. Resolving an inflammatory concept: The importance of inflammation and resolution in tendinopathy. *Vet. Immunol. Immunopathol.* **2014**, *158*, 121–127. [CrossRef]
21. Pierce, G.F.; Tarpley, J.E.; Yanagihara, D.; Mustoe, T.A.; Fox, G.M.; Thomason, A. Platelet-derived growth factor (BB Homo-dimer), transforming growth factor-β1, and basic fibroblast growth factor in dermal wound healing. *Am. J. Pathol.* **1992**, *140*, 1375–1388.
22. Yang, G.; Rothrauff, B.B.; Tuan, R.S. Tendon and ligament regeneration and repair: Clinical relevance and developmental paradigm. *Birth Defects Res. Part C Embryo Today Rev.* **2013**, *99*, 203–222. [CrossRef] [PubMed]
23. Yang, Q.Q.; Zhang, L.; Zhou, Y.L.; Tang, J.B. Morphological changes of macrophages and their potential contribution to tendon healing. *Colloids Surf. B Biointerfaces* **2022**, *209*, 112145. [CrossRef] [PubMed]
24. Citeroni, M.R.; Ciardulli, M.C.; Russo, V.; Della Porta, G.; Mauro, A.; El Khatib, M.; Di Mattia, M.; Galesso, D.; Barbera, C.; Forsyth, N.R.; et al. In Vitro Innovation of Tendon Tissue Engineering Strategies. *Int. J. Mol. Sci.* **2020**, *21*, 6726. [CrossRef] [PubMed]
25. Dimmen, S.; Engebretsen, L.; Nordsletten, L.; Madsen, J.E. Negative effects of parecoxib and indomethacin on tendon healing: An experimental study in rats. *Knee Surg. Sports Traumatol. Arthrosc.* **2009**, *17*, 835–839. [CrossRef]
26. Tang, C.; Chen, Y.; Huang, J.; Zhao, K.; Chen, X.; Yin, Z.; Heng, B.C.; Chen, W.; Shen, W. The roles of inflammatory mediators and immunocytes in tendinopathy. *J. Orthop. Transl.* **2018**, *14*, 23–33. [CrossRef]
27. Mirkin, G.; Hoffman, M. *The Sports-Medicine Book*; Little-Brown: New York, NY, USA, 1978.
28. Lovric, V.; Ledger, M.; Goldberg, J.; Harper, W.; Bertollo, N.; Pelletier, M.H.; Oliver, R.A.; Yu, Y.; Walsh, W.R. The effects of low-intensity pulsed ultrasound on tendon-bone healing in a transosseous-equivalent sheep rotator cuff model. *Knee Surg. Sports Traumatol. Arthrosc.* **2013**, *21*, 466–475. [CrossRef] [PubMed]
29. Strauch, B.; Patel, M.K.; Rosen, D.J.; Mahadevia, S.; Brindzei, N.; Pilla, A.A. Pulsed magnetic field therapy increases tensile strength in a rat Achilles' tendon repair model. *J. Hand Surg.* **2006**, *31*, 1131–1135. [CrossRef] [PubMed]
30. Dunning, J.; Butts, R.; Mourad, F.; Young, I.; Flannagan, S.; Perreault, T. Dry needling: A literature review with implications for clinical practice guidelines. *Phys. Ther. Rev.* **2014**, *19*, 252–265. [CrossRef] [PubMed] [PubMed Central]
31. Konrad, A.; Močnik, R.; Nakamura, M. Effects of Tissue Flossing on the Healthy and Impaired Musculoskeletal System: A Scoping Review. *Front. Physiol.* **2021**, *12*, 666129. [CrossRef] [PubMed] [PubMed Central]
32. Sharma, P.; Maffulli, N. Tendon injury and tendinopathy: Healing and repair. *J. Bone Jt. Surg.* **2005**, *87*, 187–202. [CrossRef]

33. Miyashita, H.; Ochi, M.; Ikuta, Y. Histological and biomechanical observations of the rabbit patellar tendon after removal of its central one-third. *Arch. Orthop. Trauma Surg.* **1997**, *116*, 454–462. [CrossRef] [PubMed]
34. Killian, M.L.; Cavinatto, L.; Galatz, L.M.; Thomopoulos, S. The role of mechanobiology in tendon healing. *J. Shoulder Elb. Surg* **2012**, *21*, 228–237. [CrossRef] [PubMed]
35. Morrison, S.; Cook, J. Putting "Heavy" into Heavy Slow Resistance. *Sports Med.* **2022**, *52*, 1219–1222. [CrossRef] [PubMed]
36. Woodley, B.L.; Newsham-West, R.J.; Baxter, G.D. Chronic tendinopathy: Effectiveness of eccentric exercise. *Br. J. Sports Med* **2007**, *41*, 188–198, discussion 199. [CrossRef] [PubMed] [PubMed Central]
37. Bolcato, V.; Franzetti, C.; Fassina, G.; Basile, G.; Martinez, R.M.; Tronconi, L.P. Comparative study on informed consent regulation in health care among Italy, France, United Kingdom, Nordic Countries, Germany, and Spain. *J. Forensic Leg. Med.* **2024**, *103*, 102674. [CrossRef]
38. Kelly, M.P.; Perkinson, S.G.; Ablove, R.H.; Tueting, J.L. Distal Biceps Tendon Ruptures: An Epidemiological Analysis Using a Large Population Database. *Am. J. Sports Med.* **2015**, *43*, 2012–2017. [CrossRef]
39. Balazs, G.C.; Brelin, A.M.; Dworak, T.C.; Brooks, D.I.; Mauntel, T.C.; Tintle, S.M.; Dickens, J.F. Outcomes and complications of triceps tendon repair following acute rupture in American military personnel. *Injury* **2016**, *47*, 2247–2251. [CrossRef]
40. Newman, P.G.; Rozycki, G.S. The History of Ultrasound. *Surg. Clin. N. Am.* **1998**, *78*, 179–195. [CrossRef]
41. Quarato, C.M.I.; Lacedonia, D.; Salvemini, M.; Tuccari, G.; Mastrodonato, G.; Villani, R.; Fiore, L.A.; Scioscia, G.; Mirijello, A.; Saponara, A.; et al. A review on biological effects of ultrasounds: Key messages for clinicians. *Diagnostics* **2023**, *13*, 855. [CrossRef]
42. Dinnes, J.; Loveman, E.; McIntyre, L.; Waugh, N. The effectiveness of diagnostic tests for the assessment of shoulder pain due to soft tissue disorders: A systematic review. *Health Technol. Assess.* **2003**, *7*, 1–166. [CrossRef]
43. Lynch, J.; Yu, C.C.; Chen, C.; Muh, S. Magnetic resonance imaging versus ultrasound in diagnosis of distal biceps tendon avulsion. *Orthop. Traumatol. Surg. Res.* **2019**, *105*, 861–866. [CrossRef] [PubMed]
44. Barber, F.A. Biodegradable materials: Anchors and interference screws. *Sports Med. Arthrosc. Rev.* **2015**, *23*, 112–117. [CrossRef] [PubMed]
45. Li, L.-H.; Kong, Y.-M.; Kim, H.-W.; Kim, Y.-W.; Kim, H.-E.; Heo, S.-J.; Koak, J.-Y. Improved biological performance of Ti implants due to surface modification by micro-arc oxidation. *Biomaterials* **2004**, *25*, 2867–2875. [CrossRef] [PubMed]
46. Cho, C.-H.; Bae, K.-C.; Kim, D.-H. Biomaterials Used for Suture Anchors in Orthopedic Surgery. *Clin. Orthop. Surg.* **2021**, *13*, 287–292. [CrossRef] [PubMed] [PubMed Central]
47. Giannicola, G.; Bullitta, G.; Rotini, R.; Murena, L.; Blonna, D.; Iapicca, M.; Restuccia, G.; Merolla, G.; Fontana, M.; Greco, A.; et al. Results of primary repair of distal triceps tendon ruptures in a general population a multicentre study. *Bone Jt. J.* **2018**, *100-B*, 610–616. [CrossRef]
48. Basile, G.; Accetta, R.; Marinelli, S.; D'Ambrosi, R.; Petrucci, Q.A.; Giorgetti, A.; Nuara, A.; Zaami, S.; Fozzato, S. Traumatology: Adoption of the Sm@rtEven Application for the Remote Evaluation of Patients and Possible Medico-Legal Implications. *J. Clin. Med.* **2022**, *11*, 3644. [CrossRef]
49. Darrieutort-Laffite, C.; Blanchard, F.; Soslowsky, L.J.; Le Goff, B. Biology and physiology of tendon healing. *Jt. Bone Spine* **2024**, *91*, 105696. [CrossRef] [PubMed]
50. Liu, C.F.; Aschbacher-Smith, L.; Barthelery, N.J.; Dyment, N.; Butler, D.; Wylie, C. What We Should Know Before Using Tissue Engineering Techniques to Repair Injured Tendons: A Developmental Biology Perspective. *Tissue Eng Part B-Rev.* **2011**, *17*, 165–176. [CrossRef]
51. Nourissat, G.; Berenbaum, F.; Duprez, D. Tendon injury: From biology to tendon repair. *Nat. Rev. Rheumatol.* **2015**, *11*, 223–233. [CrossRef]

Journal of
Clinical Medicine

MDPI

Systematic Review

Translating Biomarker Research into Clinical Practice in Orthopaedic Trauma: A Systematic Review

Alexander Baur [1,*] and Augustine Mark Saiz, Jr. [2]

[1] Liberty University College of Osteopathic Medicine, Lynchburg, VA 24502, USA
[2] Department of Orthopaedic Surgery, UC Davis Health, Sacramento, CA 95817, USA
* Correspondence: ajbaur@liberty.edu

Abstract: Background/Objectives: Orthopaedic trauma management in polytrauma patients presents challenges, particularly in selecting between damage control orthopaedics (DCO) and early appropriate care (EAC). This systematic review evaluates these approaches and explores the role of biomarkers in optimising surgical timing. The primary objective of this review was to evaluate the potential clinical utility of biomarkers in guiding surgical timing and predicting perioperative complications. The secondary objective was to compare the effectiveness of DCO and EAC approaches, focusing on their impact on patient outcomes when controlled for Injury Severity Scores (ISSs). **Methods:** A systematic search of PubMed, MEDLINE, and Google Scholar identified studies focusing on fracture management (DCO versus EAC), timing protocols, and biomarkers in polytrauma patients. Twenty-seven studies met inclusion criteria. **Results:** Among the 27 studies, 12 evaluated biomarkers and 15 compared DCO and EAC. Point-of-care (POC) biomarkers, including lactate ($p < 0.001$; OR 1.305), monocyte L-selectin ($p = 0.001$; OR 1.5), and neutrophil L-selectin ($p = 0.005$; OR 1.56), demonstrated predictive value for sepsis, infection, and morbidity. CD16bright/CD62Ldim neutrophils were significant predictors of infection ($p = 0.002$). Advanced biomarkers, such as IL-6, IL-10, RNA IL-7R, HMGB1, and leptin offered prognostic insights but required longer processing times. No clear superiority was identified between DCO and EAC, with comparable outcomes when injury severity scores (ISS) were controlled. **Conclusions:** This systematic review highlights the challenge of translating biomarker research into clinical practice, identifying several point-of-care and advanced laboratory biomarkers with significant potential to predict complications like sepsis, infection, and MODS. Future efforts should focus on refining biomarker thresholds, advancing point-of-care technologies, and validating their role in improving surgical timing and trauma care outcomes.

Keywords: orthopaedic trauma; damage control orthopaedics; early appropriate care; biomarkers; surgical timing

1. Introduction

Orthopaedic trauma management in polytrauma patients presents a multifaceted challenge, where timely and precise interventions are paramount for achieving optimal outcomes. The decision-making process surrounding fracture management in these patients is particularly complex, requiring a delicate balance between immediate stabilisation and the acute consequences of surgical intervention [1].

The global burden of orthopaedic and musculoskeletal trauma is profound, affecting millions annually and representing a significant source of morbidity and socioeconomic strain [2]. Trauma-related injuries account for substantial disability-adjusted life years, with road traffic accidents and falls being among the leading causes. Miclau et al. emphasize that while advancements in trauma care systems have improved outcomes in high-income countries, the disparities in low- and middle-income regions remain stark, where limited access to trauma systems, prehospital care, and trained surgeons exacerbates the burden [3]. Even in high-income countries, Hoogervorst et al. highlight the substantial economic toll of musculoskeletal injuries, as both direct healthcare costs and productivity losses significantly impact individuals and national economies [4]. As Stinner and Edwards discuss, there is a substantial need for coordinated and comprehensive trauma systems [5]. Implementing well-designed systems that integrate the most up-to-date research can enhance acute care outcomes while reducing both mortality and long-term disability associated with these injuries. Globally, enhancing trauma care accessibility and standardisation holds the potential to significantly mitigate the impact of musculoskeletal trauma on patients and society.

Trauma resuscitation has been a cornerstone of critical care research for decades, with a primary focus on stabilising patients and mitigating life-threatening physiological derangements [6]. Historically, metrics such as lactate clearance and base deficit have served as reliable indicators of resuscitation efficacy, correlating with outcomes such as organ dysfunction and mortality [7,8]. These foundational studies have established the importance of achieving optimal physiological stability before proceeding with surgical interventions.

The evolution of trauma care has shifted from focusing solely on achieving resuscitation endpoints that are concrete to a more comprehensive and fluid understanding of the physiological response to trauma. Recent advancements in medical science, particularly in understanding the physiologic response to trauma, offer promising avenues to refine the decision-making process in orthopaedic trauma management [9,10]. Biomarkers such as interleukin-6 (IL-6) and neutrophil L-selectin show potential in predicting postoperative complications and guiding optimal timing for surgical interventions. By integrating biomarker data into clinical practice guidelines, clinicians may enhance the precision and safety of surgical timing, thereby potentially reducing risks associated with either premature or delayed procedures [11]. Lord et al. and Weinberg et al. underscore the growing body of evidence supporting the integration of resuscitation metrics within the broader physiological context, highlighting this as a critical area of research in trauma care [12,13]. Their comprehensive systematic reviews emphasise the importance of this shift in guiding informed and adaptive decision making, particularly in determining the optimal timing for surgical interventions. This evolving focus not only underscores the relevance of this research but also lays the foundation for advancing clinical practices, supporting the central themes of this paper.

While acid–base measurements remain the most researched and primary indicators, they are now understood to function within a more fluid and dynamic context that includes systemic inflammation, immune dysregulation, and metabolic derangements. This broader understanding has significant implications for trauma management strategies, particularly in orthopaedics, where decisions about surgical timing and the approach to injury fixation—whether through temporary stabilisation or definitive repair—are critical.

Two primary strategies have emerged: damage control orthopaedics (DCO) and early appropriate care (EAC). DCO involves initial, temporary acute stabilisation without definitive reduction and fixation in order to mitigate systemic inflammatory responses and physiological stress, deferring definitive surgery until the patient's condition stabilises [9,14]. Conversely, EAC aims for prompt anatomical alignment and functional restoration through early comprehensive surgical repair. The controversy between DCO and EAC revolves around their respective benefits and risks, with extensive research exploring which approach yields superior outcomes under varying clinical scenarios. While each method has merits, the choice hinges on patient-specific factors, injury severity, and the patient's overall physiological status. Central to this decision-making process is the concept of physiological optimisation, as the patient's overall stability and response to resuscitation ultimately dictate whether to proceed with DCO for temporary stabilisation or EAC for definitive surgical repair.

The primary objective of this systematic review is to evaluate current practices in orthopaedic trauma management, focusing on the role of biomarkers in optimising surgical timing and outcomes. The secondary objective is to compare the effectiveness of DCO versus EAC in relation to patient physiology, injury severity, and clinical protocols.

2. Methods

This systematic review adhered to the Preferred Reporting Items for Systematic reviews and Meta-Analyses (PRISMA) 2020 guidelines (See supplementary checklist in Supplementary Materials) [15]. The review was registered with PROSPERO (CRD42024528619) before commencement to ensure originality and adherence to systematic review standards.

Our research questions were: (1) Can point-of-care biomarkers help predict perioperative complications in polytrauma patients undergoing orthopaedic surgery? (2) How do advanced immune biomarkers compare in their ability to predict surgical outcomes and guide timing decisions? (3) What is the comparative effectiveness of damage control orthopaedics (DCO) versus early appropriate care (EAC) when accounting for injury severity? These questions aim to clarify the role of biomarkers in clinical decision making and evaluate surgical strategies to improve patient outcomes.

The inclusion criteria for the review were determined by a two-stage screening process, where two reviewers independently screened each record and report retrieved; any discrepancies were resolved by the senior author, ensuring consensus. Inclusion criteria required studies on orthopaedic trauma in adult polytrauma patients, specifically evaluating fracture management or orthopaedic interventions and reporting on timing protocols or biomarkers. Eligible study designs included RCTs, cohort studies, and case–control studies in peer-reviewed English-language journals.

Exclusion criteria included studies on non-traumatic orthopaedic conditions, non-orthopaedic trauma, isolated spinal fractures, proximal femur fractures, or those lacking direct relevance to fracture management. Studies focused solely on imaging were also excluded.

A comprehensive search was conducted using electronic databases, including PubMed, MEDLINE, and Google Scholar. Specific search strategies for each database can be found in Supplemental File S1. For each search, the following search terms were used (Dec 2024): ((orthopedic trauma) OR (orthopedic injuries)) AND ((fracture management) OR (orthopedic surgical procedures) OR (orthopedic interventions)) AND ((optimal timing) OR (biomarkers) OR (Damage Control) OR (Early Appropriate Care)) AND ((clinical outcomes) OR (fracture nonunion) OR (complications)) AND (polytrauma) NOT (spine or imaging). The PRISMA 2020 flow diagram (Figure 1) for the systematic review details the processes used to identify and assess eligible studies. Titles were independently screened by two authors, resulting in 239 articles eligible for abstract screening across the three databases. Abstracts were then reviewed in full against the inclusion and exclusion criteria (see Figure 1 for exclusions in this stage of screening). After this screening process, 56 articles were selected for full-text retrieval. Of the 56 articles sought for retrieval, two were not retrievable, leaving 54 articles to be fully reviewed and assessed for eligibility. At this stage, reports were excluded because they focused on proximal femur fractures (2), lacked sufficient data analysis (8), did not include DCO and EAC grouping (16), or were systematic reviews (4). Additionally, reference lists of eligible articles were analysed, resulting in the inclusion of three additional studies, culminating in a final total of 27 studies for synthesis.

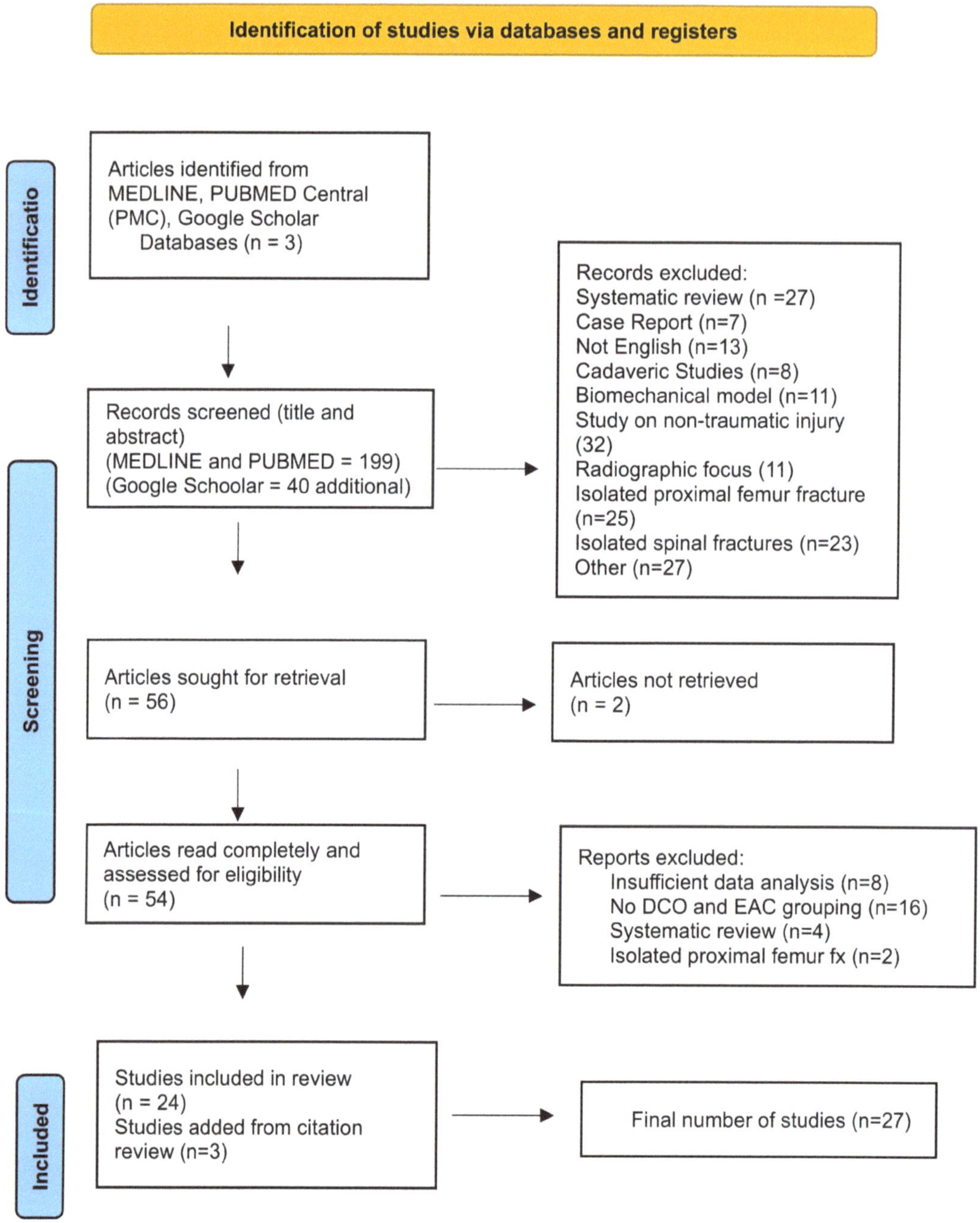

Figure 1. PRISMA flow diagram.

After selecting 27 papers for inclusion, both authors independently assessed the risk of bias for each study using the ROBINS-I tool (Table 1 for non-randomised trials and the

RoB version 2 tool (Table 2) for randomised trials [16,17]. Any discrepancies were resolved through discussion, and no automation tools were used in this process.

Table 1. Appraisal using the Cochrane ROBINS-I Risk of Bias Assessment Tool.

Author	Confouding	Selection of Participants	Deviations from Intended Interventions	Missing Data	Measurement of Outcomes	Selection of the Reported Result	Overall Bias	Notes
Li et al. 2024 [18]	+	+	+	+	+	+	Low-risk	
Vallier et al. 2010 [19]	+	?	+	+	+	+	Mod-risk	Unclear selection criteria.
Vallier et al. 2015 [20]	-	+	+	+	+	+	High-risk	Lack of matching.
Lubken et al. 2023 [21]	-	+	+	+	+	+	High-risk	Lack of matching.
Yamamoto et al. 2019 [22]	+	?	+	+	+	+	Mod-risk	Unclear selection criteria.
Enocson et al. 2023 [23]	-	+	+	+	+	+	High-risk	Lack of matching.
Gaski et al. 2019 [24]	-	-	+	+	+	+	High-risk	Lack of matching due to case-series.
Enninghorst et al. 2010 [25]	+	+	+	+	+	+	Low-risk	
Pape et al. 2001 [26]	+	+	+	+	+	+	Low-risk	
Harvin et al. 2012 [27]	-	-	+	+	+	+	High-risk	Lack of matching.
O'Toole et al. 2009 [28]	-	-	+	+	+	+	High-risk	Lack of matching.
Arnold et al. 2024 [29]	+	+	+	+	+	+	Low-risk	
Yu et al. 2023 [30]	+	?	+	+	+	+	Mod-risk	Unclear intervention criteria.
Glass et al. 2017 [31]	+	+	+	+	+	+	Low-risk	
Andruszkow et al. 2013 [32]	+	?	?	+	+	+	Mod-risk	Unclear selection methodology.
Testa et al. 2019 [33]	+	?	+	+	-	+	High-risk	Unclear intervention criteria. Missing ISS.
Frohlich et al. 2018 [34]	+	+	+	+	+	+	Low-risk	
Haupt et al. 2021 [35]	+	+	+	+	+	+	Low-risk	
Jin et al. 2022 [36]	+	+	+	+	+	+	Low-risk	

Table legend: low-risk (+); uncertain (?); **high-risk (-)**

Table 2. Appraisal of randomised control trials using the Cochrane RoB Version 2 Risk of Bias Assessment Tool.

Author	Randomisation Process	Deviations from Intended Interventions	Missing Outcome Data	Measurement of Outcomes	Selection of the Reported Result	Overall Bias	Notes
Pape et al. 2003 [37]	+	+	+	+	+	Low-risk	
Pape et al. 2007 [38]	+	+	+	+	+	Low-risk	
Rixen et al. 2016 [39]	+	+	+	+	+	Low-risk	

Table legend: low-risk (+)

We systematically extracted data on clinical, functional, intraoperative, postoperative, and additional variables to ensure a comprehensive analysis. Data from each report were collected independently by two reviewers and recorded in Microsoft (One Microsoft Way, Redmond Washington 98052 USA) Excel 365 Version 2024, with any discrepancies resolved through discussion. Clinical outcomes included infection rates, delayed union, and nonunion. Intraoperative data encompassed OR time, blood loss, and transfusion requirements. Postoperative outcomes included ICU and hospital LOS, ventilation hours, and transfusions. Functional recovery was assessed using patient-reported outcomes, while mortality was recorded at in-hospital, 28-day, and long-term intervals. Complications included DVT, sepsis, MOF, ARDS, and cardiac events. Any missing or unclear information was addressed by cross-referencing related sections of the reports or consulting with senior investigators.

Results from individual studies were tabulated to display intervention characteristics and outcomes systematically. The summary table was further divided after data extraction to provide clear comparisons between studies. These sub-groups added to the overall analysis and study heterogeneity.

3. Results

Our systematic review included 27 studies in total, 12 of which focused on biomarkers illustrated in (Table 3). The primary objective of this systematic review was to identify clinically relevant biomarkers that can guide surgical treatment and decision making in trauma patients. The aim was to determine which biomarkers have the greatest potential to inform timing and strategies for surgical interventions in this population.

Table 3. Biomarkers evaluated.

Study	Biomarker	POC vs. Delayed	Time to Results	Analysis	p-Value	Odds Ratio
Briggs [40]	Monocyte L-selectin	POC	~30 min	Sepsis	0.001	1.5
	Neutrophil L-selectin	POC	~30 min	Sepsis	0.005	1.56
Lumsdaine [41]	Neutrophil oxidative burst capacity (fMLP)	POC	~45 min	Post-op infection	0.024	
Pape [42]	IL-6	Delayed	ELISA 4–6 h	Pre vs. post op	<0.05	
	IL-8	Delayed	ELISA 4–6 h	Pre vs. post op	<0.05	
Gaski [24]	IL-10	Delayed	Bioassay 4–6 h	Nosoicomial infection	0.01	
				Degree of organ dysfunction	<0.05	
	IL-6	Delayed	Bioassay 4–6 h	Nosoicomial infection	0.15	
				Degree of organ dysfunction	<0.05	
	IL-1RA	Delayed	Bioassay 4–6 h	Nosoicomial infection	0.13	
				Degree of organ dysfunction	<0.05	

Table 3. *Cont.*

Study	Biomarker	POC vs. Delayed	Time to Results	Analysis	*p*-Value	Odds Ratio
	MCP-1	Delayed	Bioassay 4–6 h	Nosoicomial infection	0.08	
				Degree of organ dysfunction	<0.05	
	IL-8	Delayed	Bioassay 4–6 h	Nosoicomial infection	0.15	
				Degree of organ dysfunction	<0.05	
	HMGB1	Delayed	Bioassay 4–6 h	Nosoicomial infection	0.03	
				Degree of organ dysfunction	<0.05	
	MIG	Delayed	Bioassay 4–6 h	Nosoicomial infection	0.05	
				Degree of organ dysfunction	<0.05	
	IL-23	Delayed	Bioassay 4–6 h	Nosoicomial infection	0.11	
				Degree of organ dysfunction	<0.05	
Hietbrink [43]	IL-6	Delayed	ELISA 4–6 h	Degree of organ dysfunction (ISS)	0.0001	
	Active FC-gammaRII (CD32)	Delayed	ELISA 4–6 h	Degree of organ dysfunction (ISS)	0.120	
	MAC-1	Delayed	ELISA 4–6 h	Degree of organ dysfunction (ISS)	0.092	
Spijkerman [11]	CD16bright/CD62Ldim Neutrophils	POC	~30 min	Infection	0.002	
Frohlich [34]	CD144+	Delayed	Flow cytometry 2–4 h	ISS	<0.001	
	CD42B+	Delayed	Flow cytometry 2–4 h	ISS	<0.001	
Haupt [35]	Leptin	Delayed	ELISA 4–6 h	Multiple organ failure	0.027	
	IL-17A	Delayed	ELISA 4–6 h	Multiple organ failure	<0.05	
Jin [36]	RNA IL-7R	Delayed	PCR 2–4 h	Multiple organ failure	0.001	
Richards [44]	Admission lactate	POC	~30 min	Pulmonary complications	<0.001	
	Preoperative lactate	POC	~30 min	Pulmonary complications	>0.05	
Oladipo [45]	Lactate	POC	~30 min	Post-operative morbidity	0.015	1.305
	Lactate	POC	~30 min	LOS	<0.001	
Nishida [46]	Lactate	POC	~30 min	Post-op complications	0.04	2.64
	Lactate	POC	~30 min	LOS	0.78	

Table legend: Summary of biomarkers evaluated for clinical outcomes, including testing method (POC vs. delayed), result times, analyses, *p*-values, and odds ratios.

Our systematic review identified two broad categories of biomarkers: POC and advanced laboratory studies. The POC biomarkers provide rapid results, typically within 30–45 min, whereas the advanced laboratory studies such as ELISA, PCR, or flow cytometry may take much longer. When looking at the POC tests, Briggs et al. identified monocyte L-selectin as predictive of sepsis ($p = 0.001$, odds ratio [OR] = 1.5), along with neutrophil L-selectin ($p = 0.005$, OR = 1.56) [40]. Spijkerman et al. reported that CD16bright/CD62Ldim neutrophils were predictive of infection ($p = 0.002$) [11]. The most prominent POC biomarker our study identified was lactate, which was evaluated in several studies. Oladipo et al. showed that lactate was associated with post-operative morbidity ($p = 0.015$, OR = 1.305) and length of stay (LOS) ($p < 0.001$) [45]. Nishida et al. demonstrated that lactate was significantly associated with post-operative complications ($p = 0.04$, OR = 2.64), although there was no significant association with LOS ($p = 0.78$) [46].

Advanced laboratory biomarkers required specialised testing methods such as ELISA, PCR, or flow cytometry, with results taking 4–6 h to process. Gaski et al. found that IL-10 ($p = 0.01$), HMGB1 ($p = 0.03$), and MIG ($p = 0.05$) were significantly predictive of nosocomial infections [24]. IL-6, IL-8 IL-1RA, and MCP-1 were all significantly associated with the degree of organ dysfunction ($p = 0.0001$, $p = 0.015$, $p = 0.13$, and $p = 0.08$, respectively) [24]. Haupt et al. reported that leptin ($p = 0.027$) and IL-17A ($p = 0.02$) were associated with MODS [35]. Jin et al. showed that RNA IL-7R was a highly accurate predictor of MODS ($p = 0.001$) [36]. Frohlich et al. demonstrated that CD144+ and CD42B+ were significantly correlated with injury severity scores (both $p < 0.001$) [34].

The secondary objective of this study was to evaluate if DCO or EAC lead to superior outcomes in orthopaedic trauma patients, aiming to determine if the choice of strategy significantly impacts patient outcomes. Among the 15 studies comparing DCO and EAC (Table 4), 3 were randomised controlled trials, 10 were retrospective cohort studies, 5 were cohort studies (4 retrospective and 1 prospective), and 7 were case–control studies. Collectively, these studies provided comprehensive insights into the timing of orthopaedic trauma management, encompassing a total patient population of 35,026. The findings aimed to assess whether different approaches to surgical timing influence key outcomes such as complication rates, recovery trajectories, and overall patient prognosis.

Table 4. DCO vs. EAC main findings with ISS.

Study	Study Design	Sample Size	Pathology	Criteria for DCO vs. EAC	ISS	Main Findings
Li et al. 2024 [18]	CC	120	Lower extremity	Judgement of the on-scene paramedics and doctors of the emergency department.	DCO: 28.1 EAC: 21.3 $p < 0.001$	Damage control surgery is more often selected to treat patients with more severe lower limb injuries, which leads to lower complication rates.
Vallier et al. 2010 [19]	CC	645	Pelivs and acetabular fxs	Surgeon preference, delayed patient presentation to our hospital, operating room availability, severe head injuries, or inadequate resuscitation.	DCO: 24.9 EAC: 26.9 $p = 0.05$	Early fixation of unstable pelvis and acetabular fractures in multiply injured patients reduces morbidity and length of intensive care unit stay, which may decrease treatment costs. Further study to ascertain the effects of associated systemic injuries and the utility of physiologic and laboratory parameters.
Vallier et al. 2015 [20]	PC	355	Femur, pelvis, acetabular, or spine fractures	Surgeon choice 47 Intensivist choice 6 Medically unstable 5 Operating room unavailable 4 Severe head injury 2 Patient choice 2	DCO: 34 EAC: 25.1 $p < 0.001$	Our EAC protocol recommends definitive fixation within 36 h in resuscitated patients. Early fixation was associated with fewer complications and shorter length of stay. The EAC recommendations are safe and effective for the majority of severely injured patients with mechanically unstable femur, pelvis, acetabular, or spine fractures requiring fixation.

Table 4. *Cont.*

Study	Study Design	Sample Size	Pathology	Criteria for DCO vs. EAC	ISS	Main Findings
Lubken et al. 2023 [21]	**CC**	12569	Extremity or pelvic fractures	NR	DCO: 30.5 EAC: 25.9 $p < 0.001$	DCO was considerably more often associated with packed red blood cell (pRBC) transfusions (33.9% vs. 13.4%), catecholamine therapy (14.1% vs. 6.8%), lower extremity injuries (72.4% vs. 53.5%), unstable pelvic fractures (41.0% vs. 25.9%), penetrating injuries (2.8% vs. 1.5%), and shock (20.5% vs. 10.8%) and unconsciousness (23.7% vs. 16.3%) on admission.
Yamamoto et al. 2019 [22]	**CC**	19319	Extremity injury	NR	DCO: 9 EAC: 9 $p < 0.001$	DCO was associated with decreased in-hospital mortality in patients with major fractures.
Enocson et al. 2023 [23]	**CC**	419	Pelvic or acetabular fx	NR	NR	Early (within 72 h) definitive surgery of patients with pelvic or acetabular fractures seems safe with regard to risk for reoperation, other adverse events, and mortality.
Enninghorst et al. 2010 [25]	**CC**	45	Pelvic ring fx	Depending on the fracture pattern and the availability of pelvic specialist surgeon, acute temporary external or acute definitive internal fixation is performed.	DCO: 24 EAC: 30 $p > 0.05$	Acute open reduction internal fixation of unstable pelvic ring fractures within 6 h could be safely performed even in severely shocked patients with multiple injuries. The procedure did not lead to increased rates of transfusion, mortality, intensive care unit length of stay, or overall length of stay.
Pape et al. 2003 [37]	**RCT**	35	Femoral shaft	In the emergency room, all patients were randomly assigned to one treatment arm after all injuries had been categorised and the inclusion criteria were met. Patients were randomised to either femoral nailing or damage control by initial external fixation (DCO) and secondary femoral nailing.	DCO: 23.2 EAC: 21.7 $p > 0.05$	A sustained inflammatory response was measured after primary (<24 h) intramedullary femoral instrumentation, but not after initial external fixation or after secondary conversion to an intramedullary implant.
Pape et al. 2007 [38]	**RCT**	165	Femoral shaft	For all patients who met the inclusion criteria, the sealed envelope that contained the type of treatment was opened after completion of the diagnostics and grading of the patient's status to account for the exclusion criteria.	DCO: 29.0 EAC: 23.3 $p < 0.001$	In stable patients, primary femoral nailing is associated with shorter ventilation time. In borderline patients, it is associated with a higher incidence of lung dysfunctions when compared with those who underwent external fixation and later conversion to intermedullary nail.

Table 4. *Cont.*

Study	Study Design	Sample Size	Pathology	Criteria for DCO vs. EAC	ISS	Main Findings
O'Toole et al. 2009 [28]	**CC**	227	Femoral shaft	The reason why each patient was selected for DCO cannot be accurately determined.	DCO: 41.4 EAC: 36.6 $p < 0.05$	In the context of resuscitation before reamed intramedullary nailing of femoral shaft fractures, our rate of acute respiratory distress syndrome was lower ($p < 0.001$) than that of a similar study reported in the literature.
Arnold et al. 2024 [29]	**RC**	558	Femur shaft fractures	NR	DCO: 25 EAC: 16 $p < 0.001$	Early definitive fixation (≤24 h) is preferred over delayed definitive fixation (>24 h) for patients with bilateral femur shaft fractures. Although mortality does not differ, overall morbidity and deep venous thrombosis rates, as well as length of hospital and intensive care unit stay, are significantly lower.
Yu et al. 2023 [30]	**RC**	181	Long bone fractures	NR	DCO: 23.0 EAC: 21.9 $p > 0.05$	Delaying fixation may not be necessary to prevent the second hit phenomenon and has not demonstrated any clear benefits.
Rixen et al. 2016 [39]	**RCT**	34	Femoral shaft	All multiple-trauma patients who presented to the participating hospitals with femur shaft fractures were screened. If all inclusion criteria were fulfilled, the patient was randomised and documentation began.	DCO: 39.8 EAC: 38.9 $p > 0.05$	No advantage of the damage control concept could be detected in the treatment of femur fractures in multiple-trauma patients.
Andruszkow et al. 2013 [32]	**RC**	207	Femoral shaft	NR	GermanDCO: 34.4 EAC: 25.5 $p < 0.001$ Australian DCO: 41.0 EAC: 34.0 $p < 0.001$	Despite a higher ISS in the DCO group, there were no differences in posttraumatic complications and survival depending on EAC or DCO treatment.
Testa et al. 2019 [33]	**RC**	147	Femoral shaft	NR	NR	Intramedullay nail is the gold standard for definitive treatment of femoral shaft fractures. In patients with severe associated injuries, external fixation should be a good alternative.

Table legend: Overview of studies comparing damage control orthopaedics (DCO) and early appropriate care (EAC) by study design, sample size, pathology, criteria for treatment selection, Injury Severity Score (ISS), and main findings. CC: case–control study. PC: prospective cohort. RC: retrospective cohort. RCT: randomised control trial.

Across the studies reviewed, Injury Severity Scores (ISSs) were consistently higher in patients treated with DCO compared to EAC, even in studies employing matched cohorts or attempting to balance patient groups. For instance, Andruszkow et al. reported ISS values of 34.4 in the DCO group versus 25.5 in the EAC group ($p < 0.001$) in their German cohort and 41.0 versus 34.0 ($p < 0.001$) in their Australian cohort [32]. Similarly, Lubken et al., in a large cohort of over 12,000 patients, observed mean ISS values of 30.5 for DCO versus 25.9

for EAC ($p < 0.001$) [21]. These findings reflect the consistent use of DCO in patients with higher trauma severity, even when attempts were made to control for injury severity.

Interestingly, studies with lower overall ISS values in both groups still demonstrated significant differences between DCO and EAC. For example, Li et al. reported mean ISS values of 28.1 for DCO and 21.3 for EAC ($p < 0.001$) [18]. These results highlight that even in less severely injured populations, there remains a clear delineation in the severity of injuries between patients treated with DCO versus EAC, which may be institution dependent.

Of the studies reviewed, only four reported no significant difference in Injury Severity Scores (ISS) between DCO and EAC groups: two randomised controlled trials (Pape et al., 2003; Rixen et al., 2016), one retrospective cohort study (Yu et al., 2023), and one retrospective comparative study (Enninghorst et al.) [25,30,37,39]. These studies are particularly notable because they eliminate the confounding effect of differing injury severity, making their findings more relevant for guiding decision making in borderline cases where patient stability might allow for either approach.

In these studies, outcomes between DCO and EAC were generally comparable, as demonstrated by Table 5. Pape et al. (2003) found no significant differences in ICU length of stay or ARDS rates [37]. Similarly, Rixen et al. (2016) observed no significant differences in hospital LOS, transfusion requirements, or complications such as ARDS [39]. In the retrospective cohort study by Yu et al. (2023), hospital LOS was comparable between the groups, as were rates of wound complications [30]. Enninghorst et al. reported no significant differences between groups in transfusion rates, incidence of deep vein thrombosis (DVT), ICU length of stay, hospital length of stay, or mortality. These studies provide the most meaningful insights into the relative safety and efficacy of DCO and EAC, suggesting that when ISS is not a differentiating factor, the outcomes of these techniques are closely aligned.

Table 5. Comparison of DCO vs. EAC across cohort studies.

Study	Outcomes	DCO Group	EAC Group	Significance
Li [18]	Infections	2 (5%)	10 (12.5%)	NR
	Delayed union	3 (7.5%)	12 (15%)	NR
	Material failure	2 (5%)	3 (4%)	NR
	Adjusted complication rate	19.50%	30.50%	<0.01
Vallier (2010) [19]	Initial OR time	22	125	$p < 0.005$
	Total OR time	152	125	no sig
	ICU LOS	12	13	no sig
	Hospital LOS	17	21	no sig
	Pna	45	14	0.024
	ARDS	34	8	0.019
	Pulm complication	73	21	0.0024
	Any complication	81	29	0.006
Vallier (2015) [20]	Abdominal injury	31	66	0.0002
	Chest injury	42	167	no sig
	Head injury	43	149	0.08
Lubken [21]	Transfusion	2774	586	<0.001
	Number of surgical procedures	7	4	<0.001
	ICU LOS	8	3	<0.001
	Hospital LOS	26	20	<0.001
	Sepsis	804	245	<0.001
	MOF	2836	876	<0.001
	Inhospital mortality	887	167	<0.001

Table 5. *Cont.*

Study	Outcomes	DCO Group	EAC Group	Significance
Yamamoto [22]	In hospital mortality	40	66	0.011
	Mortality 28 days	35	61	0.008
	Pulm complication	17	20	no sig
	Cardiac complication	15	20	no sig
Enocson [23]	Infections	13	14	NR
	Nonunion	3	5	NR
	Nerve injury	37	26	NR
	DVT	9	7	NR
	Intraoperative bleeding	575	720	<0.01
	Hospital LOS	10	10	no sig
Enninghorst [25]	Transfusion	7	5	no sig
	DVT	2	1	no sig
	ICU LOS	4	3	no sig
	Hospital LOS	37	25	no sig
	Mortality	3	0	no sig
Pape (2003) [37]	ICU LOS	3.3	4.8	no sig
	ARDS	0	0	no sig
Pape (2001) [26]	Blood loss intraop	190	210	no sig
	ICU LOS	13.1	12.6	no sig
	Organ dysfunction	9	33	0.01
	ARDS	1	6	0.06
Pape (2007) [38]	ICU LOS (HRs)	298	197	no sig
	Hours of ventilation	209	127	no sig
	ARDS (%)	10	9	no sig
	Sepsis (%)	12	13	no sig
Harvin [27]	Hospital LOS	10	6	<0.001
	Mortality	6	4	0.01
	DVT	10	8	<0.001
	Hospital charges	97,018	59,561	<0.001
O'Toole [28]	Transfusion %	92.9	58.3	<0.05
	ARDS %	0	1.5	no sig
	Mortality	17.9	2.0	<0.05
Arnold [29]	Morbidity	63	36	0.003
	Hospital LOS	15	10	<0.001
	Post procedure LOS	14	11	0.045
	Mortality	6	5	no sig
Yu [30]	Hospital LOS	14.8	15.3	no sig
	Wound complications	5	10	no sig
Glass [31]	Hospital LOS	32	33	no sig
Andruszkow [32]	Infections requiring revision	15	1	0.002
	German-MODS	11.8%	4.6%	no sig
	German-Mortality	17.6	0	0.05
	German-Hospital LOS	54.5	29.8	<0.001
	German-ICU LOS	27.7	10.7	<0.001
	Australian-MODS	12.5	11.7	no sig
	Australian-Mortality	7.5	4.3	no sig
	Australian-Hospital LOS	24.8	20.5	0.03
	Australian-ICU LOS	12.2	7.6	0.002

Table 5. *Cont.*

Study	Outcomes	DCO Group	EAC Group	Significance
Rixen [39]	Hospital LOS	32.3	30.2	no sig
	Transfusion requirements	4.7	6.6	no sig
	ICU LOS	21.8	12.4	0.037
Testa [33]	Time to weight bearing	21.8	21.2	no sig

Table 5: Comparison of outcomes between damage control orthopaedics (DCO) and early appropriate care (EAC) across cohort studies. Outcomes include complications, mortality, hospital and ICU length of stay, transfusion requirements, and surgical metrics, with significance levels provided where applicable.

When looking at the outcomes of the other studies (Table 5) where severity of injury was not accounted for, length of stay (LOS) and complication rates followed expected patterns, with DCO patients consistently experiencing longer ICU and hospital stays and higher rates of complications. Lubken et al. reported an ICU LOS of 8 days in the DCO group versus 3 days in the EAC group ($p < 0.001$) and hospital stays of 26 days compared to 20 days ($p < 0.001$) [21]. Andruszkow et al. found similarly extended ICU LOS for DCO patients, with 27.7 days versus 10.7 days ($p < 0.001$) in their German cohort and 12.2 days versus 7.6 days ($p = 0.002$) in their Australian cohort [32]. Vallier et al. (2010) observed a hospital LOS of 17 days in the DCO group compared to 21 days in the EAC group, though this difference was not statistically significant [19]. Complication rates were also notably higher in DCO groups. Vallier et al. (2010) reported significantly higher pulmonary complications in the DCO group (73 vs. 21, $p = 0.0024$), along with higher infection rates (45 vs. 14, $p = 0.024$) and ARDS rates (34 vs. 8, $p = 0.019$) [19]. Lubken et al. observed higher rates of sepsis (804 vs. 245, $p < 0.001$) and multi-organ failure (2836 vs. 876, $p < 0.001$) in the DCO group [21]. Andruszkow et al. also reported higher rates of infections requiring revision in the DCO group (15 vs. 1, $p = 0.002$) [32]. O'Toole et al. found that transfusion rates were higher in DCO patients (92.9% vs. 58.3%, $p < 0.05$), as were mortality rates (17.9% vs. 2.0%, $p < 0.05$) [28].

The risk of bias assessment, as summarised in Table 1, reveals a spectrum of methodological rigor among the included studies, which may affect the quality and reliability of the synthesised evidence. While several studies demonstrated consistently low risk across all assessed domains, others exhibited significant vulnerabilities, particularly related to the lack of matching and robust selection criteria. These weaknesses raise concerns about potential confounding and selection bias, which could undermine the validity of their findings. Additionally, some studies had uncertain risk due to issues with participant selection, further complicating the interpretation of results

4. Discussion

Our findings build upon the foundational concepts of inflammation outlined by Gabay and Kushner, applying these principles to surgical practice, with a particular focus on fracture management in polytrauma patients [47]. Research on trauma physiology has grown significantly, aiming to enhance our understanding and improve guidance for all trauma surgery including fracture care [48]. Nauth et al. highlighted the interplay of immune dysregulation and inflammatory markers in polytrauma [9]. Our study found promising results for the potential use of biomarkers in guiding clinical decision-making frameworks. At the same time, it identifies a significant gap between basic science research and its clinical application, emphasising the need for further exploration to bridge this divide.

Notably, our systematic review is the first to address the challenge of translating academic biomarker research into practical clinical applications. It explores a broader range of biomarkers, including several that remain in the research phase but demonstrate advanced prognostic potential. Evaluating the potential of these emerging biomarkers is crucial to determine whether they warrant scaling for clinical application rather than remaining confined to academic research.

This systematic review identified multiple POC biomarkers with potential for clinical utility in trauma care, focusing on their role in predicting complications such as infection, multiple organ dysfunction syndrome (MODS), and post-operative morbidity. Lactate was particularly well-studied and emerged as a reliable predictor of morbidity and length of stay, with established thresholds enabling clinical application [44–46,49]. In addition to POC lactate, several studies demonstrated the ability to use POC tests on immune cells to predict sepsis and infection [11,40,41]. Specifically, monocyte L-selectin, neutrophil L-selectin, neutrophil oxidative burst capacity, and CD16 neutrophils showed significant predictive value in identifying patients at increased risk of these complications [11,40,41].

Our systematic review found many advanced laboratory biomarkers to have significant predictive value for infections, end organ dysfunction, and MODS [24,26,35,36,43,50]. Three studies found IL-6 to significantly predict infection [24,26,43]. Other immunoglobulins found to have significant predictive value were IL-8, IL-7R, IL-17, IL-1RA, IL-10, and IL-23 [24,26,35,36,43]. Besides immunoglobulins, Hmgb1 and leptin were also found to have significant predictive value [24,35]. These biomarkers rely on specialised techniques, such as ELISA and PCR, and they require skilled lab personnel and longer processing times, but they provide detailed insights into the inflammatory and immune responses in trauma patients. Unlike standard markers like lactate, these advanced biomarkers capture the complexity of systemic inflammation, offering significant added value. Their potential to enhance trauma care underscores the importance of further research aimed at improving accessibility and integrating them into clinical practice.

Despite advancements in biomarker research, the integration of these tools into surgical timing decisions remains underdeveloped. Surgical timing in polytrauma patients is a complex interplay of physiological stability and operative risk. Holcomb et al. emphasised the importance of timely intervention in trauma care, noting that delayed surgery in the presence of elevated inflammatory markers may predispose patients to complications like MODS or prolonged ICU stays [51]. Lactate is currently the only biomarker with established thresholds that could potentially guide timing, as supported by studies in Vincent et al.'s systematic review [49]. However, its predictive value in relation to optimal surgical windows has not been fully elucidated.

Timing decisions in trauma surgery are very complex and account for multiple organ systems, including cardiovascular, pulmonary, and renal stability. Although it would be ideal to have a definitive biomarker that provides a clear-cut indication for when to proceed with surgery, such a solution does not yet exist. Entire textbooks such as that by Bassett and Smith highlight the delicate balance required in managing anaesthesia and the decision to determine whether a patient is medically optimised [52]. They specifically address how to properly evaluate a polytrauma patient's fluid requirements, highlighting the critical role of maintaining hemodynamic stability in surgical planning. Similarly, Chong et al.'s meta-analysis further emphasises the importance of optimising patient haemodynamics prior to surgery [53]. They discuss how goal-directed fluid therapy has improved perioperative outcomes and suggest that lactate kinetics serve as a surrogate for evaluating the physiological readiness for surgery.

In addition to fluid management, the hematologic and cardiovascular systems must also be carefully evaluated, particularly in addressing traumatic coagulopathies, which are a frequent and life-threatening complication in polytrauma patients. As described by Brohi et al., these coagulopathies result from a complex interplay of trauma-induced shock, inflammation, and impaired clotting mechanisms [54]. Their work emphasises the importance of timely administration of blood products and targeted resuscitation protocols to minimise surgical risks. Tobin et al. further stress the role of timely and proper blood product administration in polytrauma patients [55].

Ultimately, a multivariate approach that integrates biomarkers, clinical scoring systems, and real-time physiological monitoring offers the greatest potential for improving trauma care. This approach aligns with the broader framework of comprehensive trauma management outlined in Schwartz's Principles of Surgery, emphasising the importance of integrating diverse data sources to guide surgical decision making [56]. Our systematic review identified 10 immune system biomarkers, including three POC and seven delayed markers, that predict important perioperative outcomes and provide valuable insights into the inflammatory cascade associated with trauma. These biomarkers hold significant promise for enhancing the understanding of systemic responses and optimising preoperative decision making. Research should focus on prospective trials that evaluate the predictive power of these markers in relation to specific surgical interventions, with an emphasis on reducing complications and optimising recovery. Furthermore, leveraging technological advancements, such as point-of-care testing and artificial intelligence, could accelerate the transition of biomarker research from bench to bedside.

The secondary objective of this review was to compare DCO and EAC and their impact on patient outcomes. Predictably, DCO was consistently associated with higher Injury Severity Scores (ISSs), longer ICU and hospital stays; and increased complication rates such as sepsis, MODS, and ARDS. This aligns with its established role in managing severely injured, unstable patients. Importantly, studies that controlled for ISS, such as Pape et al. (2003), Rixen et al. (2016), and Yu et al. (2023), reported comparable outcomes between DCO and EAC, including ICU length of stay, transfusion requirements, and complication rates. These findings highlight the subjective decision of when to pursue DCO. Ultimately, the decision is often surgeon preference and institution based.

Given this subjectivity and the variability in outcomes, national organisation guidelines and institution specific protocols play a pivotal role in standardising decision making, ensuring that both patient needs and local resources are appropriately accounted for. For example, the 2015 guidelines released by the American College of Surgeons (ACS) and Orthopaedic Trauma Association (OTA) outline specific indications for DCO, such as severe traumatic brain injury and inadequate resuscitation [57]. These guidelines also highlight the appropriateness of DCO in resource-limited settings. While they provide clear recommendations in certain scenarios, much is left open to interpretation by individual institutions. The guidelines emphasise that, although patient physiology and injury severity are key determinants, institutional factors play a critical role in shaping how these protocols are implemented.

Institutions must tailor their protocols to align with their specific resources and capabilities. This involves considering the expertise and comfort level of orthopaedic surgeons in handling complex trauma, the hospital's capacity for advanced resuscitation measures, the proficiency of anaesthesia teams in managing critically ill patients, and the availability of necessary multidisciplinary teams. For example, a Level I trauma centre with robust resources may adopt protocols emphasising aggressive resuscitation and early definitive fixation, while a smaller facility with limited resources might prioritise stabilisation and timely transfer.

Additionally, variability in patient populations served by institutions can dictate protocol design. Centres treating predominantly older populations with significant comorbidities may need to integrate additional considerations, such as optimising perioperative management and incorporating geriatric expertise into decision-making algorithms. By acknowledging these nuances, institutions can develop biomarker-guided and algorithmic protocols that provide consistency while allowing for flexibility in addressing unique clinical scenarios.

These protocols not only guide clinical decision making but also serve as a foundation for informed consent discussions, helping surgeons effectively communicate the rationale behind choosing DCO or EAC and the potential risks and benefits associated with each approach. Informed consent is a vital consideration when determining whether to pursue DCO or EAC, as both strategies carry significant risks and benefits that can impact a patient's quality of life [58]. However, trauma patients often lack the capacity to participate in these discussions due to the urgency of their condition, leaving surgeons to rely on surrogate decision-makers or act in the patient's best interest based on clinical judgment and established protocols.

These situations highlight the surgeon's responsibility to balance the ethical principles of autonomy and beneficence. While patients may later express frustration over prolonged hospitalisations, additional surgeries, or delayed recovery due to the staged nature of DCO, these measures are often necessary to manage life-threatening conditions and optimise long-term functionality. To minimise potential misunderstandings and enhance trust, preoperative discussions—when possible—should address the potential implications of both DCO and EAC, including the anticipated length of hospitalisation, surgical risks, and how these strategies align with the patient's values and goals. Surgeons should be prepared to guide these discussions by integrating their expertise; the latest evidence-based research; and an understanding of the patient's medical, surgical, and social circumstances.

In the end, surgeons must weigh numerous variables—including physiological stability, injury severity, institutional resources, and patient-specific factors—when choosing between DCO and EAC. These decisions must be informed by a thorough understanding of the current literature to ensure that the chosen strategy is the safest and most beneficial for the patient. Although input from patients or their families is invaluable, they often depend heavily on the surgeon's expertise and guidance. This underscores the importance of fostering a strong physician–patient relationship and ensuring that ethical considerations, such as informed consent, remain integral to trauma care protocols. By addressing these complexities, surgeons can not only optimise outcomes but also maintain the trust and confidence of their patients and their families.

Limitations

This review has several limitations. Variability in biomarker protocols and thresholds across studies—shaped by patient factors, laboratory differences, and timing—hinders direct comparisons. Many included studies are retrospective, introducing potential bias from confounders such as Injury Severity Score and pre-existing conditions. Heterogeneity in patient selection, institutional protocols, and clinical decision making further complicates comparisons between DCO and EAC. Additionally, differences in trauma care resources across institutions limit generalisability. Future research should prioritise standardised methodologies and multicentre collaborations to enhance consistency and external validity.

5. Conclusions

This systematic review is among the first to tackle the challenge of translating academic biomarker research into practical clinical applications. It highlights a broader range of biomarkers, including several that remain in the research phase but demonstrate promising prognostic potential. Evaluating the scalability of these emerging biomarkers is critical to determining their feasibility for clinical use beyond academic research.

Several point-of-care (POC) biomarkers, including lactate, monocyte L-selectin, neutrophil L-selectin, neutrophil oxidative burst capacity, and CD16bright/CD62Ldim neutrophils, show significant utility in predicting complications such as sepsis, infection, and multiple organ dysfunction syndrome (MODS). Among these, lactate stands out for its established thresholds, enabling actionable clinical decision making for morbidity and length of stay. Advanced laboratory biomarkers, such as IL-6, IL-10, IL-7R, HMGB1, and leptin, provide deeper insights into systemic inflammation and immune dysregulation, although their reliance on specialised techniques limits their immediate applicability in acute settings. These advanced biomarkers underscore the importance of further research to enhance accessibility and integrate their use into trauma care protocols.

Despite these advancements, the integration of biomarkers into surgical timing decisions remains underdeveloped. The complexity of determining optimal surgical timing in polytrauma patients—a dynamic interplay of physiological stability and operative risks—highlights the need for refined thresholds and prospective validation of biomarkers. While lactate remains the only biomarker with established thresholds that could potentially guide surgical timing, its role in identifying optimal surgical windows requires further exploration.

Future research should focus on bridging the gap between biomarker discovery and clinical implementation. This includes refining and validating biomarker thresholds, advancing point-of-care testing technologies, and conducting prospective trials to assess their role in improving surgical outcomes. Such efforts will be instrumental in leveraging biomarkers to optimise trauma care, reduce complications, and enhance recovery for polytrauma patients.

Supplementary Materials: The following supporting information can be downloaded at: https://www.mdpi.com/article/10.3390/jcm14041329/s1, File S1 and PROSPERO checklist.

Funding: This research received no external funding. APC was funded by Liberty University.

Conflicts of Interest: The authors declare no conflict of interest.

References

1. Pape, H.-C.; Halvachizadeh, S.; Leenen, L.; Velmahos, G.D.; Buckley, R.; Giannoudis, P.V. Timing of Major Fracture Care in Polytrauma Patients—An Update on Principles, Parameters and Strategies for 2020. *Injury* **2019**, *50*, 1656–1670. [CrossRef]
2. Mock, C.; Joshipura, M.; Arreola-Risa, C.; Quansah, R. An Estimate of the Number of Lives That Could Be Saved through Improvements in Trauma Care Globally. *World J. Surg.* **2012**, *36*, 959–963. [CrossRef] [PubMed]
3. Miclau, T.; Hoogervorst, P.; Shearer, D.W.; El Naga, A.N.; Working, Z.M.; Martin, C.; Pesántez, R.; Hüttl, T.; Kojima, K.E.; Schütz, M.; et al. Current Status of Musculoskeletal Trauma Care Systems Worldwide. *J. Orthop. Trauma* **2018**, *32*, S64–S70. [CrossRef]
4. Hoogervorst, P.; Shearer, D.W.; Miclau, T. The Burden of High-Energy Musculoskeletal Trauma in High-Income Countries. *World J. Surg.* **2020**, *44*, 1033–1038. [CrossRef] [PubMed]
5. Stinner, D.J.; Edwards, D. Surgical Management of Musculoskeletal Trauma. *Surg. Clin. N. Am.* **2017**, *97*, 1119–1131. [CrossRef] [PubMed]
6. Turen, C.H.; Dube, M.A.; LeCroy, M.C. Approach to the Polytraumatized Patient With Musculoskeletal Injuries. *J. Am. Acad. Orthop. Surg.* **1999**, *7*, 154–165. [CrossRef] [PubMed]
7. Manikis, P.; Jankowski, S.; Zhang, H.; Kahn, R.J.; Vincent, J.-L. Correlation of Serial Blood Lactate Levels to Organ Failure and Mortality After Trauma. *Am. J. Emerg. Med.* **1995**, *13*, 619–622. [CrossRef]
8. Elliott, D.C. An Evaluation of the End Points of Resuscitation. *J. Am. Coll. Surg.* **1998**, *187*, 536–547. [CrossRef] [PubMed]
9. Nauth, A.; Hildebrand, F.; Vallier, H.; Moore, T.; Leenen, L.; Mckinley, T.; Pape, H.-C. Polytrauma: Update on Basic Science and Clinical Evidence. *OTA Int. Open Access J. Orthop. Trauma* **2021**, *4*, e116. [CrossRef]
10. Wise, P.M.; Saiz, A.M.; Haller, J.; Wenke, J.C.; Schaer, T.; Schneider, P.; Morshed, S.; Bahney, C.S. Preclinical Models of Orthopaedic Trauma: Orthopaedic Research Society (ORS) and Orthopaedic Trauma Association (OTA) Symposium 2022. *OTA Int.* **2024**, *7*, e303. [CrossRef]

11. Spijkerman, R.; Hesselink, L.; Bongers, S.; Van Wessem, K.J.P.; Vrisekoop, N.; Hietbrink, F.; Koenderman, L.; Leenen, L.P.H. Point-of-Care Analysis of Neutrophil Phenotypes: A First Step Toward Immuno-Based Precision Medicine in the Trauma ICU. *Crit. Care Explor.* **2020**, *2*, e0158. [CrossRef] [PubMed]
12. Lord, J.M.; Midwinter, M.J.; Chen, Y.-F.; Belli, A.; Brohi, K.; Kovacs, E.J.; Koenderman, L.; Kubes, P.; Lilford, R.J. The Systemic Immune Response to Trauma: An Overview of Pathophysiology and Treatment. *Lancet* **2014**, *384*, 1455–1465. [CrossRef] [PubMed]
13. Weinberg, D.S.; Narayanan, A.S.; Moore, T.A.; Vallier, H.A. Assessment of Resuscitation as Measured by Markers of Metabolic Acidosis and Features of Injury. *Bone Jt. J.* **2017**, *99-B*, 122–127. [CrossRef]
14. Sears, B.W.; Stover, M.D.; Callaci, J. Pathoanatomy and Clinical Correlates of the Immunoinflammatory Response Following Orthopaedic Trauma. *J. Am. Acad. Orthop. Surg.* **2009**, *17*, 255–265. [CrossRef]
15. Page, M.J.; McKenzie, J.E.; Bossuyt, P.M.; Boutron, I.; Hoffmann, T.C.; Mulrow, C.D.; Shamseer, L.; Tetzlaff, J.M.; Akl, E.A. Brennan, S.E.; et al. The PRISMA 2020 Statement: An Updated Guideline for Reporting Systematic Reviews. *BMJ* **2021**, *372*, n71 [CrossRef] [PubMed]
16. Sterne, J.A.; Hernán, M.A.; Reeves, B.C.; Savović, J.; Berkman, N.D.; Viswanathan, M.; Henry, D.; Altman, D.G.; Ansari, M.T. Boutron, I.; et al. ROBINS-I: A Tool for Assessing Risk of Bias in Non-Randomised Studies of Interventions. *BMJ* **2016**, *355*, i4919 [CrossRef] [PubMed]
17. Sterne, J.A.C.; Savović, J.; Page, M.J.; Elbers, R.G.; Blencowe, N.S.; Boutron, I.; Cates, C.J.; Cheng, H.-Y.; Corbett, M.S.; Eldridge S.M.; et al. RoB 2: A Revised Tool for Assessing Risk of Bias in Randomised Trials. *BMJ* **2019**, *366*, l4898. [CrossRef]
18. Li, F.; Gao, L.; Zuo, J.; Wei, J. Efficacy of Damage Control Orthopedics Strategy in the Management of Lower Limb Trauma. *Surg. Open Sci.* **2024**, *19*, 101–104. [CrossRef]
19. Vallier, H.A.; Cureton, B.A.; Ekstein, C.; Oldenburg, F.P.; Wilber, J.H. Early Definitive Stabilization of Unstable Pelvis and Acetabulum Fractures Reduces Morbidity. *J. Trauma Inj. Infect. Crit. Care* **2010**, *69*, 677–684. [CrossRef]
20. Vallier, H.A.; Moore, T.A.; Como, J.J.; Wilczewski, P.A.; Steinmetz, M.P.; Wagner, K.G.; Smith, C.E.; Wang, X.-F.; Dolenc, A.J. Complications Are Reduced with a Protocol to Standardize Timing of Fixation Based on Response to Resuscitation. *J. Orthop. Surg. Res.* **2015**, *10*, 155. [CrossRef]
21. Von Lübken, F.; Prause, S.; Lang, P.; Friemert, B.D.; Lefering, R.; Achatz, G. Early Total Care or Damage Control Orthopaedics for Major Fractures? Results of Propensity Score Matching for Early Definitive versus Early Temporary Fixation Based on Data from the Trauma Registry of the German Trauma Society (TraumaRegister DGU®). *Eur. J. Trauma Emerg. Surg.* **2023**, *49*, 1933–1946. [CrossRef]
22. Yamamoto, R.; Udagawa, K.; Nishida, Y.; Ono, S.; Sasaki, J. Damage Control Orthopedics and Decreased In-Hospital Mortality: A Nationwide Study. *Injury* **2019**, *50*, 2240–2246. [CrossRef] [PubMed]
23. Enocson, A.; Lundin, N. Early versus Late Surgical Treatment of Pelvic and Acetabular Fractures a Five-Year Follow-up of 419 Patients. *BMC Musculoskelet. Disord.* **2023**, *24*, 848. [CrossRef] [PubMed]
24. Gaski, G.E.; Metzger, C.; McCarroll, T.; Wessel, R.; Adler, J.; Cutshall, A.; Brown, K.; Vodovotz, Y.; Billiar, T.R.; McKinley, T.O. Early Immunologic Response in Multiply Injured Patients With Orthopaedic Injuries Is Associated With Organ Dysfunction. *J. Orthop. Trauma* **2019**, *33*, 220–228. [CrossRef]
25. Enninghorst, N.; Toth, L.; King, K.L.; McDougall, D.; Mackenzie, S.; Balogh, Z.J. Acute Definitive Internal Fixation of Pelvic Ring Fractures in Polytrauma Patients: A Feasible Option. *J. Trauma Inj. Infect. Crit. Care* **2010**, *68*, 935–941. [CrossRef] [PubMed]
26. Pape, H.-C.; Van Griensven, M.; Rice, J.; G??nsslen, A.; Hildebrand, F.; Zech, S.; Winny, M.; Lichtinghagen, R.; Krettek, C. Major Secondary Surgery in Blunt Trauma Patients and Perioperative Cytokine Liberation: Determination of the Clinical Relevance of Biochemical Markers. *J. Trauma Inj. Infect. Crit. Care* **2001**, *50*, 989–1000. [CrossRef]
27. Harvin, J.A.; Harvin, W.H.; Camp, E.; Caga-Anan, Z.; Burgess, A.R.; Wade, C.E.; Holcomb, J.B.; Cotton, B.A. Early Femur Fracture Fixation Is Associated with a Reduction in Pulmonary Complications and Hospital Charges: A Decade of Experience with 1,376 Diaphyseal Femur Fractures. *J. Trauma Acute Care Surg.* **2012**, *73*, 1442–1449. [CrossRef] [PubMed]
28. O'Toole, R.V.; O'Brien, M.; Scalea, T.M.; Habashi, N.; Pollak, A.N.; Turen, C.H. Resuscitation Before Stabilization of Femoral Fractures Limits Acute Respiratory Distress Syndrome in Patients With Multiple Traumatic Injuries Despite Low Use of Damage Control Orthopedics. *J. Trauma Inj. Infect. Crit. Care* **2009**, *67*, 1013–1021. [CrossRef]
29. Arnold, S.C.; Lagazzi, E.; Wagner, R.K.; Rafaqat, W.; Abiad, M.; Argandykov, D.; Hoekman, A.H.; Panossian, V.; Nzenwa, I.C.; Cote, M.; et al. Two Big Bones, One Big Decision: When to Fix Bilateral Femur Fractures. *Injury* **2024**, *55*, 111610. [CrossRef]
30. Yu, T.-P.; Chen, Y.-T.; Ko, P.-Y.; Wu, C.-H.; Yang, T.-H.; Hung, K.-S.; Wu, P.-T.; Wang, C.-J.; Yen, Y.-T.; Shan, Y.-S. Is Delayed Fixation Worthwhile in Patients with Long Bone Fracture Concomitant with Mild Traumatic Brain Injury? A Propensity Score–Matched Study. *Injury* **2023**, *54*, 110804. [CrossRef]
31. Glass, N.E.; Burlew, C.C.; Hahnhaussen, J.; Weckbach, S.; Pieracci, F.M.; Moore, E.E.; Stahel, P.F. Early Definitive Fracture Fixation Is Safely Performed in the Presence of an Open Abdomen in Multiply Injured Patients. *J. Orthop. Trauma* **2017**, *31*, 624–630. [CrossRef]

32. Andruszkow, H.; Dowrick, A.S.; Frink, M.; Zeckey, C.; Krettek, C.; Hildebrand, F.; Edwards, E.R.; Mommsen, P. Surgical Strategies in Polytraumatized Patients with Femoral Shaft Fractures—Comparing a German and an Australian Level I Trauma Centre. *Injury* **2013**, *44*, 1068–1072. [CrossRef] [PubMed]
33. Testa, G.; Vescio, A.; Aloj, D.C.; Papotto, G.; Ferrarotto, L.; Massé, A.; Sessa, G.; Pavone, V. Definitive Treatment of Femoral Shaft Fractures: Comparison between Anterograde Intramedullary Nailing and Monoaxial External Fixation. *JCM* **2019**, *8*, 1119. [CrossRef] [PubMed]
34. Fröhlich, M.; Schäfer, N.; Caspers, M.; Böhm, J.K.; Stürmer, E.K.; Bouillon, B.; Maegele, M. Temporal Phenotyping of Circulating Microparticles after Trauma: A Prospective Cohort Study. *Scand. J. Trauma Resusc. Emerg. Med.* **2018**, *26*, 33. [CrossRef] [PubMed]
35. Haupt, J.; Krysiak, N.; Unger, M.; Bogner-Flatz, V.; Biberthaler, P.; Hanschen, M.; Van Griensven, M.; Haug, A.T. The Potential of Adipokines in Identifying Multiple Trauma Patients at Risk of Developing Multiple Organ Dysfunction Syndrome. *Eur. J. Med. Res.* **2021**, *26*, 38. [CrossRef] [PubMed]
36. Jin, J.; Qian, H.; Wu, G.; Bao, N.; Song, Y. Neutrophil-Derived Long Noncoding RNA IL-7R Predicts Development of Multiple Organ Dysfunction Syndrome in Patients with Trauma. *Eur. J. Trauma Emerg. Surg.* **2022**, *48*, 1545–1553. [CrossRef]
37. Pape, H.-C.; Grimme, K.; Van Griensven, M.; Sott, A.H.; Giannoudis, P.; Morley, J.; Roise, O.; Ellingsen, E.; Hildebrand, F.; Wiese, B.; et al. Impact of Intramedullary Instrumentation versus Damage Control for Femoral Fractures on Immunoinflammatory Parameters: Prospective Randomized Analysis by the EPOFF Study Group. *J. Trauma Inj. Infect. Crit. Care* **2003**, *55*, 7–13. [CrossRef]
38. Pape, H.-C.; Rixen, D.; Morley, J.; Husebye, E.E.; Mueller, M.; Dumont, C.; Gruner, A.; Oestern, H.J.; Bayeff-Filoff, M.; Garving, C.; et al. Impact of the Method of Initial Stabilization for Femoral Shaft Fractures in Patients With Multiple Injuries at Risk for Complications (Borderline Patients). *Ann. Surg.* **2007**, *246*, 491–501. [CrossRef]
39. Rixen, D.; Steinhausen, E.; Sauerland, S.; Lefering, R.; Maegele, M.G.; Bouillon, B.; Grass, G.; Neugebauer, E.A.M.; Damage Control Study Group. Randomized, Controlled, Two-Arm, Interventional, Multicenter Study on Risk-Adapted Damage Control Orthopedic Surgery of Femur Shaft Fractures in Multiple-Trauma Patients. *Trials* **2016**, *17*, 47. [CrossRef]
40. Briggs, G.D.; Lemmert, K.; Lott, N.J.; De Malmanche, T.; Balogh, Z.J. Biomarkers to Guide the Timing of Surgery: Neutrophil and Monocyte L-Selectin Predict Postoperative Sepsis in Orthopaedic Trauma Patients. *JCM* **2021**, *10*, 2207. [CrossRef] [PubMed]
41. Lumsdaine, W.; Easton, R.M.; Lott, N.J.; White, A.; Malmanche, T.L.D.; Lemmert, K.; Weber, D.G.; Balogh, Z.J. Neutrophil Oxidative Burst Capacity for Peri-Operative Immune Monitoring in Trauma Patients. *Injury* **2014**, *45*, 1144–1148. [CrossRef]
42. Pape, H.-C.; Griensven, M.V.; Hildebrand, F.F.; Tzioupis, C.T.; Sommer, K.L.; Krettek, C.C.; Giannoudis, P.V. Systemic Inflammatory Response After Extremity or Truncal Fracture Operations. *J. Trauma Inj. Infect. Crit. Care* **2008**, *65*, 1379–1384. [CrossRef] [PubMed]
43. Hietbrink, F.; Koenderman, L.; Althuizen, M.; Leenen, L.P.H. Modulation of the Innate Immune Response after Trauma Visualised by a Change in Functional PMN Phenotype. *Injury* **2009**, *40*, 851–855. [CrossRef] [PubMed]
44. Richards, J.E.; Matuszewski, P.E.; Grif, S.M.; Guillamondegui, O.D.; Obremskey, W.T.; Evans, J.M. The Role of Elevated Lactate as a Risk Factor for Pulmonary Morbidity After Early Fixation of Femoral Shaft Fractures. *J. Orthop. Trauma* **2016**, *30*, 312–318.
45. Oladipo, V.; Portney, D.; Haber, J.; Baker, H.; Strelzow, J. Lactic Acid Levels Are Associated with Morbidity, Length of Stay, and Total Treatment Costs in Urban Trauma Patients with Lower Extremity Long Bone Fractures. *Eur. J. Orthop. Surg. Traumatol.* **2024**, *34*, 1963–1970. [CrossRef]
46. Nishida, Y.; Yamamoto, R.; Ono, S.; Sasaki, J. Association between Preoperative Lactate Level and Early Complications after Surgery for Isolated Extremity Fracture. *BMC Musculoskelet. Disord.* **2024**, *25*, 314. [CrossRef] [PubMed]
47. Gabay, C.; Kushner, I. Acute-Phase Proteins and Other Systemic. *New Engl. J. Med.* **1999**, *340*, 448–454. [CrossRef]
48. Madry, H.; Grässel, S.; Nöth, U.; Relja, B.; Bernstein, A.; Docheva, D.; Kauther, M.D.; Katthagen, J.C.; Bader, R.; Van Griensven, M.; et al. The Future of Basic Science in Orthopaedics and Traumatology: Cassandra or Prometheus? *Eur. J. Med. Res.* **2021**, *26*, 56. [CrossRef] [PubMed]
49. Vincent, J.-L.; Quintairos, E.; Silva, A.; Couto, L.; Taccone, F.S. The Value of Blood Lactate Kinetics in Critically Ill Patients: A Systematic Review. *Crit Care* **2016**, *20*, 257. [CrossRef]
50. Frohlich, V.; Johandl, S.; De Zwart, P.; Stockle, U.; Ochs, B. Navigated TKA after Osteotomy versus Primary Navigated TKA: A Matched-Pair Analysis. *Orthopedics* **2016**, *39*, S77–S82. [CrossRef]
51. Holcomb, J.B.; Tilley, B.C.; Baraniuk, S.; Fox, E.E.; Wade, C.E.; Podbielski, J.M.; Del Junco, D.J.; Brasel, K.J.; Bulger, E.M.; Callcut, R.A.; et al. Transfusion of Plasma, Platelets, and Red Blood Cells in a 1:1:1 vs a 1:1:2 Ratio and Mortality in Patients With Severe Trauma: The PROPPR Randomized Clinical Trial. *JAMA* **2015**, *313*, 471. [CrossRef] [PubMed]
52. Bassett, M.D.; Smith, C.E. General Anesthesia for Trauma. In *Essentials of Trauma Anesthesia*; Varon, A.J., Smith, C., Eds.; Cambridge University Press: Cambridge, UK, 2012; pp. 76–94, ISBN 978-1-139-06133-9.
53. Chong, M.A.; Wang, Y.; Berbenetz, N.M.; McConachie, I. Does Goal-Directed Haemodynamic and Fluid Therapy Improve Peri-Operative Outcomes?: A Systematic Review and Meta-Analysis. *Eur. J. Anaesthesiol.* **2018**, *35*, 469–483. [CrossRef]

54. Brohi, K.; Singh, J.; Heron, M.; Coats, T. Acute Traumatic Coagulopathy. *J. Trauma Inj. Infect. Crit. Care* **2003**, *54*, 1127–1130. [CrossRef] [PubMed]
55. Tobin, J.M.; Barras, W.P.; Bree, S.; Williams, N.; McFarland, C.; Park, C.; Steinhiser, D.; Stone, R.C.; Stockinger, Z. Anesthesia for Trauma Patients. *Mil. Med.* **2018**, *183*, 32–35. [CrossRef]
56. Nizamuddin, J.; O'Connor, M. Chapter 46: Anesthesia for Surgical Patients. In *Schwartz's Principles of Surgery*; McGraw Hill Medical: New York, NY, USA, 2019.
57. Davis, M.L.; Rocca, G.J.D.; Brenner, M.; Cribari, C.; Cryer, H.G.; Ficke, J.R.; Hartsock, L.; Henley, M.B.; Henry, P.D.G.; Jenkins, D.H., et al. ACS Tqip Best Practices in the Management of Orthopaedic Trauma. Presented at the ACS Trauma Quality Improvement Program. 2015. Available online: https://www.google.com/url?sa=t&source=web&rct=j&opi=89978449&url=https://www.facs.org/media/mkbnhqtw/ortho_guidelines.pdf&ved=2ahUKEwjp0NXBkb-LAxWUFFkFHUbkImsQFnoECAgQAQ&usg=AOvVaw2wg6Vb-SqWCjcM2PBIKz83 (accessed on 1 February 2025).
58. Bolcato, V.; Franzetti, C.; Fassina, G.; Basile, G.; Martinez, R.M.; Tronconi, L.P. Comparative Study on Informed Consent Regulation in Health Care among Italy, France, United Kingdom, Nordic Countries, Germany, and Spain. *J. Forensic Leg. Med.* **2024**, *103*, 102674. [CrossRef]

Journal of
Clinical Medicine

MDPI

Article

Atypical Femur Fractures—An Analysis of 69 Patients from 15 Years

Cheuk Kin Kwan [1], Ning Tang [2], Man Ki Fong [1], Wing Hong Liu [2], Chi Yin Tso [1], Chaoran Liu [1], Pui Yan Wong [1], Ning Zhang [1], Wing Hoi Cheung [1] and Ronald Man Yeung Wong [1,*]

1 Department of Orthopaedics and Traumatology, The Chinese University of Hong Kong, Hong Kong, China
2 Department of Orthopaedics and Traumatology, Prince of Wales Hospital, Hospital Authority, Hong Kong, China
* Correspondence: ronald.wong@cuhk.edu.hk; Tel.: +852-3505-1654

Abstract: Background/Objectives: Bisphosphonates are effective in preventing osteoporotic fractures. However, the risk of atypical femur fractures (AFFs) increases with long-term bisphosphonate use. There are few existing publications on the analysis of clinical outcomes of atypical femur fracture cases in Chinese patients. Our objective was to review the clinical outcomes of AFF cases managed in a tertiary center in Hong Kong, China. **Methods**: Cases of AFF managed in the Prince of Wales Hospital from 2010 to 2024 were included. Data on demographics, type and duration of bisphosphonate use prior to AFF, fixation method, and mobility 1 year post-operation were retrospectively retrieved. One-way ANOVA was used to compare the duration of use prior to the development of AFF between different types of bisphosphonates. **Results**: Sixty-nine cases of AFF were included, with a mean age of 73.8 ± 9.7 years. A total of 95.6% of patients had a history of bisphosphonate use, with a mean duration of usage of 6.8 ± 5.6 years prior to the occurrence of AFF. The duration of bisphosphonate use prior to the development of AFF was comparable between alendronate, ibandronate, and a history of using more than one type of anti-resorptive agent. A non-union rate of 5.8% was observed in the current cohort, with 48.2% returning to pre-morbid mobility 1 year post-operation. **Conclusions**: AFF is more commonly seen in female patients with a history of bisphosphonate use. Considering the high success rate demonstrated in the current cohort, treating AFF with closed reduction followed by fixation with a long cephalomedullary device in dynamic locking together with immediate full-weight-bearing rehabilitation post-operation may be effective.

Keywords: atypical femur fracture; bisphosphonates; osteoporosis; rehabilitation

1. Introduction

Osteoporosis is a systemic skeletal disease involving bone tissue, leading to bone fragility and susceptibility to fractures [1,2], and it is common amongst the aging population. Fracture liaison services (FLSs) have been implemented worldwide as an effective method to reduce the risk of osteoporotic fractures [3] by actively recruiting and treating patients with osteoporosis. Their effectiveness in reducing fracture risk has been reported in previous studies [3–5].

Bisphosphonates have been widely used to treat osteoporosis since their development. In brief, bisphosphonates reduce bone resorption by inhibiting osteoclast activity [6]. Other anti-resorptive agents include denosumab, which is a monoclonal antibody that binds with the RANKL protein, preventing it from stimulating essential pathways by which osteoclast precursor cells mature into osteoclasts [7]. Rare adverse events from anti-resorptive use have been described in the literature, including atypical femoral fracture (AFF), which can occur as a result of anti-resorptive use. It typically presents as a transverse fracture of the subtrochanteric region, with minimal comminution occurring without a significant trauma history [8].

Previous studies suggested that the incidence of atypical femur fractures is low, ranging from 0.2 to 13 per 10,000 patient years, depending on duration of use [9]. However, most reported cases have been associated with oral alendronate, and whether a similar pattern is observed with other oral bisphosphonates or denosumab remains unclear [6]. It has also been reported in the literature that the risk of atypical femoral fracture drops significantly after discontinuation of bisphosphonates [9]. Therefore, "drug holidays" after every few years of treatment have been recommended for cases of long-term treatment [6].

AFFs are hypothesized to result from changes in the bone caused by decreased bone turnover [10] and microcrack formation due to impaired healing [11,12]. Reduced bone turnover is observed in anti-resorptive agent use, but it is also observed in patients with other conditions, such as diabetes and chronic kidney disease [13,14]. Previous research has suggested that Asian ethnicity is a risk factor for the development of AFF compared to Caucasian ethnicity [15]. However, a recent article also suggested that the incidence in the Korean population may be comparable to that reported for other ethnicities [16,17]. It was also reported that AFF is a challenging condition to manage, with an average time to union of 10.7 months [18], resulting in high complication rates reaching 15% [19], requiring revision surgery [20]. Currently, dedicated studies describing AFF in our locality and in the Chinese population are still scarce in the literature, and the clinical outcomes in this population may be different to those in the Western population. The primary objective of this study was to present the clinical outcomes of AFF cases managed in a tertiary unit in Hong Kong, China, and to compare the cases based on the duration, type, and practice of pharmacological agent used.

2. Materials and Methods

2.1. Patient Recruitment

This was a retrospective study approved by the Joint Chinese University of Hong Kong—New Territories East Cluster Clinical Research Ethics Committee (CRE Ref. No.: 2024.359, approval date: 20 August 2024). The study protocol was in compliance with ICH-GCP and the Declaration of Helsinki. Sixty-nine consecutive patients with atypical femur fractures (AFFs) who were admitted to the Prince of Wales Hospital in Hong Kong, China, from 2010 to 2024 were included. The inclusion criteria were (1) both male and female patients, (2) >= 18 years of age, and (3) diagnosis of atypical femur fracture based on the American Society for Bone and Mineral Research (ASBMR) guidelines. Closed reduction followed by fixation with a long cephalomedullary device is the usual practice when encountering cases of AFF. Full weight-bearing is allowed post-operatively [5,11]. Prophylactic nailing of the contralateral femur was discussed with patients when there were clinical signs or obvious stress lesions seen in radiographs. Cases of femur fracture that did not fulfill the ASBMR criteria for AFF were excluded.

2.2. Data Collection

Clinical notes of recruited cases were retrieved from the Clinical Management System (CMS) for demographics, Age-Adjusted Charlson Comorbidity Index (ACCI) [2,21], type and duration of osteoporosis medication used, documentation of "drug holidays", treatment of choice for atypical femur fracture, whether prophylactic nailing of the contralateral femur was performed, and functional mobility premorbid and 1 year post-operation were extracted [22].

2.3. Statistical Analysis

Demographic variables were presented with means ± standard deviations (SDs) and frequencies (percentages). The Kolmogorov–Smirnov test was used for normality analyses. The functional scores between cases with and without prophylactic nailing of the contralateral femur were compared using independent-sample *t*-tests. The duration of use between different types of bisphosphonates prior to the development of AFF was compared using one-way ANOVA. A post hoc Scheffe's test was performed if significant differences were obtained. Data were analyzed using IBM SPSS Statistics, version 27 (SPSS Inc., Chicago, IL, USA). Statistical significance was indicated with $p < 0.05$.

2.4. Outcome Measures

The primary outcomes of the current study were the clinical outcomes of 69 AFF cases in terms of mobility at 1 year post-operation, complication rates, and mortality. Secondary outcomes included the type and duration of anti-resorptive agent used and the practice of drug holidays.

3. Results

3.1. Patient Demographics

Clinical notes of 69 patients with a diagnosis of atypical femur fracture from 2010 to 2024 were reviewed. The patients had a mean age of 73.8 ± 9.7 years old, a BMI of 23.8 ± 3.9 kg/m^2, and a female ratio of 94.2%. A total of 21.7% had a history of diabetes mellitus, 7.2% had a documented history of smoking, 4.3% had heart failure, 4.3% had chronic kidney disease, and 8.7% had a history of malignancy. The mean Age-Adjusted Charlson Co-morbidity Index was 3.4 ± 1.2. A total of 53 out of 69 (76.8%) participants had a history of anti-resorptive agent use for primary osteoporosis, whilst 7 out of 69 (10.1%) initiated anti-resorptive treatment after fragility fracture. Six cases had a history of anti-resorptive agent use without clear documentation of the indication, and three cases had clear documentation that the participant had no previous use of anti-resorptive agents. The details of the recruited patients are shown in Table 1.

Table 1. Age distribution of cases presenting with atypical femoral fracture.

Characteristics	Total Cases (*n* = 69)
Age (years) [a]	73.8 ± 9.7
Female	65 (94.2%)
BMI	23.8 ± 3.9 kg/m^2
Current smoker	5 (7.2%)
Diabetes mellitus	15 (21.7%)
Heart failure	3 (4.3%)
Chronic kidney disease	3 (4.3%)
Malignancy [b]	6 (8.7%)
ACCI [c]	3.4 ± 1.2
History of anti-resorptive agent use	66 (95.6%)
Indication for anti-resorptive agent	
Primary osteoporosis	53 (76.8%)
Fragility fracture	7 (10.1%)

[a] Values are expressed as means ± standard deviations or n (%). [b] Documentation of any previous/active malignancy. [c] Age-Adjusted Charlson Comorbidity Index.

3.2. Fixation Method and Non-Union Rates

Amongst the 69 recruited cases, 51 (75.3%) were treated with a long cephalomedullary device (300 mm was the shortest one used). Sixteen (23.2%) were treated with a short cephalomedullary device (200 mm was the longest one used), and one (1.4%) was treated with a plate with screws.

Four out of sixty-nine cases (5.8%) resulted in non-union, requiring revision. Amongst these four cases, one case underwent fixation of AFF with a 360 mm long cephalomedullary device in static locking. The other three had initial fixation of AFF with other units: one case was initially treated with a 170 mm cephalomedullary device, one case was treated with a 200 mm cephalomedullary device, and one case was treated with plating of the proximal femur. All four cases were revised with 300–360 mm long cephalomedullary devices in dynamic locking. All cases achieved bony union after revision surgery. The non-union rates with different devices are summarized in Table 2.

Table 2. Non-union rates with different devices for fixation.

	Union	Non-Union	Total
Long cephalomedullary device	51 (98.1%)	1 (1.9%)	52
Short cephalomedullary device	14 (87.5%)	2 (12.5%)	16
Plate with screws	0 (0%)	1 (100%)	1
Total	65 (94.2%)	4 (5.8%)	69

3.3. *Location of AFFs and Non-Union Rates*

Amongst the 69 recruited cases of AFF, 22 were located in the diaphyseal region, while 47 were located in the sub-trochanteric region. Out of the four cases of non-union in this cohort, one (4.5%) case had an AFF in the diaphyseal region, while three (6.4%) cases had AFFs in the sub-trochanteric region. The non-union rates with AFFs in different locations are summarized in Table 3. There was no statistical significance in the difference between non-union rates of subtrochanteric and diaphyseal AFFs ($p > 0.05$).

Table 3. Non-union rates of AFFs in different locations.

	Union	Non-Union	Total
Subtrochanteric	44 (93.6%)	3 (6.4%)	47
Diaphyseal	21 (95.5%)	1 (4.5%)	22
Total	65 (94.2%)	4 (5.8%)	69

3.4. *Mobility Status 1 Year Post-Operation*

Amongst the 69 patients, 56 (81.8%) had information on mobility status at baseline and at 1 year post-operation documented. Twenty-seven (48.2%) cases were able to return to premorbid mobility levels at 1 year post-operation. Twenty (35.7%) cases walked unaided, twenty-nine (51.8%) cases walked with a stick, five (8.9%) cases walked with a frame, and two (3.6%) cases were wheelchair-bound (Figure 1).

3.5. *Prophylactic Nailing*

Prophylactic nailing of the contralateral femur was performed in 78.2% (54 out of 69) of recruited cases of AFF. At 1 year post-operation, there was no documented occurrence of AFF of the contralateral femur among cases without prophylactic nailing performed. There were also no significant differences in the functional mobility status of AFF cases with and without prophylactic nailing of the contralateral femur performed ($p > 0.05$).

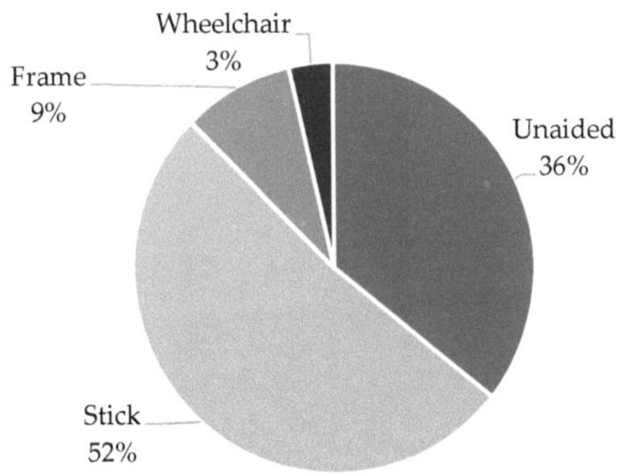

Figure 1. Mobility achieved at 1 year post-operation.

3.6. Pharmacological Agents Used for Osteoporosis

A total of 66 out of 69 (95.6%) patients had a documented history of using anti-resorptive agents, with a mean duration of 6.8 ± 5.6 years, prior to the development of AFF. Alendronate was the most common pharmacological agent used, documented in 42.0% of included cases. Ibandronate was used in 8.6%. Denosumab was used in 4.3% of cases. A total of 14.4% of AFF cases had a history of using more than one type of medication for osteoporosis prior to the development of AFF, and 26.1% cases had no clear documentation on the type of anti-resorptive agent used. The details of anti-resorptive agents used in the included population are summarized in Table 4.

Table 4. Type of anti-resorptive agent used in recruited population.

	Total Cases (n = 69)
Cases with documented use of anti-resorptive drugs	66 (95.6%)
Type of anti-resorptive agent	
Alendronate only	29 (42.0%)
Ibandronate only	6 (8.6%)
Denosumab only	3 (4.3%)
History of using more than one drug	10 (14.4%)
Unknown	18 (26.1%)

Values are expressed as n (%).

The documentation of the duration of drug use was inconsistent, with retrievable data in 53 out of 69 cases (76.8%). Missing data included the type, duration, and indication of anti-resorptive agent used. The cause of incomplete documentation was the use of over-the-counter anti-resorptive agents or the participants receiving medication from a private practice. AFF patients with sole alendronate use developed the condition after 7.6 ± 6.9 years. Patients with sole Ibandronate use developed AFF after 5.5 ± 3.5 years of treatment. Three AFF cases had a history of denosumab use, with a mean time of 3 ± 0 years use prior to development of AFF. There were no significant differences in the duration of use prior to the development of AFF observed between different types of osteoporosis medications (Figure 2).

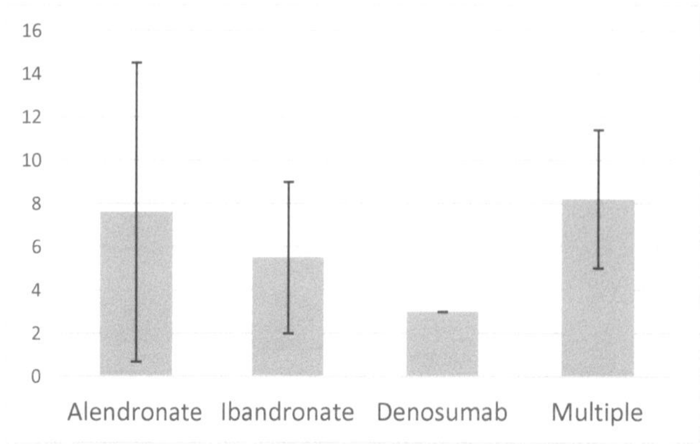

Figure 2. Years of anti-resorptive agent use prior to the development of atypical femur fractures (AFFs).

3.7. Drug Holidays

Amongst the 53 participants with available data on drug holidays, 37 cases had a history of anti-resorptive use of more than 4 years. Only 3 out of 37 (8.1%) cases practiced a drug holiday of 1–2 years after every 3 years of consecutive use of anti-resorptive agents. In these cases of AFF, the average time of consecutive anti-resorptive agent use was 8.9 ± 5.7 years.

4. Discussion

4.1. Comparable Non-Union Rates in the Literature

A previous multicenter study reported a cohort of 46 AFF cases treated with intramedullary nailing, resulting in a 4.3% non-union rate of requiring revision of intramedullary nailing [23]. In this study, 4 out of 69 (5.8%) cases of AFF required revision surgery, all of which achieved boney union after. This suggests that the non-union rate in the current study is comparable to that reported in the literature. Previous studies recommended that AFF should be treated by closed reduction followed by fixation with a long cephalomedullary device, providing adequate stability to allow immediate weight-bearing [24]. The findings of the current study support this recommendation, as non-union rates were shown to be higher in cases treated with a short cephalomedullary device (12.5%) or a plate with screws (100%). Amongst our four included cases of non-union, two cases initially attempted fixation of AFF with a short cephalomedullary device, and one case attempted fixation with plates and screws. Shorter cephalomedullary devices may not provide adequate stability, whilst extramedullary fixation methods like plates and screws may be sub-optimal as they rely on intramembranous fracture healing, which may be inhibited by anti-resorptive medications. As for the one case of failed fixation with a long cephalomedullary device, the distal locking was performed in the static position, which may have contributed to its failure (Figure 3). Static locking of cephalomedullary devices for fixation of AFF may lead to higher rates of failure due to the limited distance available for controlled subsidence. A previous study described static locking as one of the risk factors of reoperation [25].

Another explanation for the high rate of bony union in the current cohort (94.2%) could be our routine practice of dynamic locking together with immediate full weight-bearing post-operation. Comparisons of static locking and dynamic locking in the treatment of AFF are not widely reported in the existing literature. However, the potential benefits of dynamic locking were highlighted in a recent cohort study of 236 cases of AFF showing faster times for the achievement of union and lower non-union and failure rates [25].

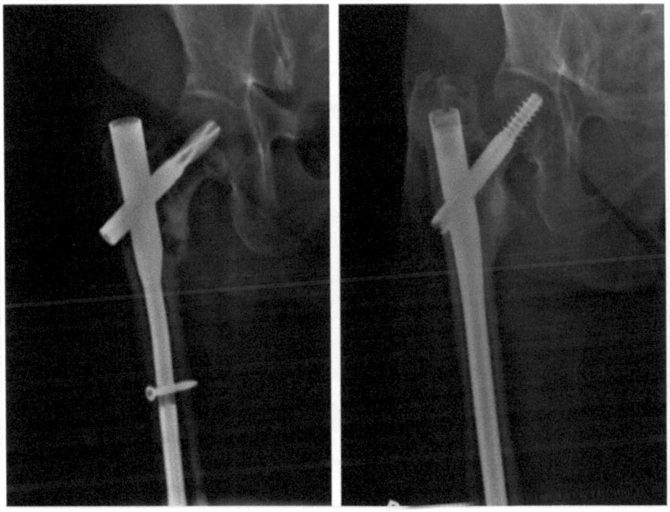

Figure 3. Case of AFF with non-union after fixation with short cephalomedullary device revised to long cephalomedullary device and achievement of bony union.

Dynamic locking is typically avoided in cases of comminuted or long oblique cases where a lack of fracture end opposition may lead to significant limb shortening [26–28] and delayed time to union [29–31], but the fracture patterns in AFFs are typically transverse or short oblique with minimal or no comminution. When adopted in suitable cases, it is believed that dynamic locking may stimulate an osteogenic response due to increased load across the fracture site [32]. No existing large-scale randomized trials compared the use of different locking options in the treatment of AFF. However, clinical trials have been performed on cases of femur fractures, showing mixed results. One study suggested that dynamic locking achieved a shorter time to union by 4 weeks [33], while another study suggested that static locking achieved a shorter time to union by 3 weeks [34]. The results from the existing literature may not be directly comparable due to differences in the recruited populations and differences in fracture patterns and rehabilitation protocols.

The results from the current study showed only one failed fixation of AFF using a long cephalomedullary device, which was fixed in static locking. There is a possibility that dynamic locking may provide superior outcomes, but further investigation is required to support this hypothesis.

4.2. Non-Union Rates Between Diaphyseal and Subtrochanteric AFFs

Previous studies suggested the classification of AFFs into diaphyseal and subtrochanteric types [8]. The clinical significance of this classification has also been highlighted in a recent systematic review showing a statistically greater non-union rate of subtrochanteric AFF at 15% versus a non-union rate of 4% in diaphyseal AFF [19]. A similar trend was observed in the cohort of the current study. Despite not reaching statistical significance, the non-union rate of subtrochanteric AFFs was higher than that of diaphyseal AFFs (6.4 vs. 4.5%). It is also noteworthy that the union rate of subtrochanteric AFFs in this study (6.4%) was lower than the non-union rate of 15% reported in the literature. Prospective studies with a larger sample size are required to support the hypothesis, but there is a possibility that the standardized AFF treatment with a long cephalomedullary device and dynamic locking followed by immediate full-weight-bearing walking may be a reasonable method to manage the challenging condition.

4.3. Mobility at 1 Year Post-Operation

In the current study, 56 (81.8%) recruited cases documented information on mobility status at baseline and at 1 year post-operation. Twenty-seven (48.2%) cases were able to return to premorbid mobility levels at 1 year post-operation. A previous multicenter study on 75 cases of AFF suggested that 80.4% of patients were able to return to pre-fracture mobility [23,35]. The discrepancy could be addressed by the relatively short follow-up time in the current study. Documentation of pre-fracture and post-fracture mobility could also be documented in a more standardized manner in future studies.

4.4. Significance of Prophylactic Nailing to the Contralateral Femur

Existing multicenter cohorts suggested the effectiveness of intramedullary nailing in treating atypical femur fractures [23,36]. Extramedullary fixation with plates and screws was also described in the literature but was suggested to be un-favourable as intramembranous fracture healing is dependent on osteoclast activity, which is inhibited in anti-resorptive therapy [5]. The management of incomplete fractures and whether to prophylactically perform intramedullary nailing of the contralateral femur remain controversial [24]. A scoring system has been described in previous literature to guide the decision on whether prophylactic nailing should be performed [37].

Prophylactic nailing of the contralateral femur was offered to all patients presenting with AFF, as there were clinical signs or radiological stress lesions. In this study, 22% of the cases presenting with AFF did not receive prophylactic nailing of the contralateral femur after discussion. The decision usually involves a balance of risks/benefits, patient preference, and discussion with the surgeon when there is a lack of significant stress lesioning suggested by radiography of the contralateral femur. An example of a significant stress lesion strongly suggestive for prophylactic nailing and a minimal stress lesion for which the patient eventually did not receive prophylactic nailing are shown in Figure 4.

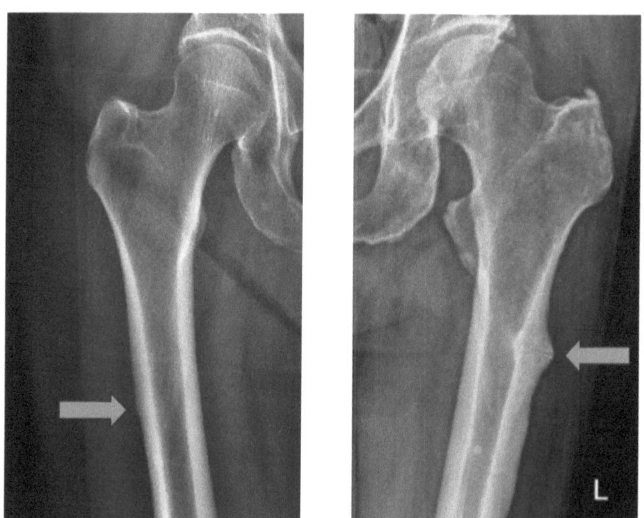

Figure 4. Example radiographs of cases where prophylactic nailing of the contralateral femur was (**right**) and was not performed (**left**). Grey arrows show the most prominent stress lesions on the radiographs.

When comparing cases with and without prophylactic nailing of the contralateral femur, there were no occurrences of AFF in the contralateral femur and no significant differences in the functional mobility status at 1 year post-operation. These results raise awareness of the fact that prophylactic nailing may not necessarily be beneficial in cases of AFF when there is a lack of significant stress lesions shown on the radiograph of the contralateral femur.

4.5. Time Leading to AFF in Different Anti-Resorptive Agents

The existing literature suggested that the majority of reported cases of AFF were associated with alendronate use, but the phenomenon was also observed in trials involving other anti-resorptive agents [6]. The etiology of AFF is yet to be fully understood. Anti-resorptive agents aim to preserve bone mineral density through suppression of bone resorption. However, resorption is part of the natural bone turnover mechanism, and it was hypothesized that its suppression may lead to the accumulation of microcracks and AFF [38,39]. Previous investigations also showed depressed levels of bone turnover markers when comparing AFFs with typical femur fractures [10]. Other studies attempted to compare the microarchitecture of bones in patients with and without atypical femur fractures, showing no significant differences [40]. Results from this study suggested that AFF cases are also observed in cases of anti-resorptive agent use other than alendronate. From the current data, there were no significant differences in the time leading to AFF between using alendronate only, ibandronate only, denosumab only, or a history of more than one type of anti-resorptive agent used prior to the development of AFF. However, the current study only included a relatively small sample of AFF patients. Population-based studies with a larger sample size may be required to further support this hypothesis.

4.6. The Importance of Stewardship in the Use of Anti-Resorptive Agents

The results from this study suggest that drug holidays were not practiced according to recommendations in the majority (92%) of cases presenting with AFF. Among these cases, the mean duration of consecutive anti-resorptive agent use was 8.9 ± 5.7 years. The importance of drug holidays has been advocated in the previous literature [41]. Existing studies demonstrated that bone turnover increases gradually over 1–2 years, leading to a drop in bone mineral density in the hips [42]. However, the bone mineral density at 2 years post-termination of anti-resorptive treatment was still higher than pre-treatment levels, suggesting lingering effects by the end of a drug holiday of 2 years [42]. Another observational cohort study assessing the fracture risks of drug holidays reported an increased risk of hip, humerus, and vertebral fractures in patients with a drug holiday of >2 years compared with patients who continued to receive anti-resorptive agents [43]. Despite evidence on the importance of drug holidays, there is currently no consensus on when and how long drug holidays should be practiced. Large, prospective, long-term observational studies may be necessary to clarify the safety of and best practice for drug holidays.

As the risk of typical fragility fracture remains high in patients with osteoporosis, five principles were described to manage patients who suffered from AFF while on bisphosphonates or denosumab [44]. The first principle suggested the termination of the anti-resorptive medication. However, it was also mentioned that extra caution is required for patients on denosumab in consideration of the risk of rebound vertebral fractures [44]. The second principle is maximizing non-pharmacological means to reduce fall and fracture risks. The third principle is to work-up and treat potential secondary causes of osteoporosis. The fourth principle is to review the drug list of the patient, eliminating candidates that may increase fracture risks. Finally, the fifth principle suggested that some patients may benefit from anabolic agents. The use of anabolic agents like teriparatide was also recommended by other authors [45]. However, it was also mentioned that there is currently no solid evidence on the indication of anabolic agents [45].

4.7. Limitations

A limitation of the current study lies in the relatively small sample size of 69 cases of AFF and the retrospective study design. Documentation of the use of medication for osteoporosis is sometimes inconsistent, and the variety of anti-resorptive agents discussed in the current study is limited to alendronate, ibandronate, and several cases of denosumab. Inconsistent documentation of anti-resorptive agent use also limited the possibility of performing a meaningful analysis of the spontaneous or non-bisphosphonate groups of AFF, as accurate identification of these groups could not be completed with the current data.

The recruited cohort of the current study only included Chinese patients. Therefore, direct comparisons between different ethnicities could not be made. The retrospective design of the current study also limited the width of the included data. Frailty measures, muscle mass, and physical function are important parameters to be considered in the geriatric population. Future prospective multicenter studies on the topic with prospective designs may be required given the rare incidence of AFF due to anti-resorptive agent use.

5. Conclusions

AFF is more commonly seen in female patients with a history of bisphosphonate use. Considering the high success rate demonstrated in the current cohort, treating AFF with closed reduction followed by fixation with a long cephalomedullary device in dynamic locking together with immediate full-weight-bearing rehabilitation post-operation may be effective.

Author Contributions: Conceptualization, C.K.K., N.T., W.H.L., C.Y.T. and R.M.Y.W.; formal analysis, C.K.K.; data curation, C.K.K. and M.K.F.; investigation, W.H.L. and C.Y.T.; methodology, N.Z. and W.H.C.; writing—original draft preparation, C.K.K.; writing—review and editing, C.K.K., N.T., M.K.F., W.H.L., C.Y.T., C.L., P.Y.W., N.Z., W.H.C. and R.M.Y.W.; visualization, C.K.K., C.L. and P.Y.W.; supervision, C.K.K., N.T., N.Z., W.H.C. and R.M.Y.W. All authors have read and agreed to the published version of the manuscript.

Funding: This research received no external funding.

Institutional Review Board Statement: This retrospective study was approved by the Joint Chinese University of Hong Kong—New Territories East Cluster Clinical Research Ethics Committee (CRE Ref No.: 2024.359, approval date 20 August 2024). All procedures performed in studies involving human participants were in accordance with the ethical standards of the institutional and/or national research committee and with the 1964 Helsinki Declaration and its later amendments or comparable ethical standards.

Informed Consent Statement: Patient consent was waived as this was a retrospective study.

Data Availability Statement: Data are contained within the article. Individual data are unavailable due to privacy or ethical restrictions.

Conflicts of Interest: Ronald Man Yeung Wong has received advisor/speaker fees from Amgen and a speaker honorarium from ZP Therapeutics—a division of the Zuellig Pharma Corporation and ZANOVEX PTE LTD. Cheuk Kin Kwan, Ning Tang, Man Ki Fong, Wing Hong Liu, Chi Yin Tso, Chaoran Liu, Pui Yan Wong, Ning Zhang, and Wing Hoi Cheung declare that they have no conflicts of interest.

Abbreviations

The following abbreviations are used in this manuscript:

ACCI	Age-Adjusted Charlson Comorbidity Index
AFF	Atypical femur fracture
CMS	Clinical Management System
FLS	Fracture liaison service

References

1. Burge, R.; Dawson-Hughes, B.; Solomon, D.H.; Wong, J.B.; King, A.; Tosteson, A. Incidence and Economic Burden of Osteoporosis-Related Fractures in the United States, 2005–2025. *J. Bone Miner. Res.* **2007**, *22*, 465–475. [CrossRef] [PubMed]
2. Wong, R.M.Y.; Zu, Y.; Chau, W.W.; Tso, C.Y.; Liu, W.H.; Ng, R.W.K.; Chow, S.K.H.; Cheung, W.H.; Tang, N.; Ho, K.K.W. High Charlson Comorbidity Index Score Is Associated with Early Fracture-Related Complication for Internal Fixation of Neck of Femur Fractures. *Sci. Rep.* **2022**, *12*, 4749. [CrossRef] [PubMed]
3. Wong, R.M.Y.; Ko, S.Y.; Chau, W.-W.; Lee, L.C.Y.; Chow, S.K.H.; Cheung, W.H.; Law, S.W. The First Reported Fracture Liaison Service (FLS) for Vertebral Fractures in China: Is Muscle the Missing Gap? *Arch. Osteoporos.* **2021**, *16*, 168. [CrossRef] [PubMed]
4. Wong, R.M.Y.; Law, S.W.; Lee, K.B.; Chow, S.K.H.; Cheung, W.H. Secondary Prevention of Fragility Fractures: Instrumental Role of a Fracture Liaison Service to Tackle the Risk of Imminent Fracture. *Hong Kong Med. J.* **2019**, *25*, 235–242. [CrossRef]
5. Wong, R.M.Y.; Cheung, W.-H.; Chow, S.K.H.; Ng, R.W.K.; Li, W.; Hsu, A.Y.-C.; Wong, K.K.; Ho, A.W.-H.; Choi, S.-H.; Fang, C.X.; et al. Recommendations on the Post-Acute Management of the Osteoporotic Fracture—Patients with "Very-High" Re-Fracture Risk. *J. Orthop. Transl.* **2022**, *37*, 94–99. [CrossRef]
6. Reid, I.R.; Billington, E.O. Drug Therapy for Osteoporosis in Older Adults. *Lancet* **2022**, *399*, 1080–1092. [CrossRef]
7. Dempster, D.W.; Brown, J.P.; Fahrleitner-Pammer, A.; Kendler, D.; Rizzo, S.; Valter, I.; Wagman, R.B.; Yin, X.; Yue, S.V.; Boivin, G. Effects of Long-Term Denosumab on Bone Histomorphometry and Mineralization in Women With Postmenopausal Osteoporosis. *J. Clin. Endocrinol. Metab.* **2018**, *103*, 2498–2509. [CrossRef]
8. Shane, E.; Burr, D.; Abrahamsen, B.; Adler, R.A.; Brown, T.D.; Cheung, A.M.; Cosman, F.; Curtis, J.R.; Dell, R.; Dempster, D.W.; et al. Atypical Subtrochanteric and Diaphyseal Femoral Fractures: Second Report of a Task Force of the American Society for Bone and Mineral Research. *J. Bone Miner. Res.* **2014**, *29*, 1–23. [CrossRef]
9. Black, D.M.; Geiger, E.J.; Eastell, R.; Vittinghoff, E.; Li, B.H.; Ryan, D.S.; Dell, R.M.; Adams, A.L. Atypical Femur Fracture Risk versus Fragility Fracture Prevention with Bisphosphonates. *N. Engl. J. Med.* **2020**, *383*, 743–753. [CrossRef]
10. Iizuka, Y.; Iizuka, H.; Kaneko, T.; Mieda, T.; Takechi, R.; Suzuki, H.; Sorimachi, Y.; Suto, T.; Tachibana, M.; Yoneyama, T.; et al. Bone Turnover Markers and the Factors Associated with Atypical Femur Fractures among Japanese Patients. *Injury* **2016**, *47*, 2484–2489. [CrossRef]
11. Black, D.M.; Abrahamsen, B.; Bouxsein, M.L.; Einhorn, T.; Napoli, N. Atypical Femur Fractures: Review of Epidemiology, Relationship to Bisphosphonates, Prevention, and Clinical Management. *Endocr. Rev.* **2019**, *40*, 333–368. [CrossRef] [PubMed]
12. Donnelly, E.; Saleh, A.; Unnanuntana, A.; Lane, J.M. Atypical Femoral Fractures: Epidemiology, Etiology, and Patient Management. *Curr. Opin. Support. Palliat. Care* **2012**, *6*, 348–354. [CrossRef] [PubMed]
13. Coen, G. Adynamic Bone Disease: An Update and Overview. *J. Nephrol.* **2005**, *18*, 117–122.
14. Haarhaus, M.; Evenepoel, P.; European Renal Osteodystrophy (EUROD) workgroup; Chronic Kidney Disease Mineral and Bone Disorder (CKD-MBD) working group of the European Renal Association–European Dialysis and Transplant Association (ERA-EDTA). Differentiating the Causes of Adynamic Bone in Advanced Chronic Kidney Disease Informs Osteoporosis Treatment. *Kidney Int.* **2021**, *100*, 546–558. [CrossRef]
15. Nguyen, H.H.; Lakhani, A.; Shore-Lorenti, C.; Zebaze, R.; Vincent, A.J.; Milat, F.; Ebeling, P.R. Asian Ethnicity Is Associated with Atypical Femur Fractures in an Australian Population Study. *Bone* **2020**, *135*, 115319. [CrossRef]
16. Lee, Y.-K.; Ahn, S.; Kim, K.M.; Suh, C.S.; Koo, K.-H. Incidence Rate of Atypical Femoral Fracture after Bisphosphonates Treatment in Korea. *J. Korean Med. Sci.* **2018**, *33*, e38. [CrossRef]
17. Abrahamsen, B.; Eiken, P.; Eastell, R. Cumulative Alendronate Dose and the Long-Term Absolute Risk of Subtrochanteric and Diaphyseal Femur Fractures: A Register-Based National Cohort Analysis. *J. Clin. Endocrinol. Metab.* **2010**, *95*, 5258–5265. [CrossRef]
18. Cho, J.-W.; Oh, C.-W.; Leung, F.; Park, K.-C.; Wong, M.K.; Kwek, E.; Kim, H.-J.; Oh, J.-K. Healing of Atypical Subtrochanteric Femur Fractures After Cephalomedullary Nailing: Which Factors Predict Union? *J. Orthop. Trauma.* **2017**, *31*, 138–145. [CrossRef]

19. Yoon, B.-H.; Kim, M.; Roh, Y.H. Does the Nonunion Rate of Atypical Femoral Fractures Differ According to Fracture Site?: A Meta-Analysis. *Clin. Orthop. Surg.* **2024**, *16*, 533–541. [CrossRef]
20. Schultz, D.S.; Gass, H.M.; Barfield, W.R.; Demos, H.A.; Hartsock, L.A. Surgical Complications Associated With Atypical Femur Fractures Attributed to Bisphosphonate Use. *J. Surg. Orthop. Adv.* **2018**, *27*, 14–20.
21. Wong, R.M.Y.; Ho, W.T.; Wai, L.S.; Li, W.; Chau, W.W.; Chow, K.-H.S.; Cheung, W.-H. Fragility Fractures and Imminent Fracture Risk in Hong Kong: One of the Cities with Longest Life Expectancies. *Arch. Osteoporos.* **2019**, *14*, 104. [CrossRef] [PubMed]
22. Wong, R.M.Y.; Qin, J.; Chau, W.W.; Tang, N.; Tso, C.Y.; Wong, H.W.; Chow, S.K.-H.; Leung, K.-S.; Cheung, W.-H. Prognostic Factors Related to Ambulation Deterioration after 1-Year of Geriatric Hip Fracture in a Chinese Population. *Sci. Rep.* **2021**, *11*, 14650. [CrossRef] [PubMed]
23. Lee, K.-J.; Yoo, J.J.; Oh, K.-J.; Yoo, J.-H.; Rhyu, K.H.; Nam, K.W.; Suh, D.-H. Surgical Outcome of Intramedullary Nailing in Patients with Complete Atypical Femoral Fracture: A Multicenter Retrospective Study. *Injury* **2017**, *48*, 941–945. [CrossRef] [PubMed]
24. Koh, A.; Guerado, E.; Giannoudis, P.V. Atypical Femoral Fractures Related to Bisphosphonate Treatment: Issues and Controversies Related to Their Surgical Management. *Bone Jt. J.* **2017**, *99-B*, 295–302. [CrossRef]
25. Fang, C.; Shen, W.Y.; Wong, J.S.H.; Yee, D.K.-H.; Yung, C.S.-Y.; Fang, E.; Lai, Y.S.; Woo, S.B.; Cheung, J.; Chau, J.Y.-M.; et al. Should Nails Be Locked Dynamically or Statically in Atypical Femoral Fractures?—A Radiological Analysis of Time to Union and Reoperations in 236 Displaced Fractures with 4 Years Average Follow-Up. *Injury* **2023**, *54*, 110909. [CrossRef]
26. Wu, C.C. The Effect of Dynamization on Slowing the Healing of Femur Shaft Fractures after Interlocking Nailing. *J. Trauma* **1997**, *43*, 263–267. [CrossRef]
27. Wu, C.C.; Shih, C.H. Effect of Dynamization of a Static Interlocking Nail on Fracture Healing. *Can. J. Surg.* **1993**, *36*, 302–306.
28. Pihlajamäki, H.K.; Salminen, S.T.; Böstman, O.M. The Treatment of Nonunions Following Intramedullary Nailing of Femoral Shaft Fractures. *J. Orthop. Trauma* **2002**, *16*, 394–402. [CrossRef]
29. Lynch, J.R.; Taitsman, L.A.; Barei, D.P.; Nork, S.E. Femoral Nonunion: Risk Factors and Treatment Options. *J. Am. Acad. Orthop. Surg.* **2008**, *16*, 88–97. [CrossRef]
30. Wolinsky, P.R.; McCarty, E.; Shyr, Y.; Johnson, K. Reamed Intramedullary Nailing of the Femur: 551 Cases. *J. Trauma* **1999**, *46*, 392–399. [CrossRef]
31. Vaughn, J.; Gotha, H.; Cohen, E.; Fantry, A.J.; Feller, R.J.; Van Meter, J.; Hayda, R.; Born, C.T. Nail Dynamization for Delayed Union and Nonunion in Femur and Tibia Fractures. *Orthopedics* **2016**, *39*, e1117–e1123. [CrossRef] [PubMed]
32. Papakostidis, C.; Psyllakis, I.; Vardakas, D.; Grestas, A.; Giannoudis, P.V. Femoral-Shaft Fractures and Nonunions Treated with Intramedullary Nails: The Role of Dynamisation. *Injury* **2011**, *42*, 1353–1361. [CrossRef] [PubMed]
33. Basumallick, M.N.; Bandopadhyay, A. Effect of Dynamization in Open Interlocking Nailing of Femoral Fractures. A Prospective Randomized Comparative Study of 50 Cases with a 2-Year Follow-Up. *Acta Orthop. Belg.* **2002**, *68*, 42–48. [PubMed]
34. Tigani, D.; Fravisini, M.; Stagni, C.; Pascarella, R.; Boriani, S. Interlocking Nail for Femoral Shaft Fractures: Is Dynamization Always Necessary? *Int. Orthop.* **2005**, *29*, 101–104. [CrossRef]
35. Kim, S.M.; Rhyu, K.H.; Lim, S.J. Salvage of Failed Osteosynthesis for an Atypical Subtrochanteric Femoral Fracture Associated with Long-Term Bisphosphonate Treatment Using a 95° Angled Blade Plate. *Bone Jt. J.* **2018**, *100-B*, 1511–1517. [CrossRef]
36. Oh, C.-W.; Oh, J.-K.; Park, K.-C.; Kim, J.-W.; Yoon, Y.-C. Prophylactic Nailing of Incomplete Atypical Femoral Fractures. *Sci. World J.* **2013**, *2013*, 450148. [CrossRef]
37. Min, B.-W.; Koo, K.-H.; Park, Y.-S.; Oh, C.-W.; Lim, S.-J.; Kim, J.-W.; Lee, K.-J.; Lee, Y.-K. Scoring System for Identifying Impending Complete Fractures in Incomplete Atypical Femoral Fractures. *J. Clin. Endocrinol. Metab.* **2017**, *102*, 545–550. [CrossRef]
38. Saita, Y.; Ishijima, M.; Kaneko, K. Atypical Femoral Fractures and Bisphosphonate Use: Current Evidence and Clinical Implications. *Ther. Adv. Chronic Dis.* **2015**, *6*, 185–193. [CrossRef]
39. Odvina, C.V.; Zerwekh, J.E.; Rao, D.S.; Maalouf, N.; Gottschalk, F.A.; Pak, C.Y.C. Severely Suppressed Bone Turnover: A Potential Complication of Alendronate Therapy. *J. Clin. Endocrinol. Metab.* **2005**, *90*, 1294–1301. [CrossRef]
40. Zanchetta, M.B.; Diehl, M.; Buttazzoni, M.; Galich, A.; Silveira, F.; Bogado, C.E.; Zanchetta, J.R. Assessment of Bone Microarchitecture in Postmenopausal Women on Long-Term Bisphosphonate Therapy With Atypical Fractures of the Femur. *J. Bone Miner. Res.* **2014**, *29*, 999–1004. [CrossRef]
41. Reid, I.R. Bisphosphonate Holidays. *Drug Ther. Bull.* **2021**, *59*, 35–36. [CrossRef] [PubMed]
42. Naylor, K.E.; Bradburn, M.; Paggiosi, M.A.; Gossiel, F.; Peel, N.F.A.; McCloskey, E.V.; Walsh, J.S.; Eastell, R. Effects of Discontinuing Oral Bisphosphonate Treatments for Postmenopausal Osteoporosis on Bone Turnover Markers and Bone Density. *Osteoporos. Int.* **2018**, *29*, 1407–1417. [CrossRef] [PubMed]
43. Curtis, J.R.; Saag, K.G.; Arora, T.; Wright, N.C.; Yun, H.; Daigle, S.; Matthews, R.; Delzell, E. Duration of Bisphosphonate Drug Holidays and Associated Fracture Risk. *Med. Care* **2020**, *58*, 419–426. [CrossRef] [PubMed]

44. Adler, R.A. Treating Osteoporosis in Patients with Atypical Femoral Fracture. *J. Bone Miner. Res.* **2024**, *39*, 1711–1715. [CrossRef]
45. van de Laarschot, D.M.; McKenna, M.J.; Abrahamsen, B.; Langdahl, B.; Cohen-Solal, M.; Guañabens, N.; Eastell, R.; Ralston, S.H.; Zillikens, M.C. Medical Management of Patients After Atypical Femur Fractures: A Systematic Review and Recommendations From the European Calcified Tissue Society. *J. Clin. Endocrinol. Metab.* **2020**, *105*, 1682–1699. [CrossRef]

Journal of
Clinical Medicine

MDPI

Article

Post-Traumatic Osteoarthritis and Functional Outcomes After Volar Plating vs. Casting of Unstable Distal Radius Fractures: A Minimum 2-Year Follow-Up of the VOLCON Randomized Controlled Trial

Daniel Wæver [1,*], Rikke Thorninger [2], Karen Larsen Romme [1], Michael Tjørnild [1] and Jan Duedal Rölfing [2,3]

1 Department of Orthopaedics, Regional Hospital Randers, Skovlyvej 15, Randers NØ, 8930 Randers, Denmark; karrom@rm.dk (K.L.R.); michael.tjornild@rm.dk (M.T.)
2 Department of Orthopaedics, Aarhus University Hospital, Aarhus N, 8200 Aarhus, Denmark; rikkthor@rm.dk (R.T.); jan.rolfing@rm.dk (J.D.R.)
3 Department of Clinical Medicine, HEALTH, Aarhus University, Aarhus C, 8000 Aarhus, Denmark
* Correspondence: daniel_waever@yahoo.dk

Abstract: Background/Objectives: Distal radius fractures (DRFs) are among the most common fractures in the elderly, with increasing incidence due to population aging. Recent evidence questions the benefits of operative treatment, particularly in elderly patients. The present study aimed to assess post-traumatic osteoarthritis (OA) and patient-reported outcome measures (PROMs) after a minimum of two years of follow-up of the previously published VOLCON randomized controlled trial (RCT), which compared operative and non-operative treatments of unstable DRFs in patients aged $\geq$ 65 years. **Methods**: This study presents a minimum two-year follow-up of a single-center, assessor-blinded RCT. A total of 100 patients with unstable DRFs were randomized to either operative treatment with volar locking plating or non-operative treatment with cast immobilization. The primary outcome was post-traumatic OA, assessed using the Knirk and Jupiter classification. Secondary outcomes included PROMs (Quick Disabilities of the Arm, Shoulder, and Hand (Quick-DASH)) and Patient-Rated Wrist/Hand Evaluation (PRWHE), complications, pain, grip strength, and range of motion (ROM). Statistical analyses were performed using two-way ANOVA. **Results**: After a median follow-up of 3.0 years, 60 patients (28 non-operative and 32 operative) were available for analysis. There was no significant difference in OA between the groups ($p = 0.57$). PROMs (Quick-DASH, PRWHE), pain, grip strength, and ROM were time-dependent ($p < 0.001$) but not treatment-dependent. Complications were more frequent in the operative group, including hardware-related issues requiring reoperation. **Conclusions**: At a minimum of two years of follow-up, no correlation was found between treatment choice and post-traumatic OA. Functional outcomes were similar between groups, suggesting that non-operative treatment remains a viable option for elderly patients with unstable DRFs.

Keywords: distal radius fractures; post-traumatic osteoarthritis; randomized controlled trial; non-operative treatment

1. Introduction

Distal radius fractures (DRFs) are among the most common fractures in the elderly with incidence rates of 190–200 per 100,000 person-years [1,2]. These incidence rates are expected to increase with the projected aging population [3].

In Denmark, operative treatment was recommended by the National Clinical Guidelines (NCG) (2017) for unstable DRFs when the following radiological criteria were fulfilled after attempted closed reduction in the emergency department (ED) [4,5]: >10° dorsal tilt of the radius, >2 mm articular step-off, >3 mm ulnar variance, incongruence of the distal radioulnar joint, and substantial dorsal comminution indicating gross instability.

For the past few decades, open reduction and internal fixation (ORIF) with volar locking plates has becoming increasingly popular [6,7] and is now the operative treatment of choice. Studies have shown that ORIF improves radiological alignment and restores the distal radius closer to normal anatomy [8,9]. However, recent high-quality studies have questioned the benefits of operative treatment for DRFs in the elderly, and evidence supporting non-operative treatment is mounting [10–14].

Three studies have had an observation period of more than one year of elderly patients with unstable DRFs randomized to either operative or non-operative treatment. However, these studies have shown conflicting results [15–17].

The present study is a minimum 2-year follow-up of a previously published randomized controlled trial (VOLCON RCT) [14] comparing operative and non-operative treatments of unstable DRF in patients $\geq$ 65 years. Given the poorer radiological parameters in terms of angulation and shortening in the non-operatively treated group at 5-week follow-up, it seemed logical to reinvite the VOLCON patients and assess their post-traumatic osteoarthritic changes and patient-related outcome measures (PROMs) after a longer follow-up period of more than one year.

In the present study, we wanted to assess the explorative outcomes of the original RCT. Therefore, we assessed PROMs as well as radiological osteoarthritis (OA) changes after non-operative and operatively treated patients after a minimum of two years of follow-up.

2. Materials and Methods

This study describes the minimum 2-year follow-up on an already published prospective, single-center, assessor-blinded, randomized, controlled superiority trial comparing non-operative versus operative treatments of unstable DRFs in patients $\geq$ 65 years [14]. A study protocol was also published [18]. The primary study took place between November 2019 and March 2022.

Interventions and randomization

Patients with DRFs aged 65 years and above admitted to the ED at Randers Regional Hospital, Denmark, were screened for eligibility. Exclusion criteria were high-energy fractures, open fractures, concomitant injuries, previous ipsilateral DRFs, and the inability to give written consent for participation in the study.

DRFs were diagnosed on radiographs of the wrist (posterior–anterior and lateral projections), and closed reduction was performed with a hematoma block by the attending physician in the ED. A maximum of two attempts at closed reduction were allowed to obtain an acceptable reduction in the fracture. If the NCG criteria [4] for operation were fulfilled, the patient was randomized to either operative or non-operative treatment.

According to sample size calculations from the primary study, 100 patients were included. Thus, patients were blindly randomized by picking one of 100 identical sealed envelopes, each containing a note stating "operative" or "non-operative" written. The envelopes were non-transparent, and the concealment of allocation was therefore effective.

Patients allocated to operation were treated with ORIF with volar locking plate fixation (AcuLoc, Acumed, Hillsboro, OR, USA or VariAx, Stryker, Kalamazoo, MI, USA). All patients were operated on using a standard Henry approach for the distal radius. The repair of the pronator quadratus was performed when possible. Patients were operated under regional or general anesthesia. Post-operatively, the wrist was immobilized with a dorsal plaster cast for 2 weeks, followed by 3 weeks of immobilization with a removable wrist orthosis. A single session of hand therapy instruction took place.

Patients allocated to the non-operative treatment were immobilized with a dorsal plaster cast for 5 weeks. A single session of hand therapy instruction took place after cast removal. No radiographs were performed before the 5-week follow-up.

Outcomes

Primary and secondary outcomes were assessed for the primary study at day 0, 2 weeks, 5 weeks, 6 months, and 12 months after injury. For the present study, patients were followed-up at minimum 2 years after the injury. Patients were contacted by telephone and invited to participate. At the 2-year follow-up, the observers DW and KLR were blinded as all measurements were performed with the wrist covered by a glove to mask potential surgical scars.

Explorative Outcomes of the Original RCT

The degree of post-traumatic OA in the radiocarpal and distal radioulnar joints was assessed by an orthopedic trauma specialist according to the Knirk and Jupiter classification [19] on a scale from 0 to 3 (0: none, 1: slight joint-space narrowing, 2: marked joint-space narrowing and osteophyte formation, and 3: bone-on-bone osteophyte formation and cyst formation) on standard radiographs of the wrist (posterior–anterior and lateral projections).

PROMs included a Danish version of the Quick Disabilities of the Arm, Shoulder, and Hand (Quick-DASH). A difference of 16–20 points in Quick-DASH was considered the minimum clinically important difference (MCID) [20–22]. The validated Danish version of the Patient-Rated Wrist/Hand Evaluation (PRWHE) was also reported [23]. The MCID for PRWHE was defined as a difference of 11.5 [24].

Complications were reported as follows:

- Sensory disturbance, including carpal tunnel syndrome and chronic regional pain syndrome;
- Flexor tendon rupture and irritation;
- Extensor tendon rupture and irritation;
- Hardware failure, e.g., osteosynthesis loosening;
- Infection: superficial (treated with antibiotics only) or deep (requiring a surgical intervention);
- Reoperation with hardware replacement;
- Reoperation with hardware removal (partial or total), which is not routinely performed in our country.

Pain was reported using the 0–10 numeric rating scale (NRS). Grip strength was measured using a calibrated dynamometer (EH101 CAMRY, by Camry® Scales, South El Monte, CA, USA). The grip strength of both the left and right hands was estimated as the mean score of three repetition of each hand. Range of motion (ROM) was measured by one of the investigators using a goniometer.

Statistics

Basic demographic statistics were used to describe the study population. Two-way ANOVA was applied to determine if the observed effects were time-dependent, subject-dependent, or treatment-dependent. The significance level was set to $p < 0.05$.

The present trial was approved by the Danish Scientific Ethical Committee (ID: 1-10-72-420-17) and registered at Clinicaltrials.gov (ID: NCT03716661).

3. Results

After a median follow-up time of 3.0 (range 2.0–4.3) years, a total of 60 patients (28 non-operatively and 32 operatively treated DRFs) were available for data analysis at a minimum follow-up time of 2 years. Of the 85 patients available for the 1-year analysis of the published VOLCON RCT [14], 25 patients were lost to follow-up: a total of 5 patients were deceased, while 6 patients were lost to follow-up as they could not be contacted by telephone, and 14 patients did not want to participate in the study due to illness or a lack of time/interest (Figure 1).

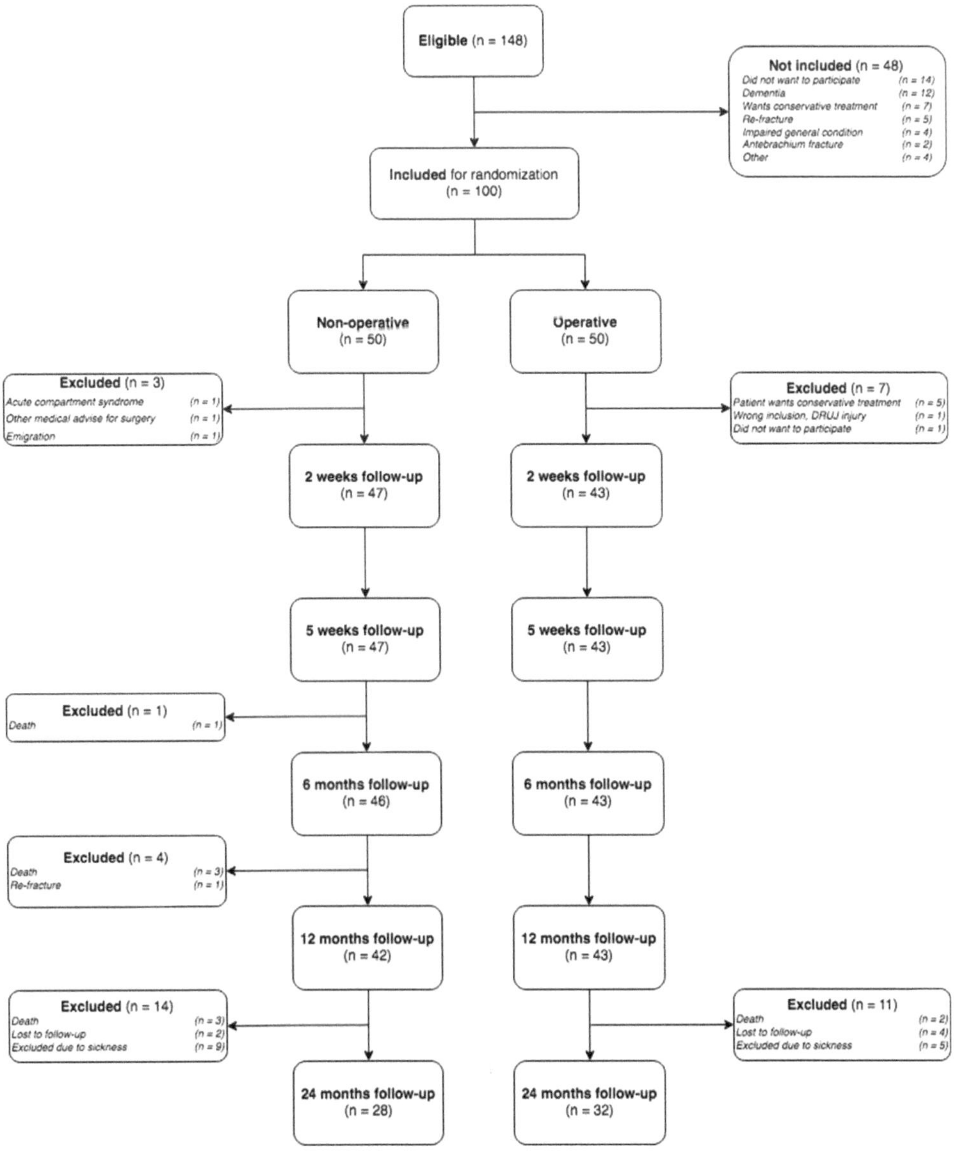
Eligible (n = 148)
Not included (n = 48)
Did not want to participate (n = 14)
Dementia (n = 12)
Wants conservative treatment (n = 7)
Re-fracture (n = 5)
Impaired general condition (n = 4)
Antebrachium fracture (n = 2)
Other (n = 4)
Included for randomization (n = 100)
Non-operative (n = 50)
Operative (n = 50)
Excluded (n = 3)
Acute compartment syndrome (n = 1)
Other medical advise for surgery (n = 1)
Emigration (n = 1)
Excluded (n = 7)
Patient wants conservative treatment (n = 5)
Wrong inclusion, DRUJ injury (n = 1)
Did not want to participate (n = 1)
2 weeks follow-up (n = 47)
2 weeks follow-up (n = 43)
5 weeks follow-up (n = 47)
5 weeks follow-up (n = 43)
Excluded (n = 1)
Death (n = 1)
6 months follow-up (n = 46)
6 months follow-up (n = 43)
Excluded (n = 4)
Death (n = 3)
Re-fracture (n = 1)
12 months follow-up (n = 42)
12 months follow-up (n = 43)
Excluded (n = 14)
Death (n = 3)
Lost to follow-up (n = 2)
Excluded due to sickness (n = 9)
Excluded (n = 11)
Death (n = 2)
Lost to follow-up (n = 4)
Excluded due to sickness (n = 5)
24 months follow-up (n = 28)
24 months follow-up (n = 32)

Figure 1. Consort flowchart.

Baseline demographics (age, gender, dominant hand fractured (yes/no), working status, and ASA class 1–6 (American Society of Anaesthesiologists Classification)) for the patients available for data analysis at a minimum 2-year follow-up and patients lost to follow-up between the 1- and 2-year follow-ups are given in Table 1, while the population at large from the VOLCON study can be found in the 1-year follow-up [14]. From years 1 to 2, the 25 patients lost to follow-up seemed to be slightly older but otherwise comparable to the included patients in terms of gender, occupational status, and ASA groups.

Table 1. Patient demographics for patients available for 2-year analysis and patients lost to follow-up from 1 to 2 years of follow-up.

	Available at Follow-Up at 2 Years		Lost to Follow-Up 1–2 Years	
	n = 60		n = 25	
	Non-Operative n = 32	Operative n = 28	Non-Operative n = 14	Operative n = 11
Women [n/N (%)]	26/32 (81%)	22/28 (78%)	11/14 (79%)	8/11 (73%)
Fractured dominant side [n/N (%)]	13/32 (41%)	13/28 (46%)	8/14 (57%)	4/11 (36%)
Median age (range) [years]	73 (66–92)	72 (65–87)	78 (65–91)	78 (69–91)
Retired	31/32 (97%)	28/28 (100%)	14/14 (100%)	11/11 (100%)
ASA 1/ASA 2/ASA 3 [n]	10/19/3	11/16/1	2/9/3	3/7/1

ASA: American Society of Anaesthesiologists Classification.

Explorative outcomes of the original RCT:

Radiological post-traumatic OA was assessed using pairs of radiographs at the 5-week follow-up and the latest follow-up at 2 years. The post-traumatic osteoarthritis grades are given in Table 2. Knirk and Jupiter describe these as follows: 0: none, 1: slight joint-space narrowing, 2: marked joint-space narrowing and osteophyte formation, and 3: bone-on-bone osteophyte formation and cyst formation [19]. According to two-way ANOVA analysis, time accounted for 25% ($p < 0.001$), the subject for 47% ($p = 0.004$), and treatment only for 0.3% ($p = 0.57$) of total variation.

Table 2. Post-traumatic osteoarthritis grade according to Knirk et al. [19].

PA Grade	Non-Operative 5 Weeks	Non-Operative 2 Years	Operative 5 Weeks	Operative 2 Years
0	22	14	30	7
1	4	7	1	16
2	1	5	0	6
3	0	1	0	2

PA: Post-traumatic osteoarthritis.

The dorsal angulation was statistically significantly different between the treatment groups ($p < 0.001$), while time did not have a statistically significant impact when comparing immediate post-operative or closed reduction radiographs to radiographs after 5 weeks and 2 years ($p = 0.978$) (Figure 2). Notably, the AO/OTA classification was comparable with the AO type A/B/C distributed as follows: (19/4/9) in the operative group and (11/5/12) in the non-operative group.

The Quick-DASH from pre-injury, 2 weeks, 5 weeks, 6 months, 1 year, and 2 years was dependent on time ($p < 0.001$) and participant ($p < 0.001$) but not treatment ($p = 0.56$). If treatment had no effect overall, there was thus a 56% chance of randomly observing our results.

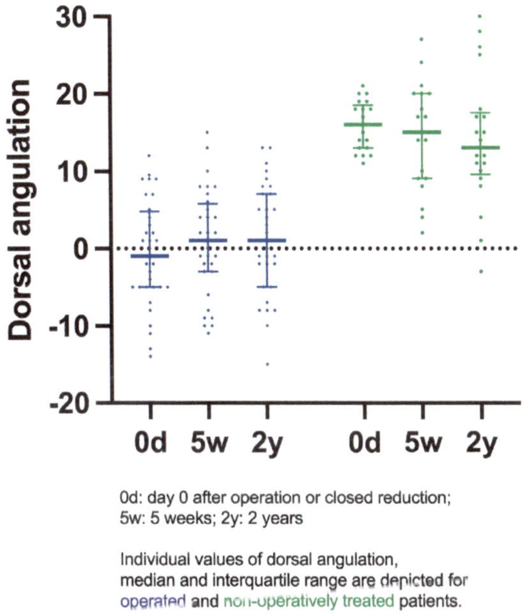

Figure 2. Dorsal angulation on day 0, 5 weeks, and 2 years.

Likewise, PRWHE scores at 6 months, 1 year, and 2 years were dependent on time ($p = 0.01$) and participant ($p < 0.001$) but not treatment ($p = 0.96$) (Figure 3). The mean Quick-DASH and PRWHE scores are presented in Table 3. Pain was also not treatment-dependent ($p = 0.43$), but it was time-dependent (Table 3). Likewise, ROM was not treatment-dependent, and the combined active movements, namely flexion–extension, ulnar–radial deviation, and supination–pronation, were all solely time-dependent. Combined flexion–extension ROM in the non-operative group vs. the operative group had a median of 105 (35–170) and 110 (45–170) degrees at the latest follow-up ($p > 0.05$). ROM in the other directions was also similar between groups; i.e., median combined pronation–supination scores of 180 (125–180) vs. 180 (135–180) and median combined deviation scores of 65 (35–75) vs. 55 (30–75) degrees ($p > 0.05$).

Table 3. Quick-DASH, PRWHE, and pain scores 6 months, 1 year, and 2 years after the injury.

	Quick-DASH		PRWHE		Pain (NRS 0–10)	
	Non-Operative	**Operative**	**Non-Operative**	**Operative**	**Non-Operative**	**Operative**
6 months	**2.3** (0.0; 0.0–6.8; 25)	**2.3** (0.0; 0.0–6.8; 59)	**6.5** (0.0; 0.5–16; 42)	**7.0** (0.0; 0.0–15; 87)	**0** (0; 0–1; 5)	**0** (0; 0–1; 5)
1 year	**0.0** (0.0; 0.0–4.5; 75)	**0.0** (0.0; 0.0–6.2; 64)	**0.5** (0.0; 0.0–13; 54)	**0.0** (0.0; 0.0–10; 93)	**0** (0; 0–0; 5)	**0** (0; 0–0; 7)
2 years	**0.5** (0.0; 0.0–8.5; 55)	**0.0** (0.0; 0.0–2.3; 50)	**0.0** (0.0; 0.0–8; 68)	**0.0** (0.0; 0.0–3; 89)	**0** (0; 0–0; 5)	**0** (0; 0–0; 5)

Quick-DASH: Quick Disabilities of the Arm, Shoulder, and Hand. PRWHE: The Patient-Rated Wrist/Hand Evaluation. NRS: numerical rating scale.

The mean grip strength of the fractured wrist was time-dependent ($p < 0.001$) but not treatment-dependent ($p = 0.72$). The mean grip strength of the fractured wrist was 15.4 kg, 17.3 kg, and 17.6 kg after 6 months, 1 year, and 2 years, respectively. The mean grip strength of the healthy side was not time-dependent (21.8 kg, 21.1 kg, and 20.5 kg; $p = 0.07$).

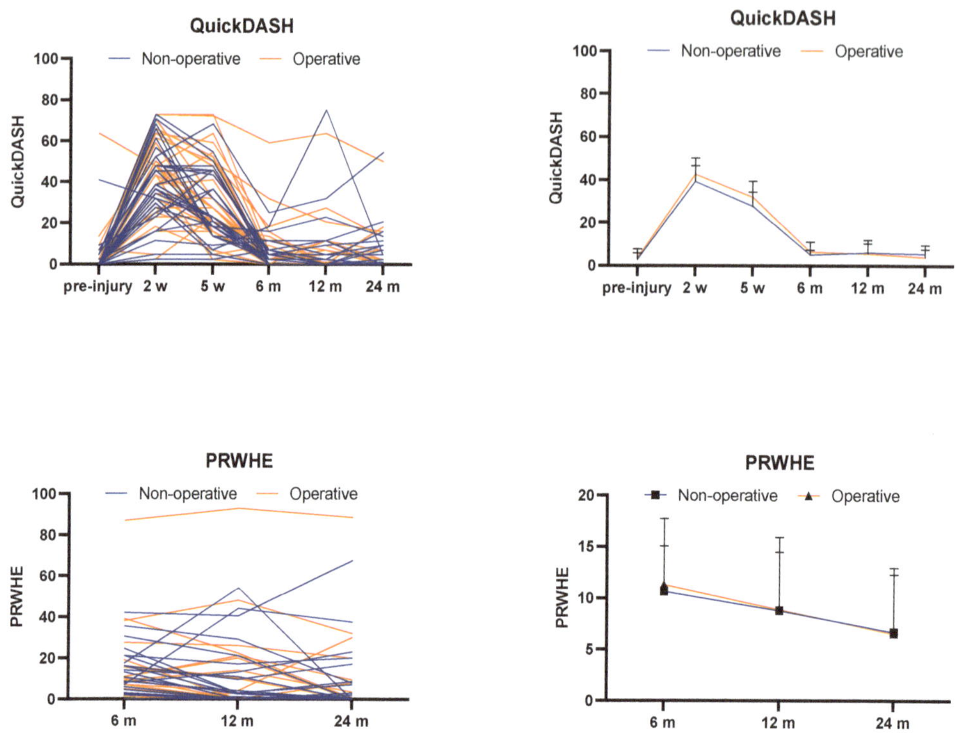

Figure 3. Mean Quick-DASH and PRWHE scores and mean scores at different time points.

Complications between the 1- and 2-year follow-ups occurred predominantly in the operative group. For two non-operatively treated patients, one underwent surgery for carpal tunnel syndrome, while another one was diagnosed with De Quervain's tenosynovitis and trigger finger, both of which required surgery. These complications were in addition to those observed within the first year, as reported in the VOLCON RCT [14]: two cases of superficial wounds at cast removal, two cases of surgically treated carpal tunnel syndromes, and three cases of nonspecific sensory disturbances within the first year.

In the operative group, two additional surgeries were performed between the 1- and 2-year follow-ups: one plate was removed due to extensor tendon irritation, and one patient underwent wrist arthrodesis. Furthermore, one proximal screw loosened but was not removed, and one patient had broken screws; however, the bone healed with increased dorsal angulation without requiring reoperation. Notably, the fluctuating sensory disturbances reported at 1 year were no longer present in the same patients at 2 years.

4. Discussion

In this minimum 2-year follow-up of an RCT investigating operative versus non-operative treatments of displaced DRFs in patients ≥65 years, we found no correlation between treatment choice and the development of post-traumatic OA. Furthermore, we found no difference in Quick-DASH, PRWHE, the pain score, ROM, or grip strength at the 2-year follow-up. As expected, there was significantly greater dorsal angulation in the non-operative group. Implant-related complications such as screw loosening and plate removal due to protruding screws causing tendon irritation were still observed between 1 and 2 years. Given the greater dorsal angulation in the non-operative group, it was surprising that one arthrodesis surgery was performed in a volar-plated DRF patient, while none of the non-operatively treated patients had bony surgery. However, a carpal tunnel release surgery for De Quervain's tenosynovitis and trigger finger was performed in two non-operatively treated patients.

Our results regarding post-traumatic OA are comparable to Südow et al. [15] who also published an extension of an RCT comparing operative versus non-operative treatments of displaced DRFs in elderly patients. Similarly, they found no significant difference in OA at the 3-year follow-up. In contrast, another study found a significantly higher degree of post-traumatic OA in non-operatively treated DRFs with an indication for surgery. However, this study was retrospective, thus not randomized, and included a relatively small population of 50- to 70-year-old patients [25].

Several studies have found a correlation between malunion and articular step-off and the development of OA [19,26,27]. These studies, published in 1986, 1990, and 2011, included relatively young patients. However, Lutz et al. [27] concluded that there was no correlation between OA and the DASH score and grip strength and the pain score at the 9-year follow-up in a population with a mean age of 38 years. The relevance of these findings for an older population, such as in the present study, is unclear. We found a greater degree of dorsal angulation in the non-operative group compared to the operative group. According to these studies, this malunion could result in a higher degree of OA. However, we found similar OA rates in both groups. Additionally, functional outcomes were comparable between the two groups

The etiology of post-traumatic OA in the wrist is believed to be multifactorial. A review on the topic suggests that ligament injuries and fractures are major contributing factors [28]. Injuries in other joints, such as the knee, have been associated with accelerated OA, particularly in the elderly [29,30]. Some have proposed intra-articular steroid injections to reduce the development of OA in DRFs post-operatively, but these failed to show any effect [31]. Interestingly, preexisting wrist or carpometacarpal OA did not affect postoperative functional outcomes (PRWHE or DASH) after DRFs in a retrospective case–control study including 61 patients [32].

We found no difference in Quick-DASH or PRWHE scores between the operative and non-operative groups at the 2-year follow-up, which aligns with findings from several meta-analyses and RCTs on operatively versus non-operatively treated DRFs [10,12,13,33–36]. However, these studies all had a maximum follow-up of 1 year. In contrast to our findings, some studies report better PROM scores in the operative group [37,38]. One of these meta-analyses found a lower Quick-DASH score of −5.22 (95% CI −8.87 to −1.57) in the operative group in the first year. However, in a subgroup analysis including elderly patients (>60 years), this difference diminished and was no longer significant [38]. Saving et al. [37] found a difference of 11.6 (8.3 vs. 19.9) in DASH scores favoring the operative group. Given that the MCID is defined as 16–20 points, the clinical relevance of this difference remains uncertain [20–22].

Three RCTs comparing operative versus non-operative treatments of DRFs with a minimum of two years of follow-up were identified [15–17]. Südow et al. concluded that the operative group had a small but statistically significant improvement in PRWHE scores (9-point difference) [15]. However, given that the MCID for PRWHE is 11.5, this difference is unlikely to be clinically relevant [24]. Additionally, they found no difference in DASH scores, which aligns with our findings. Likewise, Martinez-Mendez et al. [16] investigated operative versus non-operative treatments in patients > 60 years with intra-articular DRFs and found evidence of better PROM scores in the operative group at the 2-year follow-up. However, DASH scores remained below the MCID.

In another extension of a previously published RCT with a 2-year follow-up, Lawson et al. [17] found no difference in the pain score, PRWHE, the EuroQol−5 Domain (EQ5D), or complications supporting our results. Similar to another study [10], they found a higher degree of patient-reported treatment success in the operative group. The authors speculate whether this was due to earlier mobilization in the operative group or due to patients generally having a presumption that surgery is superior. Our study did not record patient expectations, but this may have been important, as patient expectations have been correlated to outcomes 12 months post-injury [39].

The Quick-DASH scores measured in the present study did not vary considerably from 6 to 24 months (Figure 3). This may be due to the inability of the PROMs to detect differences in patients rating themselves in the lower range of the instrument or due to patients adapting to a "new normal" and accepting decreased wrist function post-injury through adaptation and coping strategies. However, neither DASH nor PRWHE scores have been reported to show floor effects up to 9 months post-injury [40].

We found no difference in grip strength in the two groups. This finding is consistent with a comparable RCT with long-term follow-up [15] but contradicts most RCTs and meta-analyses with a one-year follow-up [13,33,35,37,38].

In this study, we had a small study population with a relatively high loss to follow-up, which is a considerable limitation. Of the 100 originally included patients, only 60 remained available for the final follow-up at a minimum of 2 years, resulting in a dropout rate of 40%. However, this is comparable to other RCTs [41–43]. Additionally, the sample size analysis for the original study was estimated to detect complication rates rather than post-traumatic OA [18]. While few studies have a follow-up period of at least 2 years, this may still be too short to detect post-traumatic OA development. Therefore, studies with larger sample sizes and longer follow-ups of up to 5–10 years are warranted. Finally, we used the classification of OA of the wrist proposed by Knirk and Jupiter [19], who included 43 patients with a mean age of 27 years. Our study population consisted of elderly patients > 65 years, and the applicability of this classification system to this age group is uncertain.

5. Conclusions

This study found no difference in post-traumatic OA or functional outcomes between operatively or non-operatively treated displaced DRFs in elderly patients > 65 years of age after 2 years of follow-up. This adds to the compiling evidence that the choice of treatment contributes little to the variability in functional and radiological outcomes after DRFs. However, longer follow-up studies are warranted to better assess the detection of post-traumatic OA as this study contributes to highlight short- to medium-term results.

Author Contributions: Conceptualization, J.D.R. and R.T.; methodology, J.D.R., R.T. and D.W.; formal analysis, J.D.R.; investigation, D.W., K.L.R. and R.T.; resources, M.T.; data curation, J.D.R.; writing—original draft preparation, D.W.; writing—review and editing, D.W., J.D.R. and R.T.; visualization, D.W. and J.D.R.; supervision, J.D.R. and R.T.; project administration, J.D.R. and R.T.; funding acquisition, M.T. All authors have read and agreed to the published version of the manuscript.

Funding: This research received no external funding.

Institutional Review Board Statement: The study was conducted in accordance with the Declaration of Helsinki, approved by the Danish Scientific Ethical Committee (ID: 1-10-72-420-17), and registered at Clinicaltrials.gov (ID: NCT03716661) date: 1 November 2018.

Informed Consent Statement: Informed consent was obtained from all subjects involved in the study. Written informed consent has been obtained from the patient(s) to publish this paper.

Data Availability Statement: Data are unavailable due to privacy and ethical restrictions.

Acknowledgments: The authors would like to thank radiographer Jacob Nielsen for his contribution to this work.

Conflicts of Interest: The authors declare no conflicts of interest.

Abbreviations

The following abbreviations are used in this manuscript:

DRF	Distal radius fracture
NCG	National clinical guideline
ED	Emergency department
ORIF	Open reduction internal fixation
PROMs	Patient-related outcome measures
OA	Osteoarthritis
Quick-DASH	Quick-disabilities of the arm, shoulder and hand
PRWHE	Patient-rated wrist/hand evaluation
MCID	Minimal clinical important difference
NRS	Numeric rating scale
ROM	Range of motion
ASA	American Society of Anaesthesiologists
EQ5D	EuroQol-5 Domain
RCT	Randomized controlled trial

References

1. Bäßgen, K.; Westphal, T.; Haar, P.; Kundt, G.; Mittlmeier, T.; Schober, H.-C. Population-based prospective study on the incidence of osteoporosis-associated fractures in a German population of 200 413 inhabitants. *J. Public Health* **2012**, *35*, 255–261. [CrossRef] [PubMed]
2. Court-Brown, C.M.; Caesar, B. Epidemiology of adult fractures: A review. *Injury* **2006**, *37*, 691–697. [CrossRef] [PubMed]
3. Nellans, K.W.; Kowalski, E.; Chung, K.C. The epidemiology of distal radius fractures. *Hand Clin.* **2012**, *28*, 113–125. [CrossRef]
4. Sundhedsstyrelsen. National Klinisk Retningslinje for Behandling af Håndledsnære Brud (Distal Radiusfraktur) 2017. 2022. Available online: https://www.sst.dk/-/media/Udgivelser/2014/NKR-H%C3%A5ndledsn%C3%A6re-underarmsbrud/National-klinisk-retningslinie-for-behandling-af-haandledsnaere-brud.ashx?la=da&hash=7CB223E245904E51A3B96DB08180CB01A17D229A (accessed on 10 January 2025).
5. (AAOS) AA of, OS. Management of Distal Radius Fractures Evidence-Based Clinical Practice Guideline 2020. Available online: www.aaos.org/drfcpg (accessed on 10 January 2025).
6. Mellstrand-Navarro, C.; Pettersson, H.J.; Tornqvist, H.; Ponzer, S. The operative treatment of fractures of the distal radius is increasing: Results from a nationwide Swedish study. *Bone Joint J.* **2014**, *96-b*, 963–969. [CrossRef]
7. Chung, K.C.; Shauver, M.J.; Birkmeyer, J.D. Trends in the United States in the treatment of distal radial fractures in the elderly. *J. Bone Joint Surg. Am.* **2009**, *91*, 1868–1873. [CrossRef] [PubMed]
8. Egol, K.A.; Walsh, M.; Romo-Cardoso, S.; Dorsky, S.; Paksima, N. Distal radial fractures in the elderly: Operative compared with nonoperative treatment. *J. Bone Joint Surg. Am.* **2010**, *92*, 1851–1857. [CrossRef]
9. Wæver, D.; Madsen, M.L.; Rölfing, J.H.D.; Borris, L.C.; Henriksen, M.; Nagel, L.L.; Thorninger, R. Distal radius fractures are difficult to classify. *Injury* **2018**, *49* (Suppl. 1), S29–S32. [CrossRef]
10. Hassellund, S.S.; Williksen, J.H.; Laane, M.M.; Pripp, A.; Rosales, C.P.; Karlsen, Ø.; Madsen, J.E.; Frihagen, F. Cast immobilization is non-inferior to volar locking plates in relation to QuickDASH after one year in patients aged 65 years and older: A randomized controlled trial of displaced distal radius fractures. *Bone Joint J.* **2021**, *103-b*, 247–255. [CrossRef] [PubMed]
11. Luokkala, T.; Laitinen, M.K.; Hevonkorpi, T.P.; Raittio, L.; Mattila, V.M.; Launonen, A.P. Distal radius fractures in the elderly population. *EFORT Open Rev.* **2020**, *5*, 361–370. [CrossRef]
12. Lawson, A.; Naylor, J.M.; Buchbinder, R.; Ivers, R.; Balogh, Z.J.; Smith, P.; Xuan, W.; Howard, K.; Vafa, V.; Perriman, D.; et al. Surgical Plating vs Closed Reduction for Fractures in the Distal Radius in Older Patients: A Randomized Clinical Trial. *JAMA Surg.* **2021**, *156*, 229–237. [CrossRef]
13. Li, Q.; Ke, C.; Han, S.; Xu, X.; Cong, Y.X.; Shang, K.; Liang, J.D.; Zhang, B.F. Nonoperative treatment versus volar locking plate fixation for elderly patients with distal radial fracture: A systematic review and meta-analysis. *J. Orthop. Surg. Res.* **2020**, *15*, 263. [CrossRef] [PubMed]
14. Thorninger, R.; Wæver, D.; Tjørnild, M.; Lind, M.; Rölfing, J.D. VOLCON: A randomized controlled trial investigating complications and functional outcome of volar plating vs casting of unstable distal radius fractures in patients older than 65 years. *J. Orthop. Traumatol.* **2022**, *23*, 54. [CrossRef] [PubMed]

15. Südow, H.; Severin, S.; Wilcke, M.; Saving, J.; Sköldenberg, O.; Navarro, C.M. Non-operative treatment or volar locking plate fixation for dorsally displaced distal radius fractures in patients over 70 years—A three year follow-up of a randomized controlled trial. *BMC Musculoskelet. Disord.* **2022**, *23*, 447. [CrossRef]
16. Martinez-Mendez, D.; Lizaur-Utrilla, A.; de-Juan-Herrero, J. Intra-articular distal radius fractures in elderly patients: A randomized prospective study of casting versus volar plating. *J. Hand Surg. Eur. Vol.* **2018**, *43*, 142–147. [CrossRef]
17. Lawson, A.; Naylor, J.; Buchbinder, R.; Ivers, R.; Balogh, Z.J.; Smith, P.; Xuan, W.; Howard, K.; Vafa, A.; Perriman, D.; et al. Plating vs Closed Reduction for Fractures in the Distal Radius in Older Patients. *JAMA Surg.* **2022**, *157*, 563. [CrossRef]
18. Pedersen, J.; Mortensen, S.O.; Rölfing, J.D.; Thorninger, R. A protocol for a single-center, single-blinded randomized-controlled trial investigating volar plating versus conservative treatment of unstable distal radius fractures in patients older than 65 years *BMC Musculoskelet. Disord.* **2019**, *20*, 309. [CrossRef]
19. Knirk, J.L.; Jupiter, J.B. Intra-articular fractures of the distal end of the radius in young adults. *J. Bone Joint Surg. Am.* **1986**, *68*, 647–659. [CrossRef] [PubMed]
20. Franchignoni, F.; Vercelli, S.; Giordano, A.; Sartorio, F.; Bravini, E.; Ferriero, G. Minimal clinically important difference of the disabilities of the arm, shoulder and hand outcome measure (DASH) and its shortened version (QuickDASH). *J. Orthop. Sports Phys. Ther.* **2014**, *44*, 30–39. [CrossRef]
21. Mintken, P.E.; Glynn, P.; Cleland, J.A. Psychometric properties of the shortened disabilities of the Arm, Shoulder, and Hand Questionnaire (QuickDASH) and Numeric Pain Rating Scale in patients with shoulder pain. *J. Shoulder Elbow Surg.* **2009**, *18*, 920–926. [CrossRef]
22. Schønnemann, J.O.; Eggers, J. Validation of the Danish version of the Quick-Disabilities of Arm, Shoulder and Hand Questionnaire. *Dan. Med. J.* **2016**, *63*, A5306.
23. Hansen, A.Ø.; Knygsand-Roenhoej, K.; Ardensø, K. Danish version of the Patient-Rated Wrist/Hand Evaluation questionnaire: Translation, cross-cultural adaptation, test–retest reliability and construct validity. *Hand Ther.* **2018**, *24*, 22–30. [CrossRef]
24. Walenkamp, M.M.; de Muinck Keizer, R.J.; Goslings, J.C.; Vos, L.M.; Rosenwasser, M.P.; Schep, N.W. The Minimum Clinically Important Difference of the Patient-rated Wrist Evaluation Score for Patients With Distal Radius Fractures. *Clin. Orthop. Relat. Res.* **2015**, *473*, 3235–3241. [CrossRef] [PubMed]
25. Visser, D.; Mathijssen, N.M.C.; van Outeren, M.V.; Colaris, J.W.; de Vries, M.R.; Kraan, G.A. Long-term follow-up of distal radius fractures, an evaluation of the current guideline: The relation between malunion, osteoarthritis and functional outcome. *Eur. J. Orthop. Surg. Traumatol.* **2020**, *30*, 1357–1362. [CrossRef]
26. Home, J.G.; Devane, P.; Purdie, G. A Prospective Randomized Trial of External Fixation and Plaster Cast Immobilization in the Treatment of Distal Radial Fractures. *J. Orthop. Trauma.* **1990**, *4*, 30–34. [CrossRef]
27. Lutz, M.; Arora, R.; Krappinger, D.; Wambacher, M.; Rieger, M.; Pechlaner, S. Arthritis predicting factors in distal intraarticular radius fractures. *Arch. Orthop. Trauma. Surg.* **2011**, *131*, 1121–1126. [CrossRef]
28. Andersson, J.K.; Hagert, E.; Brittberg, M. Cartilage Injuries and Posttraumatic Osteoarthritis in the Wrist: A Review. *Cartilage* **2021**, *13*, 156S–168S. [CrossRef]
29. Driban, J.B.; Eaton, C.B.; Lo, G.H.; Ward, R.J.; Lu, B.; McAlindon, T.E. Association of Knee Injuries With Accelerated Knee Osteoarthritis Progression: Data From the Osteoarthritis Initiative. *Arthritis Care Res.* **2014**, *66*, 1673–1679. [CrossRef] [PubMed]
30. Driban, J.B.; Harkey, M.S.; Barbe, M.F.; Ward, R.J.; MacKay, J.W.; Davis, J.E.; Lu, B.; Price, L.L.; Eaton, C.B.; Lo, G.H.; et al. Risk factors and the natural history of accelerated knee osteoarthritis: A narrative review. *BMC Musculoskelet. Disord.* **2020**, *21*, 332. [CrossRef]
31. Logli, A.L.; Evans, C.H.; Duryea, J.; Larson, D.R.; Bakri, K.; Carlsen, B.T.; Dennison, D.G.; Karim, K.E.; Pulos, N.A.; Rhee, P.C.; et al. Investigation Into the Effects of Intra-Articular Steroid on Post-Traumatic Osteoarthritis in Distal Radius Fractures: A Randomized Controlled Pilot Study. *J. Hand Surg. Am.* **2024**, *49*, 757–765. [CrossRef]
32. Davies, J.; Centomo, H.; Leduc, S.; Beaumont, P.; Laflamme, G.-Y.; Rouleau, D. Preexisting Carpal and Carpometacarpal Osteoarthritis Has No Impact on Function after Distal Radius Fractures. *J. Wrist Surg.* **2017**, *6*, 301–306. [CrossRef]
33. Arora, R.; Lutz, M.; Deml, C.; Krappinger, D.; Haug, L.; Gabl, M. A prospective randomized trial comparing nonoperative treatment with volar locking plate fixation for displaced and unstable distal radial fractures in patients sixty-five years of age and older. *J. Bone Joint Surg. Am.* **2011**, *93*, 2146–2153. [CrossRef] [PubMed]
34. Woolnough, T.; Axelrod, D.; Bozzo, A.; Koziarz, A.; Koziarz, F.; Oitment, C.; Gyemi, L.; Gormley, J.; Gouveia, K.; Johal, H. What Is the Relative Effectiveness of the Various Surgical Treatment Options for Distal Radius Fractures? A Systematic Review and Network Meta-analysis of Randomized Controlled Trials. *Clin. Orthop. Relat. Res.* **2021**, *479*, 348–362. [CrossRef] [PubMed]
35. Chen, Y.; Chen, X.; Li, Z.; Yan, H.; Zhou, F.; Gao, W. Safety and Efficacy of Operative Versus Nonsurgical Management of Distal Radius Fractures in Elderly Patients: A Systematic Review and Meta-analysis. *J. Hand Surg. Am.* **2016**, *41*, 404–413. [CrossRef]
36. Bell, K.; Oliver, W.; White, T.; Molyneux, S.; Clement, N.; Duckworth, A. OPERATIVE VERSUS NONOPERATIVE MANAGEMENT OF DISTAL RADIUS FRACTURES IN ADULTS: A SYSTEMATIC REVIEW AND META-ANALYSIS OF RANDOMIZED CONTROLLED TRIALS WITH AN ELDERLY SUBGROUP ANALYSIS. *Orthop. Proc.* **2023**, *105-B*, 50. [CrossRef]

37. Saving, J.; Severin Wahlgren, S.; Olsson, K.; Enocson, A.; Ponzer, S.; Sköldenberg, O.; Wilcke, M.; Navarro, C.M. Nonoperative Treatment Compared with Volar Locking Plate Fixation for Dorsally Displaced Distal Radial Fractures in the Elderly: A Randomized Controlled Trial. *J. Bone Joint Surg. Am.* **2019**, *101*, 961–969. [CrossRef]
38. Ochen, Y.; Peek, J.; van der Velde, D.; Beeres, F.J.P.; van Heijl, M.; Groenwold, R.H.H.; Houwert, R.M.; Heng, M. Operative vs Nonoperative Treatment of Distal Radius Fractures in Adults: A Systematic Review and Meta-analysis. *JAMA Netw. Open* **2020**, *3*, e203497. [CrossRef] [PubMed]
39. Fang, C.; Chen, Y.-J.; Fang, E.; Wong, T.-M.; Liu, Z.-H.; Lau, T.-W.; Fok, M.W.M.; Yee, D.K.; Pun, T.; Luo, C.-F.; et al. Patient expectations predict outcomes following distal radius fracture: A prospective cohort study using the TEFTOM questionnaire. *Injury* **2021**, *52*, 877–882. [CrossRef]
40. Jayakumar, P.; Teunis, T.; Vranceanu, A.-M.; Lamb, S.; Williams, M.; Ring, D.; Gwilym, S. Construct Validity and Precision of Different Patient-reported Outcome Measures During Recovery After Upper Extremity Fractures. *Clin. Orthop. Relat. Res.* **2019**, *477*, 2521–2530. [CrossRef]
41. van Leerdam, R.H.; Huizing, F.; Termaat, F.; Kleinveld, S.; Rhemrev, S.J.; Krijnen, P.; Schipper, I.B. Patient-reported outcomes after a distal radius fracture in adults: A 3–4 years follow-up. *Acta Orthop.* **2019**, *90*, 129–134. [CrossRef]
42. Bhandari, M.; Guyatt, G.H.; Tong, D.; Adili, A.; Shaughnessy, S.G. Reamed versus nonreamed intramedullary nailing of lower extremity long bone fractures: A systematic overview and meta-analysis. *J. Orthop. Trauma.* **2000**, *14*, 2–9. [CrossRef]
43. Bhandari, M.; Guyatt, G.H.; Swiontkowski, M.F.; Schemitsch, E.H. Treatment of open fractures of the shaft of the tibia. *J. Bone Joint Surg. Br.* **2001**, *83*, 62–68. [CrossRef] [PubMed]

MDPI AG
Grosspeteranlage 5
4052 Basel
Switzerland
Tel.: +41 61 683 77 34

Journal of Clinical Medicine Editorial Office
E-mail: jcm@mdpi.com
www.mdpi.com/journal/jcm

www.ingramcontent.com/pod-product-compliance
Lightning Source LLC
Chambersburg PA
CBHW041412210926
51850CB00013B/3249